Gastrointestinal Emergencies

Gastrointestinal Emergencies

Tony C.K. Tham

Consultant Gastroenterologist, The Ulster Hospital, Dundonald, Belfast, Northern Ireland, UK

John S.A. Collins

Consultant Gastroenterologist, Royal Victoria Hospital, Belfast, Northern Ireland, UK

Roy M. Soetikno

Chief, GI Section, VA Palo Alto Health Care System; Associate Professor, Stanford University

SECOND EDITION

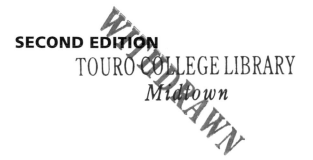
WILEY-BLACKWELL

This edition first published 2009, © 2000, 2009 by Blackwell Publishing Ltd

Blackwell Publishing was acquired by John Wiley & Sons in February 2007.
Blackwell's publishing program has been merged with Wiley's global Scientific, Technical and Medical business to form Wiley-Blackwell.

Registered office: John Wiley & Sons Ltd, The Atrium, Southern Gate, Chichester, West Sussex, PO19 8SQ, UK

Editorial offices: 9600 Garsington Road, Oxford, OX4 2DQ, UK
The Atrium, Southern Gate, Chichester, West Sussex, PO19 8SQ, UK
111 River Street, Hoboken, NJ 07030-5774, USA

For details of our global editorial offices, for customer services and for information about how to apply for permission
to reuse the copyright material in this book please see our website at www.wiley.com/wiley-blackwell

The right of the author to be identified as the author of this work has been asserted in accordance with the Copyright, Designs and Patents
Act 1988.

Wiley also publishes its books in a variety of electronic formats. Some content that appears in print may not be available in electronic books.

Designations used by companies to distinguish their products are often claimed as trademarks. All brand names and product names used in
this book are trade names, service marks, trademarks or registered trademarks of their respective owners. The publisher is not associated
with any product or vendor mentioned in this book. This publication is designed to provide accurate and authoritative information in regard
to the subject matter covered. It is sold on the understanding that the publisher is not engaged in rendering professional services. If
professional advice or other expert assistance is required, the services of a competent professional should be sought.

The contents of this work are intended to further general scientific research, understanding, and discussion only and are not intended and
should not be relied upon as recommending or promoting a specific method, diagnosis, or treatment by physicians for any particular patient.
The publisher and the author make no representations or warranties with respect to the accuracy or completeness of the contents of this
work and specifically disclaim all warranties, including without limitation any implied warranties of fitness for a particular purpose. In view of
ongoing research, equipment modifications, changes in governmental regulations, and the constant flow of information relating to the use of
medicines, equipment, and devices, the reader is urged to review and evaluate the information provided in the package insert or instructions
for each medicine, equipment, or device for, among other things, any changes in the instructions or indication of usage and for added warn-
ings and precautions. Readers should consult with a specialist where appropriate. The fact that an organization or Website is referred to in this
work as a citation and/or a potential source of further information does not mean that the author or the publisher endorses the information
the organization or Website may provide or recommendations it may make. Further, readers should be aware that Internet Websites listed
in this work may have changed or disappeared between when this work was written and when it is read. No warranty may be created or
extended by any promotional statements for this work. Neither the publisher nor the author shall be liable for any damages arising herefrom.

ISBN: 978-1-4051-4634-0

Library of Congress Cataloging-in-Publication Data

Gastrointestinal emergencies / [edited by] Tony Tham, John Collins, Roy Soetikno. — 2nd ed.
    p. ; cm.
    Rev. ed. of: Gastrointestinal emergencies / C.K. Tham and John S.A. Collins. 2000.
    Includes bibliographical references and index.
    ISBN 978-1-4051-4634-0
    1. Gastrointestinal system—Surgery. 2. Gastrointestinal emergencies. I. Tham, Tony C. K. II. Collins, John S. A. III. Soetikno,
Roy. IV. Tham, Tony C. K. Gastrointestinal emergencies.
    [DNLM: 1. Gastrointestinal Diseases—therapy. 2. Emergency Treatment. 3. Endoscopy, Gastrointestinal. WI 140 T366g 2008]
RD540.G3754 2008
617.4'3—dc22

                                                                                          2008000427

A catalogue record for this book is available from the British Library.

Set in 8.75/12pt Meridien by Charon Tec Ltd., A Macmillan Company. (www.macmillansolutions.com)
Printed and bound in Singapore by Fabulous Printers Pte Ltd

First published 2000
Second edition 2009

1 2009

Contents

CONTENTS

List of Contributors

Aijaz Ahmed MD
Division of Gastroenterology and Hepatology, Stanford University School of Medicine, Stanford, CA, USA

Patrick Allen MB, MRCP
Specialist Registrar, Ulster Hospital, Belfast, UK

Andrés Cárdenas MD, MMSc
Institute of Digestive Diseases, Hospital Clinic, IDIBAPS, University of Barcelona, Barcelona, Spain

Stephen Attwood MCh, FRCS, FRCSI
Clinical Director for General Surgery, Northumbria Healthcare Trust; Consultant Upper GI and Laparoscopic Surgeon, North Tyneside General Hospital, Tyne & Wear, UK

Kenneth F. Binmoeller MD
Director, Interventional Endoscopy Services, California Pacific Medical Centre, San Francisco, CA, USA

David Carr-Locke MB, Bchir, FRCP, FASGE
Director, The Endoscopy Institute, Brigham & Women's Hospital, Boston, MA, USA

Victor K. Chen MD, MSPH
Fellow, Division of Gastroenterology, University Hospitals Case Medical Center, Cleveland, Ohio, USA

Ramsey C. Cheung MD
Associate Professor of Medicine, Division of Gastroenterology and Hepatology, Stanford University School of Medicine, Stanford, CA, USA

John S.A. Collins MD
Consultant Gastroenterologist, Royal Victoria Hospital, Belfast, Northern Ireland, UK

Andrew B.C. Crumley MRCS
Research Fellow, Glasgow Royal Infirmary, Glasgow, UK

Wallace Dinsmore MD, FRCP, FRCPI, FRCPEd
Professor of Medicine, Department of GU Medicine, Royal Victoria Hospital, Belfast, UK

Shai Friedland MD
Assistant Professor, Stanford University School of Medicine and VA Palo Alto, Stanford, CA, USA

Subrata Ghosh MD, FRCP, FRCP(E)
Professor of Gastroenterology, Imperial College London, Hammersmith Hospital, London, UK

Pere Ginès MD
Chairman, Liver Unit, Institute of Digestive Diseases Hospital Clinic, IDIBAPS, University of Barcelona, Spain

Tonya Kaltenbach MD
Staff Physician, Veteran Affairs, Palo Alto, Stanford University School of Medicine, Stanford, CA, USA

Emmet B. Keeffe MD
Professor of Medicine, Stanford University School of Medicine, Stanford, CA, USA

Bee Chan Lee MB, MRCP
Specialist Registrar in Gastroenterology, Royal Victoria Hospital, Belfast, UK

David R. Lichtenstein MD
Director of Endsocopy & Associate Professor of Medicine, Boston Medical Center, Boston University School of Medicine, Boston, MA, USA

Ian McAllister MD
Consultant Surgeon, Ulster Community & Hospitals Trust, Belfast, UK

John Moorehead MD, FRCS
Consultant Surgeon, Ulster Community & Hospitals Trust; Honorary Senior Lecturer in Surgery, Queen's University of Belfast, Belfast, UK

Bhavani Moparty MD, MS
Therapeutic Endoscopy Fellow, Department of Gastroenterology, Brigham and Women's Hospital/Massachusetts General Hospital, Boston, MA, USA

Graham Morrison MB, MRCP
Specialist Registrar, Royal Victoria Hospital, Belfast, UK

Afshin A. Nasoodi MD, MRCP
Specialist Registrar, Department of Radiology, Royal Victoria Hospital, Belfast, UK

Colm J. O'Loughlin MB, MRCP (UK)
Assistant Professor, Division of Gastroenterology and Hepatology, Medical College of Wisconsin, Milwaukee, WI, USA

Kelvin Palmer FRCP Edin
Consultant Gastroenterologist, Western General Hospital, Edinburgh, UK

David Patch MBBS, FRCP
Consultant Hepatologist, Department of Hepatology, Royal Free Hospital, London, UK

Andres Sanchez Yagüe MD, PhD
California Pacific Medical Center, San Francisco, CA, USA

Stefan Seewald MD
Professor of Internal Medicine, Department for Interdisciplinary Endoscopy, University Medical Center Hamburg-Eppendorf, Hamburg, Germany

Reza Shaker MD, FACP
Professor and Chief, Division of Gastroenterology and Hepatology; Director, Digestive Disease Center, Medical College of Wisconsin, Milwaukee, WI, USA

Peter D. Siersema MD, PhD
Professor of Gastroenterology and Chief, Department of Gastroenterology and Hepatology, University Medical Center, Utrecht, The Netherlands

Cecilia Sison MD
Stanford University School of Medicine, Stanford, CA, USA

Nib Soehendra MD
Professor of Surgery, Department for Interdisciplinary Endoscopy, University Medical Center Hamburg-Eppendorf, Hamburg, Germany

Roy M. Soetikno MD, MS
Chief, GI Section, VA Palo Alto Health Care System; Associate Professor, Stanford University

Robert C. Stuart MCh, FRCS (Gen)
Senior Lecturer in Surgery, Glasgow Royal Infirmary, Glasgow, UK

Tony C. K. Tham MD, FRCP, FRCPI
Consultant Gastroenterologist, The Ulster Hospital, Dundonald, Belfast, Head of School of Medicine, Northern Ireland deanery, UK

George Triadafilopoulos MD, DSc
Clinical Professor of Medicine, Division of Gastroenterology and Hepatology, Stanford University School of Medicine, Stanford, CA, USA

Sybile Van Lierde MD
Department of Gastroenterology, A.Z. St-Elisabeth, Zottegem, Belgium

Freddy Vandenbussche MD
Department of Gastroenterology, Onze-Lieve-Vrouw Ziekenhuis, Aalst, Belgium

Jo Vandervoort MD
Department of Gastroenterology, Onze-Lieve-Vrouw Ziekenhuis, Aalst, Belgium

Richard C. K. Wong MBBS, FACP, FACG, FASGE
Associate Professor of Medicine, Case Western Reserve University; Head, Section of Gastrointestinal Endoscopy, University Hospitals Case Medical Center, Cleveland, Ohio, USA

Yan Zhong MD
Department for Interdisciplinary Endoscopy, University Medical Center Hamburg-Eppendorf, Hamburg, Germany

1 Approach to Specific Presentations

1 Approach to Dysphagia

John S. Collins

Definitions

Dysphagia refers to the sensation of food passage being hindered in its passage from mouth to stomach. Patients most frequently complain that food "sticks" in the retrosternal area or simply will "not go down." Patients may complain of a feeling of choking and chest discomfort. In some cases food material is rapidly regurgitated to relieve symptoms.

Dysphagia can be divided into two types:
• *oropharyngeal dysphagia* where there is an inability to *initiate* the swallowing process and may involve disorders of striated muscle;
• *esophageal dysphagia* which involves disorders of the smooth muscle of the esophagus.

Odynophagia is the sensation of pain on swallowing which is usually felt in the chest or throat.

Globus is the sensation of a lump, fullness or tightness in the throat.

Differential diagnosis

The causes of the above types of dysphagia are shown in Tables 1.1 and 1.2.

History and examination

Acute dysphagia is a relatively uncommon but dramatic presenting symptom and constitutes a gastrointestinal emergency. The patient will complain of difficulty inititiating swallowing or state that food is readily swallowed but results in the rapid onset of chest discomfort

Gastrointestinal Emergencies, 2nd edition. Edited by Tony Tham, John Collins and Roy Soetikno. © 2009 by Blackwell Publishing, ISBN: 978-1-4051-4634-0.

Table 1.1 Etiology of oropharyngeal dysphagia.

Neurological disorders
Cerebrovascular disease
Amyotrophic lateral sclerosis
Parkinson's Disease
Multiple sclerosis
Bulbar poliomyelitis
Wilson's Disease
Cranial nerve injury
Brainstem tumours
Striated muscle disorders
Polymyositis
Dermatomyositis
Muscular dystrophies
Myasthenia gravis
Structural lesions
Inflammatory – pharyngitis, tonsillar abscess
Head and neck tumors
Congenital webs
Plummer-Vinson syndrome
Cervical osteophytes
Surgical procedures to the oropharynx
Pharyngeal pouch (Zenker diverticulum)
Cricopharyngeal Bar
Metabolic disorders
Hypothyroidism
Hyperthyroidism
Steroid myopathy

or pain which is only relieved by passage or regurgitation of the swallowed food bolus. The latter sensation can result after swallowing a mouthful of liquid. In the acute case it is important to ask the patient about the presence of other neurological symptoms.

If oropharyngeal dysphagia is suspected, the following points are important:
• The patient may complain of nasal regurgitation of liquid, coughing or choking during swallowing or a

Table 1.2 Etiology of esophageal dyphagia.

Neuromuscular/dysmotility disorders
Achalasia
CRST syndrome
Diffuse esophageal spasm
Nutcracker esophagus
Hypertensive lower esophageal shincter
Nonspecific esophageal dysmotility
Chaga disease
Mixed connective tissue disease
Mechanical strictures – intrinsic
Peptic related to GERD
Carcinoma
Esophageal webs
Esophageal diverticula
Lower esophageal ring (Schatzki)
Benign tumors
Foreign bodies
Acute esophageal mucosal infections
Pemphigus/pemphigoid
Crohn's disease
Mechanical lesions – extrinsic
Bronchial carcinoma
Mediastinal nodes
Vascular compression
Mediastinal tumors
Cervical osteoarthritis/spondylosis

change in voice character which may indicate nasal speech due to palatal weakness.
• Patients may describe repeated attempts at the initiation of swallowing.
• Symptoms are noticed within a second of swallowing.
• Patients with cerebrovascular disease may give a history of symptoms of transient ischaemic attacks (TIA) – these would include visual disturbance, dysphasia or transient facial or limb weakness.
• There may be progressive muscular weakness and dysphagia is only part of the symptom complex, in contrast to esophageal dysphagia where swallowing disorder is the most prominent symptom.
• Patients should have a careful neurological examination and evaluation of the pharynx and larynx including direct laryngoscopy.
In cases of esophageal dyphagia, the following points are important:
• Is the sensation of dysphagia worse with liquids or solids? If a progressive obstructive lesion is the cause of symptoms, the patient will notice difficulty swallowing

solids initially and liquids later. Difficulty with both solids and liquids suggests dysmotility.
• Is the dysphagia intermittent or progressive? Intermittent dysphagia may indicate a motility disorder such as diffuse esophageal spasm whereas a progressive course is more characteristic of an esophageal tumor.
• How long have symptoms been present? A long history usually greater that 12 months suggests a benign cause whereas a short history less than 4 weeks suggests a malignant etiology.
• Has the patient a history of heartburn suggesting gastroesophageal reflux disease (GERD)? While a history of heartburn does not rule out gastroesophageal cancer as a cause of dysphagia, a long history in the presence of slow onset, non-progressive symptoms may point to a benign peptic stricture as the cause.
A diagnostic algorithm for the symptomatic assessment of the patient with dysphagia is shown in Fig. 1.1.

The etiology of esophageal dysphagia is summarized in Table 1.2.

While acute dysphagia may be painful, especially in relation to foreign body or food bolus impaction above an existing stricture, a history of odynophagia usually suggests an inflammatory condition or disruption of the esophageal mucosa leading to the irritation of pain receptors. The causes of odynophagia are summarized in Table 1.3.

Clinical signs in patients who present with dysphagia are uncommon. On examination, the following signs should be noted:
• loss of weight
• signs of anemia
• cervical lymphadenopathy
• hoarseness
• concomitant neurological especially bulbar signs
• respiratory signs if history of cough/choking
• hepatomegaly
• oral ulcers or signs of *Candida*
• goitre.

Investigation

Dysphagia is considered to be an "alarm symptom" and should be investigated as a matter of urgency in all cases. Upper gastrointestinal endoscopy is a safe investigation in experienced hands provided the intubation is carried out under direct visualization of the oropharynx and upper esophageal sphincter. The endoscopist

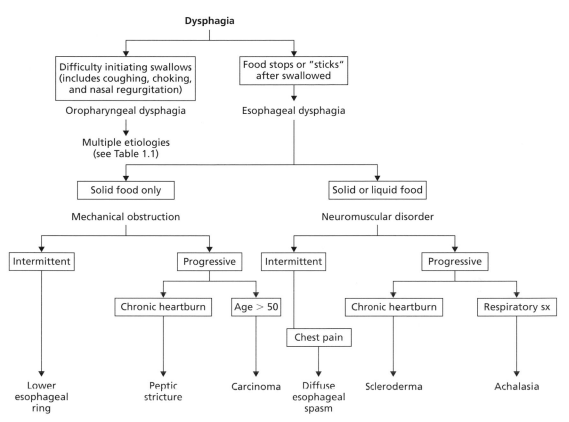

Figure 1.1 Diagnostic algorithm for the symptomatic assessment of the patient with dysphagia. (From Castell DO. Approach to the patient with dysphagia. In: Yamada et al., 1995 with permission.)

Table 1.3 Etiology of odynophagia.

Infectious esophagitis
Candida
Herpes simplex
Cytomegalovirus
Pill-induced ulceration
Reflux disease/stricture
Radiation esophagitis
Caustic injury
Motility disorders stimulated by swallowing
Cancer
Graft-versus-host disease
Foreign body

should be alert to the possibility of a high obstruction and the likelihood of retained food debris or saliva if dysphagia has been present for some time. If there is a history of choking, the patient should have a liquid-only diet for 24 hours followed by a 12-hour fast prior to the procedure. In some cases, the careful passage of a nasoesophageal tube to aspirate retained luminal contents may be necessary. At endoscopy, obstructing lesions can be biopsied and peptic strictures can be dilated with a balloon or bougie.

The presence of a dilated food and saliva-filled esophagus in the absence of a stricture raises the possibility of achalasia.

Barium studies are not a prerequisite for endoscopy but should be considered complementary in dysphagia. Barium swallow may give additional information in the following situations:
• in cases of suspected oropharyngeal dysphagia, especially if videofluoroscopy is employed;
• where a high esophageal obstruction is suspected prior to endoscopy;
• where a motility disorder is suspected as a method to assess lower esophageal relaxation.

Esophageal manometry is indicated if both endoscopy and barium studies are inconclusive in the presence of persistent symptoms. Manometry requires intubation of the esophagus with a multilumen recording catheter attached to a polygraph. Pressure changes are recorded during water bolus swallows along the esophageal body and at the upper and lower esophageal sphincters.

Management of dysphagia

The management of dysphagia depends on the underlying cause. In a patient presenting with total dysphagia who is unable to swallow even small amounts of liquid or saliva, urgent treatment is indicated (Fig. 1.2).

The management of oropharyngeal dysphagia can be treated by control of the underlying neurological or metabolic disorder. Dietary modification under the supervision of a speech and language therapist may maintain oral swallowing and avoid gastrostomy tube placement in patients with stroke and pseudobulbar or bulbar palsy. Gastrostomy tube placement may be the only management option in patients with inoperable mouth or throat tumors or in cases where recurrent pulmonary aspiration is life threatening.

Peptic stricture

When the endoscopic appearances are characteristic of a benign peptic stricture, dilatation can usually be carried out at the time of the procedure using either wire-guided bougies or a balloon. If the stricture is complex, very tight or associated with esophageal scarring, it may be safer to carry out wire guided dilatation

using graded bougies. The majority of patients will gain symptomatic relief and the risk of complications is low (See chapter on oesophageal perforation).

It is essential that all patients are treated with an adquate dose of a proton pump inhibitor to prevent recurrence. Repeat dilatations are necessary in some cases and repeat inspection and biopsy is advised if there is any concern about mucosal dysplasia or malignancy.

Esophageal carcinoma

Suspected carcinoma which is detected at endoscopy requires biopsy confirmation and subsequent staging so that a management plan can be formulated. The most accurate modality for staging is endoscopic ultrasound which can assess depth of local invasion and regional lymph node status. Chest and abdominal CT is a less accurate technique but CT/PET scanning enhances staging accuracy, especially in adenocarcinomas.

Surgery offers the only chance of cure but only 30% of tumors are resectable and 5-year survival is 10% in European studies. Contraindications to surgery include invasion of vascular structures, metastatic disease and patients with comorbidity and high operative risk.

Palliative management will be indicated in 70% of patients following staging. Esophageal dilatation followed by the endoscopic placement of a metal stent gives adequate swallowing relief in the majority of cases. In situations where there is complete obstruction of the esophageal lumen by tumor, endoscopic LASER therapy can provide adequate palliation of dysphagia. The prognosis is poor with a mean survival of 10 months after diagnosis with a 5-year survival of 5%. Where surgical resection is completed after staging and selection, 5-year survival can be up to 25%.

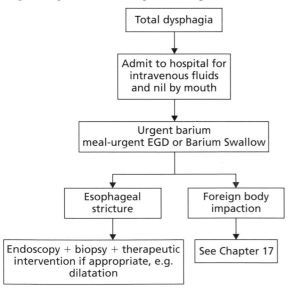

Figure 1.2 Approach to management of total dysphagia.

Further reading

Castell DO. Approach to the patient with dysphagia. In: Yamada T, Alpers DH, Owyang C, Powell DW, Silverstein FE, eds. *Textbook of Gastroenterology*. Philadelphia: Lippincott, 1995.

Falk GW, Richter JE. Approach to the patient with acute dysphagia, odynophagia, and non-cardiac chest pain. In: Taylor MB, ed. *Gastrointestinal Emergencies* 2nd edition. Baltimore: Williams & Wilkins, 1997; 65–84.

Yamada T, Alpers DH, Owyang C, Powell DW, Silverstein FE, eds. *Textbook of Gastroenterology*. Philadelphia: Lippincott, 1995.

2 Approach to Vomiting

Bee Chan Lee, John S. Collins

Definition

Acute nausea with or without vomiting is a common symptom. Nausea is described as an unpleasant sensation of imminent vomiting. Vomiting is defined as the forceful expulsion of gastric contents through the mouth and it should be differentiated from retching and regurgitation. Retching is the term which describes the labored, rhythmic respiratory activity and abdominal muscular contractions which usually precede vomiting. Regurgitation is the effortless propulsion of gastric contents into the mouth without abdominal diaphragmatic muscular contractions.

The act of vomiting is initiated by the vomiting center in the medulla or the chemoreceptor trigger zone (CTZ) in the floor of the fourth ventricle via a combination of motor and autonomic responses. Vomiting starts with salivation and then reverse peristalsis in the small intestines and a relaxed pyloric sphincter. Subsequent glottis closure (to prevent aspiration), abdominal and gastric muscular contractions and relaxation of the lower esophageal sphincter result in the final act of vomiting.

Etiology

The causes of acute nausea and vomiting are extensive and are summarized in Table 2.1.
• **Visceral (gut and peritoneum)** – visceral pain from a variety of intraabdominal causes often is associated with an acute abdomen including sepsis and mechanical obstruction. Gastric outlet obstruction leads to prolonged vomiting of the projectile nature.

Gastrointestinal Emergencies, 2nd edition. Edited by Tony Tham, John Collins and Roy Soetikno. © 2009 by Blackwell Publishing, ISBN: 978-1-4051-4634-0.

Table 2.1 Causes of acute vomiting.

Visceral stimuli	Peritonitis
	Small bowel obstruction
	Pseudo-obstruction
	Acute pancreatitis
	Acute cholecystitis
	Acute appendicitis
	Gastric outlet obstruction
	Mesenteric ischemia
CNS	Vestibular disorders
	CNS tumours
	Meningitis
	Cerebral abscess
	Subarachnoid hemorrhage
	Head injury
	Migraine
	Reye's Syndrome
Drugs	Chemotherapeutic agents
	Antibiotics/antivirals
	Narcotics
	Analgesics
	Digoxin
Infections	Sporadic viral infections
	Gastroenteritis (bacterial/viral)
	Hepatitis viruses
	Non-gastrointestinal infections
Endocrine/metabolic	Diabetic ketoacidosis
	Adrenal insufficiency
	Hypercalcemia
	Uremia
	Acute intermittent porphyria
Miscellaneous	Psychogenic
Ethanol abuse	Radiotherapy
	Pregnancy
	Carcinomatosis
	Postoperation
	Cyclical vomiting

- **CNS causes** – these include head injuries, intracranial infections/inflammation and raised intracranial pressure. Stimulation or disorders of the vestibular system such as motion sickness should not be overlooked.
- **Drugs** – nausea and vomiting are common side effects of chemotherapeutic agents, antibiotics, analgesics and narcotics but the list of other offending drugs is endless. It is also important to enquire about recreational drug use, of which the commonest is alcohol abuse. Acetaminophen/Paracetamol and salicylate toxicity also result in nausea or vomiting and this needs to be excluded.
- **Infections** – food poisoning (bacterial and viral) is the commonest. Others include epidemic viral infections, e.g. Norwalk agent and non-gastrointestinal infections such as otitis media and urinary tract infection.
- **Endocrine and metabolic** – commoner ones are hypercalcemia and uremia; less common cause includes acute intermittent porphyria.
- **Miscellaneous** – pregnancy (hyperemesis gravidarum), postoperation, cardiac causes (myocardial infarction and congestive cardiac failure), psychogenic vomiting and cyclical vomiting syndrome.

History

A detailed history is crucial in elucidating the cause of vomiting. The above causes should be considered. Constitutional symptoms of fever, myalgia, headache or possible infectious contacts in the family, school, workplace or institutions should alert the clinicians to an infectious etiology. Foreign travel and ingestion of inadequately cooked meat raise the suspicion of gastroenteritis. In these situations, a stool sample may reveal Norwalk agent, *Salmonella*, *Campylobacter*, *Staphylococcus aureus* or *Bacillus cereus*.

Any associated abdominal pain with guarding points to an acute abdomen. Bilious vomiting suggests a proximal intestinal obstruction while feculant vomiting is due to a more distal obstruction. Gastric outlet obstruction usually leads to postprandial projectile vomiting. When vomiting is associated with jaundice, anorexia and nausea, a hepatic etiology should be considered.

If there are no obvious symptoms of infection or acute abdomen, pregnancy should be excluded in female patients who are in their reproductive years.

A thorough drug history, including over-the-counter medication and herbal remedies, may reveal the cause. Patients should also be asked about recent relevant CNS symptoms of vertigo, headache, blurred vision or head injury. If no organic causes are obvious, then consider psychogenic or functional vomiting.

Examination

- Signs of dehydration – dry tongue, decreased skin turgor, postural hypotension.
- Smell of alcohol or ketones on the breath.
- Confusion may be present due to hypercalcemia or hypernatremia.
- Abdominal examination for signs of peritonism, gastric stasis or acute intestinal obstruction. A succussion 'splash' is suggestive of gastric outlet obstruction.
- CNS signs of meningism, nystagmus or papilledema. Other important clinical features to look out for include:
- Signs of uremia – sallow appearance, pericardial rub.
- Signs of hypoadrenalism – pigmentation, postural hypotension.
- Characteristic skin blisters of acute intermittent porphyria.

Investigations

In all cases, basic laboratory tests such as full blood count, urea, electrolytes and inflammatory markers are essential. A pregnancy test should be performed in any female of reproductive age, preferably before any radiographic studies are performed. Subsequent investigations will be directed towards the suspected cause elicited from the history.

If infection is suspected:
- liver function tests
- viral hepatitis serology
- stool culture
- urinalysis and urine culture (particularly in elderly patients).

If a visceral cause is suspected:
- serum pancreatic enzymes (amylase and lipase) – if acute epigastric tenderness suggests acute pancreatitis.
- plain abdominal radiographs (erect and supine) – in the presence of peritonism, they may show an ileus, small bowel obstruction or free gas due to perforation.

• abdominal ultrasound – may show gallstones and a thickened gallbladder wall if biliary signs are present.
• Upper endoscopy or barium meal – to confirm gastric outlet obstruction, preferably *after* the residual gastric contents have been emptied using a nasogastric tube.

If a CNS cause is suspected:
• CT or MRI of brain;
• lumbar puncture – should be avoided until the presence of raised intracranial pressure has definitely been excluded;
• vestibular testing.

Other tests to consider: synacthen test, urinary porphyrins.

Management of acute nausea and vomiting

A three-step approach is advocated:
1. Correction of any complications of vomiting such as dehydration and acid/electrolyte abnormalities.
2. Targeted therapy of identified cause of vomiting.
3. Symptomatic treatment if necessary.

Fluid replacement

If the patient is dehydrated and cannot tolerate oral fluids, intravenous fluid replacement using normal saline should be started. Potassium supplements may be required in patients with gastric outlet obstruction or if the vomiting has been associated with prolonged diarrhea. Management of diabetic ketoacidosis should be tailored according to local hospital guidelines.

Antiemetic drugs

These agents are useful in the acute phase in the majority of cases of acute vomiting where the underlying etiology is not clear but urgent symptomatic relief is necessary. In some cases, more than one agent may be required. The main types of antiemetic drugs are summarized in Table 2.2 and their clinical uses in Table 2.3.
• **Prochlorperazine (Stemetil®):** Particularly effective in vestibular vomiting. Its main side effects are extrapyramidal symptoms. It must be cautiously used in patients with Parkinson disease, narrow angle glaucoma and a history of phenothiazine sensitivity.

Oral prochlorperazine – 20 mg initially followed by 10 mg after 2 hours. For prevention, give 5–10 mg 2–3 times daily.

Table 2.2 Classes of antiemetic drug.

Antimuscarinic	Scopalamine (hyoscine)
Antihistamine	Cyclizine
	Promethazine
	Meclozine
	Cinnarazine
Antidopaminergic	Prochlorperazine
	Domperidone
	Metoclopramide
Antiserotoninergic	Ondansetron
	Granisetron
	Tropisetron

Table 2.3 Clinical uses of different antiemetics.

Antimuscarinic	Motion sickness
Antihistamine	Motion sickness, vestibular causes
Antidopaminergic	Extensive indications including gastroenteritis, postoperative, chemo/radiotherapy-induced vomiting, medication
Antiserotoninergic	As above indications

Sublingual (Buccastem®) – a 3 mg tablet can be placed high up between the upper lip and gums and left to dissolve. Recommended dosage is 1–2 tablets twice daily.

Suppository – a 25 mg suppository can be placed rectally stat, followed by oral dose after 6 hours if necessary.

Injection – give 12.5 mg stat by deep intramuscular injection, followed by oral dose after 6 hours if necessary.
• **Cyclizine (Valoid®):** This is a histamine H1 receptor antagonist and is effective in patients where there is a contraindication to the above. It can cause drowsiness and should be used with caution in the elderly. For severe vomiting or in patients who cannot tolerate oral medication, give 50 mg stat either by intramuscular or intravenous injection and this can be repeated 8-hourly. For less severe vomiting, oral dose 50 mg 8-hourly can be given.
• **Domperidone (Motilium®) and metoclopramide (Maxolon®):** These drugs are dopamine receptor antagonists and also function as prokinetic agents. Domperidone has not been approved for use in the

US. Metoclopramide is contraindicated in gastrointestinal obstruction and perforation. Domperidone can be given orally (10–20 mg) or rectally (30–60 mg) every 4–8 hours. Alternatively, give metoclopramide 10 mg, either oral or injections (intramuscular/intravenous) every 8 hours.

• **Ondansetron (Zofran®):** If all above fail, this serotonin 5-HT3 receptor antagonist can be given as a 4 mg dose either by intramuscular or intravascular injection. It can also be given as 16 mg suppositories.

If vomiting is controlled after the initial dose, the oral form can be given up to a daily maximum dose of 32 mg in the 4 or 8 mg tablet form. 5-HT3 receptor antagonists are regarded as first line anti-emetics for chemotherapy-induced vomiting and they are generally well tolerated.

Management of specific causes of acute vomiting is described in detail in relevant chapters in this book.

3 Approach to Upper Gastrointestinal Bleeding

Patrick Allen, Tony C.K. Tham

Introduction

Upper gastrointestinal bleeding is broadly divided into two main patient groups, nonvariceal and variceal upper gastrointestinal bleeding.

The initial assessment and aggressive resuscitation of patients who present with an episode of upper gastrointestinal bleeding are important before endoscopy and have been shown to reduce mortality [1]. This chapter will discuss the background, initial assessment and management of patients who present with suspected upper gastrointestinal bleeding.

Pathophysiology

Nonvariceal upper gastrointestinal bleeding

Peptic ulcer is the most common cause of nonvariceal upper gastrointestinal bleeding. These ulcers are mainly caused by *Helicobacter pylori* or by nonsteroidal antiinflammatory drugs. *H. pylori* can be found in the stomach in 95% of patients with a duodenal ulcer and in most patients with a gastric ulcer not associated with NSAID use. Daily NSAID usage causes an estimated 40-fold increase in gastric ulcer creation and an 8-fold increase in duodenal ulcer creation [2]. As the peptic ulcer defect invades deeper into the gastroduodenal mucosa, the arterial wall weakens and necrosis develops. This leads to the development of a pseudoaneurysm which can rupture and then bleeding may result. Duodenal ulcers are more common

Gastrointestinal Emergencies, 2nd edition. Edited by Tony Tham, John Collins and Roy Soetikno. © 2009 by Blackwell Publishing, ISBN: 978-1-4051-4634-0.

than gastric ulcers, but the incidence of bleeding is comparable for both. Bleeding vessels larger than 1.5 mm in diameter are associated with an increased mortality rate. There is evidence that therapy with high-dose proton pump inhibitors may decrease the rate of rebleeding after endoscopic therapy; this is thought to be due to its effect on increasing the gastric pH above 6, thereby stabilizing the clot.

Variceal hemorrhage

The portal vein carries approximately 1500 mL/min of blood from the intestines, spleen and stomach to the liver. Obstruction of portal venous flow, whatever the etiology, results in a raised portal venous pressure. An elevated portal venous pressure (>10 mmHg) causes distension to proximal veins and increase in the intracapillary pressure in organs drained by the obstructed veins.

Gastroesophageal varices have two main inflows, the first being the left gastric or coronary vein, and the other is the splenic hilus, through the short gastric veins.

The bleeding risk for esophageal varices becomes significant once the intravariceal pressure reaches a threshold value. The increased tension (T) within the varices is directly related to its intravascular pressure (P) and radius (R) and is inversely related to its wall thickness (W), i.e. $T = P \times R/W$. The life-threatening bleeding that occurs is the result of the high intravascular tension. Of the patients newly diagnosed with cirrhosis each year, 30% will have decompensated disease; however, it is the 60% with uncompensated disease who have varices [2]. Estimates from prospective studies indicate that the overall incidence of esophageal varices in patients with cirrhosis is 8% each year.

Elevated portal venous pressure can lead to uncontrolled variceal hemorrhage and therefore provides

Table 3.1 Major causes of upper gastrointestinal bleeding (% frequency) [4].

Source of bleeding	Frequency (%)
Peptic ulcer	35–62%
Gastroesophageal varices	4–31%
Mallory–Weiss tear	4–13%
Gastroduodenal erosions	3–11%
Erosive esophagitis	2–8%
Malignancy	1–4%
Unidentified source	7–25%

the rationale for the use of transjugular intrahepatic portosystemic shunts (TIPS). The goal of the procedure is to reduce the portal-to-atrial pressure to less than 12 mmHg. Another measurement of portal pressure is the portal–hepatic vein gradient (PHVG). Measurement of the free hepatic and wedged hepatic pressures before and after the procedure should document a decrease of the PHVG to less than 12 mmHg. The TIPS procedure controls variceal bleeding in more than 90% of patients [3].

Causes of upper gastrointestinal hemorrhage

The major causes of upper GI hemorrhage are summarized in Table 3.1 [4]. Bleeding from peptic ulcers accounts for over half of all cases of upper gastrointestinal bleeding.

Morbidity/mortality from upper gastrointestinal bleeding

Non variceal upper gastrointestinal bleeding

Patients usually present with an ulcer that has bled or is actively bleeding, but approximately 80% of ulcers stop bleeding. The overall mortality is approximately 10%. The presence of rebleeding or continued bleeding is strongly associated with a high mortality. The presence of comorbidities has been shown to increase the risk of rebleeding in patients after endoscopic therapy. The

cause of mortality is usually due to the patient's preexisting comorbidity rather than due to exsanguinations.

Variceal hemorrhage

Patients who bleed from esophageal varices have a 70% risk of rebleeding and of these approximately 30% of further bleeding episodes are fatal. Mortality is highest in the first 24–48 hours after a bleeding episode and decreases slowly over the next 6 weeks. Again the presence of comorbidities (i.e. renal, pulmonary, cardiovascular) predicts the highest mortality (20–65%).

History

The symptoms and signs of patients presenting with upper gastrointestinal bleeding may include:
- dyspepsia
- epigastric pain
- heartburn
- weakness
- syncope
- hematemesis (e.g. coffee-ground vomitus, bright red vomitus, etc.)
- melena (black stools)
- hemotochezia (bright red rectal bleeding)
- weight loss
- dysphagia.

Past medical history

It is necessary to document the recent use of aspirin or NSAIDs. As ulcers can recur, it is important to elicit a past medical history of peptic ulcer disease. Patients may present subacutely with a vague dyspeptic history or an incidental finding of iron deficiency anemia. A history of chronic alcohol abuse or chronic hepatitis (B or C) increases the likelihood of variceal hemorrhage or portal gastropathy.

Examination and assessment

Primary assessment

The amount of blood loss should be estimated. The patient's hemodynamic status should be determined. Clinical signs such as tachycardia >100 beats/min (bpm), systolic blood pressure <90 mmHg, cool extremities, syncope and other signs of shock such as ongoing hematemesis or hematochezia should alert the clinician

Table 3.2 Estimated fluid and blood losses in shock [5].

	Class 1	Class 2	Class 3	Class 4
Blood loss, mL	<750	750–1500	1500–2000	>2000
Blood loss, % blood volume	<15%	15–30%	30–40%	>40%
Pulse rate	<100	>100	>120	>140
Blood pressure	normal	normal	decreased	decreased
Respiratory rate	normal or increased	decreased	decreased	decreased
Urine output mL/h	14–20	20–30	30–40	>35
Mental status	slightly anxious	mildly anxious	confused	lethargic
Fluid replacement	crystalloid	crystalloid	crystalloid and blood	crystalloid and blood

to properly triage these patients to a high dependency setting.

Patients who present with upper gastrointestinal bleeding associated with hemorrhagic shock have been shown to have a mortality of up to 30%. Hemorrhage may be classified based on the amount of blood loss, as noted in the Table 3.2 [5]. This classification scheme aids understanding of the clinical manifestations of hemorrhagic shock. In early class 1 shock seen with a 15% loss of total blood volume, the patient may have normal vital signs. As the amount of blood loss increases the clinical signs and symptoms become more obvious.

Secondary assessment

• Signs of chronic liver disease should be sought on further examination, including ascites, splenomegaly, spider nevi.
• Signs suggestive of malignancy indicate a poorer prognosis, i.e. a nodular or enlarged liver, ascites or lymphadenopathy.
• The finding of telangiectasia may indicate a case of hereditary hemorrhagic telangiectasia.

Initial management: resuscitation

Despite recent advances in diagnosis and therapeutic endoscopic techniques the mortality of patients with upper gastrointestinal bleeding has remained relatively constant. In one prospective study patients who received early intensive resuscitation were more quickly stabilized hemodynamically and the hematocrit was corrected sooner, resulting in a lower incidence of myocardial infarction and reduction in mortality [1].

The approach to a hemodynamically unstable patient begins initially with assessing the airway, breathing and circulation, i.e. ABC. Some patients who present with severe blood loss and hypovolemic shock can present with mental status changes; in these circumstances the patients are at increased risk for aspiration. This is a potentially preventable complication and one that if present may increase morbidity and mortality in these patients. This situation should be recognized early and patients electively intubated in a controlled setting using cricoid pressure.

When the airway has been secured it is necessary to obtain intravenous access. It is adequate to insert bilateral 16-gauge upper extremity intravenous lines for volume resuscitative measures. An estimated guideline for fluid replacement to correct the hypovolemia is the *3 for 1 rule*. This rule aims to replace each millilitre (mL) of blood loss with 3 mL of crystalloid (or colloid) fluid. This regime is commonly the initial fluid replacement until cross-matched or type-specific blood becomes available. Patients with comorbidities, e.g. cardiovascular diseases, may require pulmonary artery catheter insertion to evaluate cardiac performance profiles and resuscitation adequacy in the early stages.

Risk assessment

Several validated risk stratification scores have been published; many of these are composite scoring systems including both clinical and endoscopic parameters. Such a score should aid clinical decisions, e.g. by triaging patients to a high dependency unit if they are

Table 3.3 Rockall risk score scheme [6].

Value	Score			
	0	1	2	3
Age (years)	<60	60–79	>80	–
Shock	None (systolic BP >100, pulse <100)	Tachycardia (systolic BP >100, pulse >100)	Hypotension (systolic BP <100)	–
Comorbidity	No major comorbidity	–	Cardiac failure, ischemic heart disease, any major comorbidity	Renal failure, liver failure, disseminated malignancy
Diagnosis	Mallory-Weiss tear, no lesion identified and no SRH	All other diagnoses	Malignancy of upper gastrointestinal tract	–
Major stigmata of recent haemorrhage	None or dark spot only	–	Blood in upper gastrointestinal tract, adherent clot, visible or spurting vessel	–

The total score is calculated by simple addition of each variable. Maximum additive score prior to endoscopy is 7, maximum additive score following endoscopy is 11. BP blood pressure, SRH stigmata of recent hemorrhage.

at high risk. If they are low risk, these patients can be discharged sooner.

The *Rockall score* (see Table 3.3 [6]) is based on age, comorbidities, the presence of shock, and endoscopic findings. A total score of 3 or less is associated with an excellent prognosis, while a score of 8 or more is associated with a high risk of mortality. To date, the Rockall score is one of the most widely used methods for risk assessment in upper gastrointestinal bleeding and it has been validated by several studies.

In a study designed to validate the Rockall risk score, admissions to a gastrointestinal bleeding unit were scored prospectively for upper gastrointestinal bleeding secondary to both peptic ulcer and variceal hemorrhage. The results showed that if an initial (clinical) Rockall score was less than or equal to 2, the risk of mortality for esophageal variceal bleeding was 2.6% and for peptic ulcer bleeding no patients died. If the complete Rockall score (i.e. total score post-endoscopy) was less than or equal to 4 the risk of rebleeding in the variceal group was 1.8%, and 7.5% in the peptic ulcer group. See Table 3.4 for relationship between Rockall score and risk of rebleeding and mortality [7].

Another risk assessment tool is the *Blatchford score* (see Table 3.5). This utilizes simple clinical and

Table 3.4 Relationship between Rockall score, rebleeding and mortality [7].

Score	% Rebleeding	% Mortality
0	5	0
1	3	0
2	5	0
3	11	3
4	14	5
5	24	11
6	33	17
7	44	27
8+	42	41

biochemical parameters to derive a score that predicts the need for intervention to control recurrent bleeding. This has an advantage over the Rockall score in that it does not require endoscopic parameters to derive a score. The risk factors – elevated blood urea, reduced hemoglobin, a drop in systolic blood pressure, a tachycardia, the presence of melena or syncope, and evidence of hepatic or cardiac disease – are assigned numerical values. The full score can be used to determine the required level of care on admission and to

Table 3.5 Blatchford admission risk markers [8].

Admission risk marker	Score component value
Blood urea (mmol/L)	
6.5–8	2
8.0–10.0	3
10.0–25.0	4
>25	6
Hemoglobin (g/dL) for men	
12–13	1
10–12	3
<10	6
Hemoglobin (g/dL) for women	
10–12	1
<10	6
Systolic blood pressure (mmHg)	
100–109	1
90–99	2
<90	3
Other markers	
Pulse >100 bpm	1
Presenting with melena	1
Presentation with syncope	2
Hepatic failure	2
Cardiac failure	2

Table 3.6 Need for intervention (i.e. transfusion, endoscopic therapy, surgery) and total Blatchford score.

Total score	Need for intervention (approx %)
<3	<10
4	25
5	40
6	50
7–9	75
>10	95

Table 3.7 The Child–Pugh classification [9].

Parameter	1 point	2 points	3 points
Bilirubin	<2	2–3	>3
Albumin	>35	28–35	<28
Increase in PT	1–3	4–6	>6
Ascites	None	Slight	Moderate
Encephalopathy	None	1–2	3–4

Total score: grade A: 5–6 (well-compensated disease), grade B: 7–9 (significant functional compromise), grade C: 10–15 (decompensated disease). These grades correlate with 1- and 2-year survival: grade A 100% and 85%; grade B 80% and 60%; and grade C 45% and 35%, respectively. PT prothrombin time.

women, systolic blood pressure >110 mmHg or higher and pulse less than 100 bpm [8].

The following are independent risk factors for variceal upper gastrointestinal bleed and include:
- variceal size: the larger the varix, the higher the risk of rupture and bleeding;
- the presence of endoscopic red colour signs (e.g. red wale markings, cherry red spots);
- the Child–Pugh classification;
- active alcohol intake in patients with chronic alcohol-related diseases;
- local changes in the distal oesophagus (e.g. gastroesophageal reflux disease).

The *Child–Pugh classification* (Table 3.7) can aid in assessing prognosis following an acute variceal hemorrhage. A total score of less than or equal to 3 is associated with a good prognosis, while a score of 8 or more is associated with a high risk of death [9].

Investigations

Initial investigations are necessary to determine baseline indices in evaluating patients with an upper GI bleed and include:
- **Full blood count with platelet count:** this is required to assess the level of blood loss, although this can be normal in the early stages. The hemoglobin should be monitored serially in order to follow the progress of the bleed as falling hemoglobin may signify ongoing hemorrhage requiring further intervention.

identify those patients who need urgent treatment (see Table 3.6). A simplified fast-track risk screening procedure has been developed to identify patients at low risk of needing clinical intervention for upper gastrointestinal bleeding. This states that if all of the following variables are present then the patient is at low risk for requiring intervention, i.e. blood urea <6.5 mmol/L, hemoglobin >13.0 g/dL for men or >12.0 g/dL for

However, hemoglobin may fall in the initial 72 hours after a bleed due to hemodilution rather than continued bleeding. The presence of a hemodynamic stability would suggest hemodilution rather than continued bleeding. A platelet count of <50 with active acute hemorrhage requires a platelet transfusion and fresh frozen plasma in an attempt to restore clotting factors.

- **Liver profile:** can identify hepatic comorbidity.
- **Urea and electrolytes:** useful to evaluate presence of renal disease. An elevated urea with a normal creatinine (in a patient without chronic kidney disease) is suggestive of an upper gastrointestinal hemorrhage.
- **Coagulation profile:** the prothrombin time (PT), activated partial thromboplastin time (APTT) and international normalized ratio (INR) should be checked to determine the presence of coagulopathy either as primary (e.g. chronic liver disease) or secondary, i.e. consumptive which is associated with thrombocytopenia.
- **Group and screen/cross-match:** based on the patient's condition (i.e. presence or absence of shock) or the initial hemoglobin level, a group type and screen or cross-match should be requested. The patient should be cross-matched 2–6 units depending on the rate of active bleeding.
- **ECG:** to exclude cardiac arrhythmias and acute coronary syndromes.
- **Chest radiograph:** to exclude pneumonia (particularly secondary to aspiration) and pulmonary oedema.

Medical management of suspected nonvariceal upper gastrointestinal hemorrhage

A study from India showed a benefit from omeprazole for the treatment of peptic ulcer bleeding. A total of 220 patients were randomized to receive either oral omeprazole 40 mg twice daily or placebo for 5 days after endoscopic confirmation of a bleeding peptic ulcer. Endoscopic therapy was not applied. Patients whose ulcers had a nonbleeding visible vessel or a clot were less likely to have further bleeding. A reduction in recurrent bleeding was not evident in those patients with ulcers with spurting or oozing hemorrhage who were given oral omeprazole [10].

In a landmark study from Hong Kong, Lau et al. included 240 patients with peptic ulcer bleeding who received endoscopic therapy and were then randomized to receive either placebo or an intravenous omeprazole with a loading dose of 80 mg followed by an infusion of omeprazole 8 mg/h for 72 h. Those who received omeprazole had significantly lower rates of rebleeding, the mean units of blood transfused, and shorter hospital stay. However there was no statistically significant difference in mortality [11].

A recent Cochrane systematic review of the use of proton pump inhibitors for peptic ulcer bleeding compared 21 randomized controlled trials with a total of 2195 participants. They concluded that there were no significant differences in mortality between patients receiving proton pump inhibitors and controls. However, proton pump inhibitors significantly reduced the rate of recurrent bleeding and surgical intervention compared with control. The result was independent of the route of administration of proton pump inhibitors – oral or intravenous – as long as a high dose was given [12].

The benefit of pre-endoscopic use of proton pump inhibitors was supported by a large randomized controlled trial involving 638 patients. Patients admitted with upper gastrointestinal bleeding randomly received either intravenous omeprazole (80 mg bolus followed by 8 mg infusion per hour) or placebo. The need for endoscopic treatment and hospital stay were lower in the omeprazole compared to the placebo group. At endoscopy, fewer patients in the omeprazole group had actively bleeding ulcers and more omeprazole-treated patients had ulcers with clean bases. There was no differences between the groups in the mean amount of blood transfused, recurrent bleeding, need for emergency surgery, or 30-day mortality [13].

In summary, patients presenting with an acute upper gastrointestinal bleed should receive a proton pump inhibitor prior to endoscopy. These can be administered at a high dose (e.g. omeprazole 40 mg twice daily) either orally or intravenously depending on the clinical circumstances, e.g. intravenous if the patient is vomiting or is fasting for endoscopy. If they require endoscopic therapy for bleeding ulcers, they should receive high-dose intravenous omeprazole (80 mg stat then 8 mg per hour), esomeprazole or pantoprazole (available intravenous proton pump inhibitor preparations) for 72 hours postendoscopic therapy.

Management of variceal upper gastrointestinal hemorrhage

Prophylactic antibiotics

A recent Cochrane systematic review evaluated the effectiveness of prophylactic antibiotics in hospitalised cirrhotic patients with variceal hemorrhage. There was an overall reduction in infectious complications and possibly decreased mortality. Antibiotics may also reduce the risk of recurrent bleeding in hospitalised patients who bleed from esophageal varices. Thus, cirrhotic patients who present with upper gastrointestinal hemorrhage should be prescribed broad-spectrum prophylactic antibiotics [14].

Vasopressin analogues

Somatostatin inhibits the release of vasodilator hormones, indirectly causing splanchnic vasoconstriction and decreased portal inflow. Octreotide is a long-acting analogue of somatostatin. A metaanalysis of trials comparing somatostatin to vasopressin found two benefits with somatostatin, i.e. a higher relative risk of achieving initial control of the bleeding, and lower risk of adverse effects. However, these initial beneficial effects

Presentation with suspected upper gastrointestinal hemorrhage

Assessment of:

- **Airway**
  If compromised e.g. reduced level of consciousness or inability to protect airway

- **Breathing**
  Record respiratory rate, quality of respirations and oxygen saturations

- **Circulation**
  Assess blood pressure, pulse, capillary refill time (sec)

Resuscitation:

- Restore circulating blood volume eg colloid, crystalloid, until crossmatched/type-specific blood available (use 3-for-1 rule i.e. replace each 1 mL of blood lost with 3 mL of crystalloid/colloid)
- Establish airway protection in patients with massive upper gastrointestinal hemorrhage and/or reduced level of consciousness
- If indicated, correct clotting factor deficiencies, e.g. fresh frozen plasma

Medical therapy:

- Suspected non-variceal upper gastrointestinal hemorrhage
  o IV or oral high-dose PPI

- Suspected variceal upper gastrointestinal hemorrhage
  o Intravenous terlipressin (if available), or octreotide/somatostatin,
  o Broad-spectrum antibiotics

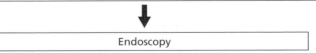

Endoscopy

Figure 3.1 Approach to patient with acute upper gastrointestinal bleed.

on bleeding have not been shown to improve survival. Somatostatin (250 µg bolus followed by 250 µg/h by intravenous infusion for 5 days) is more effective for controlling bleeding than placebo or vasopressin and has fewer side effects than vasopressin [15].

Although the role of octreotide is less well established, it is the current drug of choice in the US because of its easy availability compared to somatostatin, but despite their use neither drug has been shown to reduce mortality compared with placebo.

Terlipressin (triglycyl lysine vasopressin) is a synthetic analogue of vasopressin that is released in a slow and sustained manner. This is not yet available in the US but is used in other parts of the world. At least 20 clinical trials have demonstrated its efficacy and a recent Cochrane metaanalysis found a statistically significant reduction in all-cause mortality with terlipressin compared with placebo (RR 0.66). In comparison to somatostatin or endoscopic treatment, terlipressin has been shown to be as efficacious in the control of acute bleeding [16].

Summary

• The commonest cause of upper gastrointestinal bleeding is peptic ulceration.
• Approx. 80% of upper gastrointestinal bleeding from peptic ulceration ceases spontaneously.
• Early intensive resuscitation of those presenting with upper gastrointestinal bleeding decreases mortality.
• For variceal hemorrhage terlipressin (or octreotide in the US) and prophylactic antibiotics should be administered as these may reduce mortality.
• The use of risk assessment scores e.g. Rockall, Blatchford, aids risk stratification in those presenting with upper gastrointestinal hemorrhage and may help predict prognosis. See Fig. 3.1 for summary algorithm of our suggested approach to suspected upper gastrointestinal bleeding.

References

1. Baradarian R, Ramdhaney S, Chapalamadagu R et al. Early intensive resuscitation of patients with upper GI bleeding decreases mortality. Am J Gastroenterol 2004; 99(4):619–22.

2. Corson JD, Williamson RCN, eds. Surgery. London, Mosby Year Book; 2001.

3. Sarin SK, Agarwal SR. Gastric varices and portal hypertensive gastropathy. Clin Liver Dis 2001; 5(3):727–67.

4. Laine L. Gastrointestinal bleeding, in: Braunwalde E, Fauci A, Kasser D, eds. Harrison's Principles of Internal Medicine. 15th edn. New York, McGraw Hill; 2001:252.

5. American College of Surgeons Committee on Trauma. American College of Surgeons. 1997.

6. Rockall TA, Logan RF, Devlin HB et al. Selection of patients for early discharge or outpatient care after acute upper gastrointestinal haemorrhage. Lancet 1996; 347:1338–40.

7. Sanders DS, Carter MJ, Goodchap RJ, Cross SS, Gleeson DC, Lobo AJ. Prospective validation of the Rockall risk scoring system for upper GI hemorrhage in subgroups of patients with varices and peptic ulcers. Am J Gastroenterol 2002; 97:630–5.

8. Blatchford O, Murray WR, Blatchford M. A risk score to predict need for treatment for upper gastrointestinal haemorrhage. Lancet 2000; 356: 1318–21

9. Pugh RNH, Murray-Lyon IM, Dawson JL et al. Transection of the oesophagus for bleeding oesophageal varices. Br J Surg 1973; 60:649–9.

10. Khuroo MS, Yattoo GN, Javid G, Khan BA, Shah AA, Gulzar GM, Sodi JS. A comparison of omeprazole and placebo for bleeding peptic ulcer. N Engl J Med 1997; 336:1054–8.

11. Lau JY, Sung JJ, Lee KK et al. Effect of intravenous omeprazole on recurrent bleeding after endoscopic treatment of bleeding peptic ulcers. N Engl J Med 2000; 343:310–16.

12. Leontiadis GI, McIntyre L, Sharma VK, Howden CW. Proton pump inhibitor treatment for acute peptic ulcer bleeding. Cochrane Database Syst Rev 2004; (3): CD002094.

13. Lau JY, Wai KL, Justin CY et al. Omeprazole before endoscopy in patients with gastrointestinal bleeding. N Engl J Med 2007; 356:1631–40.

14. Soares-Weiser K, Brezis M, Tur-Kaspa R, et al. Antibiotic prophylaxis for cirrhotic patients with gastrointestinal bleeding. Cochrane Database Syst Rev 2002; (2):CD002907.

15. Imperiale TF, Teran JC, McCullough AJ. A metaanalysis of somatostatin versus vasopressin in the management of acute oesophageal haemorrhage. Gastroenterology 1995; 109:1289.

16. Ioannou G, Doust J, Rockey DC. Terlipressin for acute esophageal variceal haemorrhage. Cochrane Database Syst Rev 2003; CD002147.

4 Approach to Acute Abdominal Pain

Tony C.K. Tham

Introduction

The term acute abdomen describes a syndrome of sudden abdominal pain with accompanying symptoms and signs that focus attention on the abdominal region. The causes of an acute abdomen can be abdominal (Table 4.1) or extraabdominal (Table 4.2). In the majority of cases in adults, the diagnosis of acute abdominal pain can be established on clinical grounds without resort to extensive investigation.

The following pathophysiological mechanisms can cause acute abdominal pain (Table 4.3): peritoneal, obstructive, hemorrhage, and non-specific.

Peritoneal

This symptom complex is a consequence of an inflamed intraabdominal viscus. The inflamed viscus causes irritation of the visceral peritoneum, initially causing vague central abdominal pain which may be difficult for the patient to localize. Continued inflammation or localized perforation leads to involvement of the parietal peritoneum. Pain becomes localized and is then associated with tenderness, guarding and rebound tenderness on local palpation. Spread of infection generally throughout the abdominal cavity leads to generalized abdominal wall rigidity, often associated with a rigid or board-like abdomen. Generalized systemic signs of sepsis are apparent at this stage with pyrexia, tachycardia and pallor.

Obstructive

In this situation, a hollow viscus has a lumenal blockage which interferes with its normal motility pattern and its

Table 4.1 Abdominal causes of acute abdomen [1].

Gastrointestinal	Appendicitis
	Perforated peptic ulcer
	Intestinal obstruction
	Intestinal perforation
	Intestinal ischemia
	Colonic diverticulitis
	Meckel diverticulitis
	Inflammatory bowel disease
Pancreatic, biliary, hepatic, splenic	Acute pancreatitis
	Acute cholecystitis
	Hepatic abscess
	Ruptured or hemorrhagic hepatic tumour
	Acute hepatitis
	Acute cholangitis
	Splenic rupture
Urological	Ureteral stone
	Pyelonephritis
Retroperitoneal	Aortic aneurysm
	Retroperitoneal hemorrhage
Gynecological	Ruptured ovarian cyst
	Ovarian torsion
	Ectopic pregnancy
	Acute salpingitis
	Pyosalpinx
	Endometritis
	Uterine rupture
Abdominal wall	Rectus muscle hematoma

ability to deal with lumenal contents or secretions. This results in often severe crampy pain as in cases of biliary colic where the cystic duct is obstructed by a gallstone or renal colic due to an obstructing ureteric calculus.

Gastrointestinal Emergencies, 2nd edition. Edited by Tony Tham, John Collins and Roy Soetikno. © 2009 by Blackwell Publishing, ISBN: 978-1-4051-4634-0.

Table 4.2 Extraabdominal causes of acute abdomen [1].

Thoracic	Myocardial infarction
	Acute pericarditis
	Lower lobe pneumonia
	Pneumothorax
	Pulmonary infarction
Hematological	Sickle cell crisis
	Acute leukemia
Neurological	Herpes zoster
	Tabes dorsalis
	Nerve root compression
Metabolic	Diabetic ketoacidosis
	Addisonian crisis
	Acute porphyria
	Hyperlipoproteinemia
Drug related	Lead toxicitiy
	Narcotic withdrawal

Table 4.3 Causes of abdominal pain based on pathophysiological mechanisms.

Infective/inflammatory	Acute cholecystitis
	Acute pancreatitis
	Acute appendicitis
	Pelvic inflammatory disease
Hemorrhagic	Ruptured aneurysm
	Ruptured ectopic pregnancy
	Mesenteric thrombosis
	Ruptured spleen
Obstructive	Intestinal obstruction
	Biliary obstruction
	Renal colic
Miscellaneous	Referred from chest, spine
	Diabetes
	Porphyria
	Psychogenic

When the bowel itself is obstructed the result is the classical clinical triad of:
- abdominal colic
- vomiting (due to failure of transit)
- increasing constipation.

Intestinal obstruction if left untreated will lead to perforation with signs of an acute abdomen. In the early stages of acute obstruction, bowel sounds are often high pitched or 'tinkling' in character, but the sounds disappear when prolonged obstruction leads to perforation and peritonitis.

Hemorrhagic

Although this is not the commonest cause of acute abdominal pain, it must be considered because of its serious and often rapid progression. It is due to bleeding into the peritoneal cavity or retroperitoneum either due to a leaking major vessel (e.g. aortic aneurysm) or a ruptured organ (e.g. spleen or ectopic tubal pregnancy). Onset of the pain may be insidious and poorly localized at first. Soiling of the peritoneum with blood may simulate peritonitis. The bowel sounds may diminish and ileus may be present. The patient's circulatory system will show signs of shock and the abdomen will distend as bleeding progresses.

Nonspecific acute abdominal pain

This presentation is common and may present with colicky abdominal pain or even progressive generalized pain. Pain may result from:
- parietal pleura in pneumonia
- subphrenic sepsis
- myocardial ischemia
- due to diabetic ketoacidosis
- hypercalcemia
- porphyria
- psychogenic factors.

In this scenario, the abdomen is usually generally tender with guarding. Bowel sounds are preserved and there may be no signs of systemic sepsis or bleeding.

History

A careful history can often lead to an accurate diagnosis of abdominal pain. Several important features need to be determined. A comparison of the symptoms of common causes of acute abdominal pain is shown in Table 4.4.

Site

A diagnosis based on site alone is difficult because of the phenomenon of referred pain. However, such an approach is commonly used with most clinicians dividing the abdomen into quadrants (Table 4.5).

Temporal characteristics

Immediate pain is suggestive of an acute obstruction of a hollow viscus (e.g. bile duct obstruction by a stone), perforation or acute ischemia. The more common

Table 4.4 Comparison of symptoms of common causes of acute abdominal pain [2].

Condition	Onset	Location	Character	Descriptor	Radiation	Intensity
Appendicitis	Gradual	Periumbilical early; RIF late	Diffuse early, localized late	Ache	RIF	+ +
Cholecystitis	Rapid	RUQ	Localized	Constricting	Scapula	+ +
Pancreatitis	Rapid	Epigastric, back	Localized	Boring	Midback	+ + to + + +
Diverticulitis	Gradual	LIF	Localized	Ache	None	+ to + +
Perforated peptic ulcer	Sudden	Epigastric	Localized early, diffuse late	Burning	None	+ + +
Small bowel obstruction	Gradual	Periumbilical	Diffuse	Crampy	None	+ +
Mesenteric ischemia/infarct	Sudden	Periumbilical	Diffuse	Agonising	None	+ + +
Ruptured abdominal aortic aneurysm	Sudden	Abdominal, back, flank	Diffuse	Tearing	Back, flank	+ + +
Gastroenteritis	Gradual	Periumbilical	Diffuse	Spasmodic	None	+ to + +
Pelvic inflammatory disease	Gradual	Either LIF, pelvic	Localized	Ache	Upper thigh	+ +
Ruptured ectopic pregnancy	Sudden	Either LIF, pelvic	Localized	Light headed	None	+ +

RIF, right iliac fossa; RUQ, right upper quadrant; LIF, left iliac fossa; +, mild; + +, moderate; + + +, severe

situation is a relatively gradual onset of pain which may take hours or days. This is typical of inflammatory conditions such as appendicitis, diverticulitis, pancreatitis and cholecystitis. Abrupt spontaneous cessation of pain suggests the relief of an obstructed organ, e.g. passage of a stone. Intermittent or waxing and waning pain is typical of colic which is usually intestinal in origin. Biliary pain actually shows less variability than is commonly thought. Some other causes of intermittent abdominal pain with periodicity, i.e. long duration of pain-free intervals, are shown in Table 4.6.

Character and intensity of pain

Rating the severity or describing the nature of the pain seldom helps in distinguishing the cause of the pain. The pain of colic refers to a characteristic wave-like build-up in intensity, culminating in severe pain often associated with other symptoms such as sweating, nausea and dizziness. Colicky abdominal pain is due to obstructive causes as described above. Causes of colicky abdominal pain are listed in Table 4.3 (obstructive causes).

Relieving and aggravating factors

The pain of duodenal ulcer tends to improve with food or antacids. The pain of gastric ulcer may be worsened by food. Relief after vomiting suggests a pyloric or proximal small bowel lesion. In contrast, recurrent and progressive vomiting usually results from mechanical intestinal obstruction. Colonic pain may be relieved by a bowel movement. Retroperitoneal processes, e.g. pancreatitis, tend to be relieved by maneuvers that increase the volume of this space, i.e. sitting up and bending forward. Obstructive pain tends to induce restlessness. Peritoneal pain is aggravated by motion, coughing or straining.

Associated symptoms

Anorexia accompanies almost all acute abdominal processes but is not specific to any pathological process. Anorexia is found less frequently with urological or gynaecological causes. Abdominal distension usually signifies accumulation of swallowed gas in the bowel as a result of mechanical obstruction or ileus. Constipation may be a sign of previous health habits, a disease process such as obstruction or the development of a complication, e.g. perforation. Obstipation refers to the cessation of intestinal movements or flatus coinciding with the development of acute abdominal pain. Obstipation is associated with

Table 4.5 Localization of common causes of acute abdominal pain [3].

Right upper quadrant	Acute cholecystitis
	Biliary colic
	Acute hepatic inflammation or distention
Left upper quadrant	Splenic infarct
	Splenic flexure ischemia
Right lower quadrant	Appendicitis
	Infective terminal ileitis
	Crohn's disease
	Tubo-ovarian disorders
	Ectopic pregnancy
	Ruptured ovarian cyst
	Salpingitis
	Renal disorders
	Right ureteric calculus
	Pyelonephritis
	Pyogenic sacroileitis
Left lower quadrant	Acute diverticulitis
	Infectious of inflammatory colitis
	Pyogenic sacroileitis
	Tubo-ovarian disorders
Central abdominal pain	Gastroenteritis
	Peptic ulcer disease
	Small intestinal colic
	Acute pancreatitis
Diffuse abdominal pain	Acute infectious peritonitis
	Appendicitis
	Diverticulitis
	Inflammatory bowel disease and toxic megacolon
	Perforated ulcer
	Spontaneous bacterial peritonitis in cirrhosis
	Ischemic bowel
	Acute non infectious peritonitis
	Familial Mediteranean Fever
	Hemorrhagic pancreatitis
	Postoperative pain
	Perforated ulcer

Table 4.6 Causes of intermittent abdominal pain with periodicity [3].

Physical or obstructive	Cholelithiasis
	Ampullary stenosis
	Intermittent intestinal obstruction, e.g.
	– intussusception
	– internal hernia
	– abdominal wall hernia
Metabolic or genetic	Acute intermittent porphyria
	Familial Mediterranean fever
Neurological	Abdominal epilepsy
	Abdominal migraine
	Diabetic and other forms of radiculopathy
	Nerve entrapment syndromes
Miscellaneous	Irritable bowel syndrome
	Endometriosis
	Heavy metal poisoning
	Mesenteric ischemia
	Acute recurrent pancreatitis

Other aspects of history

Recent symptoms of dyspepsia, jaundice, amenorrhea, dysuria or renal colic can suggest a possible etiology. A past history of peptic ulcer, gallstones, abdominal trauma or peripheral vascular disease can also suggest a possible etiology. A history of peripheral vascular disease could suggest an aortic aneurysm or mesenteric ischemia. Recent NSAID or aspirin use could suggest an ulcer. Other aspects of the history such as presence of diabetes, alcohol or drug abuse may be relevant in determining the cause.

Examination

Inspection

A patient with serious intraperitoneal disease usually has an anxious, pale face, sweating, dilated pupils and shallow breathing. The patient should be assessed for pyrexia, signs of shock, fetor and ketones on the breath. With peritonitis, the patient tends to lie immobile. Knees may be flexed. Inhaling or coughing aggravates the pain. With colic, the patient may appear restless with frequent changes in posture to relieve discomfort. The location of all surgical scars, masses, external hernias

mechanical obstruction or ileus. Watery diarrhea suggests acute gastroenteritis. Bloody diarrhea may be associated with exacerbation of inflammatory bowel disease, mesenteric ischemia or mesenteric venous thrombosis.

and stomas should be determined. Bruising in the flanks will indicate possible acute pancreatitis (Grey-Turner's sign). This is due to exudation of fluid stained by pancreatic necrosis into the subcutaneous tissue. Similar discoloration in the periumbilical area is known as the Cullen sign. A distended abdomen should suggest ascites or intestinal obstruction.

Palpation

Light and deep palpation of the abdomen will indicate areas of local tenderness, rebound or guarding or whether generalized tenderness is present. Point tenderness, caused by the movement of parietal peritoneum against the inflamed surface of a diseased viscus, gives good evidence of a localized inflammatory process. The Carnett test may help to determine whether chronic abdominal pain arises from the abdominal wall or has an intraabdominal origin. If a tender spot is identified, the patient is asked to raise his or her head, thus tensing the abdominal muscles. If there is greater tenderness on repeat palpation, the Carnett test is positive and suggests a cause in the abdominal wall. The Murphy sign may indicate the presence of an acute cholecystitis. The right upper quadrant is palpated and, during the palpation, the patient is asked to take a deep breath. If the patient complains of increased pain during this maneuver due to the movement of the gallbladder towards the peritoneum, this sign is positive suggesting the presence of an inflamed gallbladder. If a mass is palpable, this could be due to a neoplasm or hernia. A palpable tender mass in the right iliac fossa could also be due to Crohn's disease or an appendix abscess. A pulsatile abdominal mass usually indicates the presence of an abdominal aortic aneurysm.

Auscultation

Bowel sounds will be high pitched in impending obstruction, absent in ileus or the presence of peritonitis. Bowel sounds are considered absent if no tones are heard over a 2-minute period.

A *digital rectal examination* should be performed. If an inflamed appendix lies deep within the pelvis, point tenderness may be elicited by palpation through the right rectal wall.

A *pelvic examination* should be performed if a gynaecological cause is suspected.

Investigation

Investigations should reflect the clinical suspicion raised during the history and clinical examination. They must be tailored to answer specific questions arising from the differential diagnosis.

• **Full blood picture and differential white cell count:** Hemoglobin will be reduced in the presence of acute intraabdominal bleeding. White cell count will rise in the presence of sepsis with a neutrophilia in cases of bacterial infection

• **Serum amylase** will be elevated in acute pancreatitis (usually three or four times greater than normal), perforated peptic ulcer and in some cases of ruptured abdominal aortic aneurysm, small bowel obstruction and ischemia and ectopic pregnancy.

• **Serum lipase** has a superior sensitivity and specificity for acute pancreatitis and where available is preferable to serum amylase for the diagnosis of acute pancreatitis.

• **Urea, electrolytes and blood glucose:** Sodium will be low in cases of pain associated with prolonged vomiting and decreased fluid intake.

• **Liver function tests:** Should be performed in patients with upper abdominal pain.

• **Urine pregnancy testing:** Should be performed in women of reproductive age with lower abdominal pain.

• **Other blood tests:** These are obtained on the basis of clinical history, e.g. prothrombin time in those with suspected liver disease, blood cultures if pyrexia is present.

• **Plain abdominal radiography (erect and supine)** will demonstrate bowel fluid levels in cases of obstruction, free intraabdominal gas. It is important to determine if a patient has complete or partial small bowel obstruction. Complete obstruction is characterized by dilated loops of small intestine with air-fluid levels and no gas within the colon. Those with partial obstruction usually show clear evidence of gas in the colon in addition to dilated loops of small intestine. Only 10% of abdominal radiographs reveal diagnostic findings but the examination is readily available, inexpensive and should be obtained in most circumstances.

• **Chest radiography** may demonstrate a basal pneumonia or a pleural effusion or pneumoperitoneum (air under the diaphragm).

• **Ultrasound of abdomen** if ruptured aortic aneurysm, ectopic pregnancy or acute pancreatitis are suspected. Ultrasound is the preferred initial test for acute cholecystitis. It can detect gallstones with 95% sensitivity and also provides information regarding other abdominal organs, e.g. ectopic pregnancy, ovarian cyst. A positive sonographic Murphy sign in the presence of gallstones predicts acute cholecystitis in 90% of cases.

• **CT abdomen and pelvis:** CT of the abdomen and pelvis provides information about the presence of pneumoperitoneum, abnormal bowel gas patterns and calcifications. CT can also detect inflammatory lesions, e.g. appendicitis, diverticulitis, pancreatitis and abscess. CT can detect neoplastic lesions (e.g. obstructing colon cancer, pancreatic tumors and trauma (e.g. spleen, liver and kidney injury). CT also provides information about vascular lesions, e.g. portal vein thrombosis, pyelophlebitis, aneurysms and intraabdominal or retroperitoneal hemorrhage. CT is rapidly displacing traditional contrast radiography in the evaluation of small bowel obstruction. CT is useful when diverticular complications are suspected as it can confirm diverticulitis (sensitivity 65%) and also perforation, abscess or fistula (sensitivity 90–100%).

• **Endoscopy:** Endoscopy can be useful in evaluation of the stomach, duodenum and colon for ulceration, neoplasia and inflammation.

• **Diagnostic laparoscopy:** This is a safe and accurate tool that can be used to rule out acute intraabdominal disease thus avoiding the need for a laparotomy. This technique is appealing in critically ill patients, in whom the morbidity and mortality associated with a nontherapeutic laparotomy can be substantial. In some cases, definitive therapy can also be undertaken using minimally invasive techniques. Also if conversion to a laparotomy is required, the information obtained from the laparoscopy allows the surgeon to appropriately place and minimize the size of a laparotomy incision.

• **Laparotomy:** This is reserved for patients with intraabdominal catastrophe whose diagnosis is obvious from the clinical history and examination, e.g. ruptured aortic aneurysm or patients in extremis in whom delay in therapy would be life-threatening. The placement of the incision is influenced strongly by the presumed pathological process and by the certainty of diagnosis. In many instances, the precise diagnosis is not known at the time of laparotomy and a vertical midline incision may be performed.

Management

• If the patient is shocked, he or she will need the following:

– vigorous fluid resuscitation, initially via a peripheral intravenous line with colloid 500 mL over 15–30 minutes and then guided by measurement of the central venous pressure;

– monitor urine output with a urinary catheter;

– antibiotic therapy with cefotaxime 1 g 8-hourly intravenously plus gentamicin 80 mg 8-hourly intravenously (reduce dose in renal impairment) plus metronidazole 500 mg 8-hourly intravenously;

– an urgent surgical consult.

• Give oxygen if the patient has severe pain, is breathless, or if oxygen saturation by pulse oximetry is <90%.

• Relieve severe pain with diamorphine or pethidine.

• Further management will be determined by clinical assessment and the results of the investigations. The treatment of specific causes of acute abdominal pain are dealt with in the specific sections relating to intraabdominal emergencies.

References

1. Mulholland MW, Sweeney JF. Approach to the patient with acute abdomen. Textbook of Gastroenterology, 4th edition, Yamada T. Lippincott Williams & Wilkins, Philadelphia, 2003; 813–28.
2. Glasgow RE, Mulvihill SJ. Abdominal pain, including the acute abdomen. Sleisenger & Fordtran's Gastrointestinal and Liver Disease, 7th edition, Feldman M, Friedman LS, Sleisenger MH (eds). Saunders, Philadelphia, 2003; 71–83.
3. Pasricha PJ. Approach to the patient with abdominal pain. Textbook of Gastroenterology, 4th edition, Yamada T. Lippincott Williams & Wilkins, Philadelphia, 2003; 781–801.

5 Approach to Jaundice

Tony C.K. Tham

Definition

Jaundice is the abnormal accumulation of bilirubin in body tissues which occurs when the serum bilirubin level exceeds 50 μmol/L (3 mg/dL). Excess bilirubin causes a yellow tinting to the skin, sclera and mucous membranes. A basic knowledge of bilirubin metabolism is necessary to understand the investigations of jaundice (Fig. 5.1). *Bile acids* or *bile salts* are soluble, amphipathic end products of cholesterol metabolism formed in the pericentral hepatocytes and accounts for approximately 85% of the constituents of bile. *Cholestasis* is characterized by the constellation of physiological, morphological and clinical manifestations that result from the impairment of the bile excretory system in the liver and biliary tree. Reduced bile flow results in the accumulation of conjugated bilirubin, bile salts and cholesterol in the blood. *Obstructive jaundice* usually applies to extrahepatic causes. About 20% of patients with features of cholestasis have hepatocellular disease.

Differential diagnosis

Conditions which cause jaundice can be classified under the broad categories of (1) isolated disorder of bilirubin metabolism (*prehepatic jaundice*), (2) liver disease (*hepatic jaundice*) and (3) obstruction of the bile ducts (*obstructive/cholestatic jaundice*) (see Table 5.1). A mixed pattern

Gastrointestinal Emergencies, 2nd edition. Edited by Tony Tham, John Collins and Roy Soetikno. © 2009 by Blackwell Publishing, ISBN: 978-1-4051-4634-0.

of conjugated and unconjugated bilirubin is usually present. Normally about 95% of bilirubin is conjugated unless there is an enzyme deficiency or transport defect (prehepatic jaundice).

History and examination

When first evaluating a patient with jaundice, a quick assessment of the emergency of the situation must be made. Fever, leukocytosis and hypotension point to ascending cholangitis which requires immediate therapy. Asterixis, confusion or decreased level of consciousness may indicate severe hepatocellular dysfunction or fulminate hepatic failure and requires immediate therapy. After immediate life-threatening causes of jaundice have been excluded, a systematic approach to the patient helps to make the diagnosis. An algorithm for assessing the patient with jaundice is shown in Fig. 5.2 [1]. The history and examination provide important clues regarding the cause of the jaundice (see Table 5.2).

History

A simplified aide memoire to help in remembering specific questions to ask to ascertain the cause of jaundice is as follows:

A: **A**lcohol – ask about alcohol use, present and past.

B: **B**lood transfusion – ask about previous transfusions of blood, plasma factors or tattoos.

C: **C**ontact with jaundice.

D: **D**rugs – ask about prescribed, over-the-counter or alternative medicines such as homeopathic treatment. Hepatotoxicity can be divided into those that occur in most patients given a sufficiently high dose of the drug

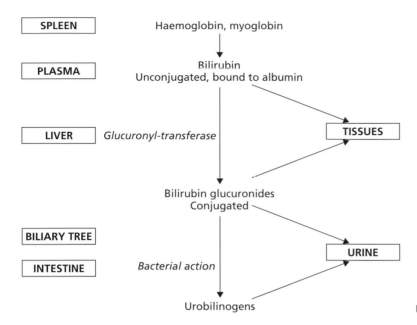

Figure 5.1 Bilirubin metabolism.

(dose-related) and idiosyncratic (dose-independent) reactions. Dose-related hepatotoxicity can be due to paracetamol/acetaminophen (>10 g/24 h, but as little as 6 g/24 h in those with alcoholic liver disease), anabolic steroids, halothane, methotrexate (fibrosis is unusual if total dose <2 g). Drugs which can cause dose-independent hepatoxicity are listed in Table 5.3. The diagnosis is suspected if jaundice occurs within 3 months of starting any new drug. Occasionally, liver damage can present 1 year or more after starting the drug (minocycline, methotrexate, methyldopa).

E: **E**nvironment – ask about animal contact, e.g. rats; industrial exposure.

F: **F**oreign travel – hepatitis-endemic areas, malaria. **F**amily history – e.g. hemochromatosis.

G: **G**allstones – ask about right upper quadrant abdominal pain.

H: **H**epatitis – ask about intravenous drug abuse and sexual relations.

Ask about associated symptoms. The time sequence of symptoms may be helpful in distinguishing hepatitis from cholestatic causes. Dark urine, pale stools and pruritus indicates cholestasis. Anorexia, nausea, distaste for cigarettes may indicate hepatitis. Weight loss may indicate malignancy or chronic pancreatitis. Pyrexia and rigors suggest cholangitis or abscess.

Examination

Look for signs suggesting acute or chronic liver disease or cholestasis/obstruction (Table 5.2). Physical signs in *chronic liver disease* include [2]:
- leukonychia/telangiectasia
- loss of muscle bulk
- spider nevi
- splenomegaly
- ascites
- peripheral edema
- loss of axillary/pubic hair
- testicular atrophy
- Dupuytren contracture
- small or large liver.

Physical signs in cholestatic/obstructive jaundice include [2]:
- pale stools
- dark urine
- scratch marks (excoriation)
- polished nails (itching)
- xanthelasma (eyelids)
- xanthomas (rarely palmar creases, tendons)
- hepatomegaly (alcohol, malignancy)
- palpable gallbladder (especially malignancy) – Courvoisier sign states that if the gallbladder is palpable in the right upper quadrant, then jaundice is

Table 5.1 Differential diagnosis of jaundice[†].

Prehepatic jaundice: isolated disorders of bilirubin metabolism
Unconjugated hyperbilirubinemia
1. Increased bilirubin production, e.g. *hemolysis, ineffective erythropoiesis*, blood transfusion, resorption of hematomas
2. Decreased hepatocellular uptake, e.g. rifampicin
3. Decrease conjugation, e.g. *Gilbert syndrome*, Crigler–Najjar syndrome, physiologic jaundice of the newborn

Conjugated or mixed hyperbilirubinemia
1. Dubin–Johnson syndrome
2. Rotor syndrome

Hepatic jaundice: liver disease
Acute or chronic hepatocellular dysfunction
1. Acute or subacute
   - *Viral hepatitis*
   - Toxins (*alcohol*, amanita)
   - Drugs (*paracetamol/acetominophen*, isoniazid, methyldopa)
   - Ischemia (hypotension, vascular occlusion)
   - Metabolic disorders (Wilson disease, Reye syndrome)
   - Pregnancy related (acute fatty liver of pregnancy, pre-eclampsia)
2. Chronic
   - *Viral hepatitis*
   - Toxins (*ethanol*, vinyl chloride, vitamin A)
   - *Autoimmune hepatitis*
   - Metabolic (*hemachromatosis*, Wilson disease, α_1-antitrypsin deficiency)

Obstructive/cholestatic jaundice: obstruction of the bile ducts
Extrahepatic
1. *Choledocholithiasis*
2. Diseases of the bile ducts
   - Neoplasms (*cholangiocarcinoma*)
   - Inflammation/infection (primary sclerosing cholangitis, AIDS cholangiopathy, hepatic arterial chemotherapy, post-surgical strictures)
3. Extrinsic compression of the biliary tree
   - Neoplasms (*pancreatic carcinoma*, metastatic lymphadenopathy, hepatoma)
   - Chronic pancreatitis
   - Vascular enlargement (aneurysm, portal cavernoma)

Intrahepatic: hepatic disorders with prominent cholestasis
1. Diffuse infiltrative disorders
   - Granulomatous diseases (mycobacterial infections, *sarcoidosis, lymphoma*, drug toxicity, Wegener granulomatosis)
   - Amyloidosis
   - Malignancy
2. Inflammation of intrahepatic bile ductules and/or portal tracts
   - *Primary biliary cirrhosis*
   - Graft-versus-host disease
   - Drug toxicity (*chlorpromazine*, *erythromycin*)
3. Miscellaneous
   - Benign recurrent intrahepatic cholestasis
   - Drug toxicity
   - Estrogens, anabolic steroids
   - Total parenteral nutrition
   - Bacterial infections
   - Uncommon manifestations of viral or alcoholic hepatitis
   - Intrahepatic cholestasis of pregnancy
   - Postoperative cholestasis

[†]Common disorders are in *italics*.

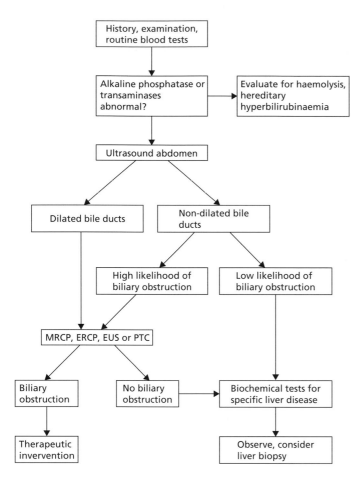

Figure 5.2 Diagnostic algorithm for assessment of the patient with jaundice. From Lidofsky S and Scharschmidt BF. Jaundice. In: *Sleisenger and Fordtran's Gastrointestinal and Liver Disease*, 6th ed., Feldman M, Scharschmidt BF, Sleisenger MH (eds), WB Saunders & Co., Philadelphia, 1998; 220–23. ERCP endoscopic retrograde cholangiopancreatography, EUS endoscopic ultrasound, MRCP magnetic resonance cholangiopancreatography, PTC percutaneous transhepatic cholangiogram.

unlikely to be due to stones. By implication, it is more likely to be due to malignancy. However, one in four patients has obstruction due to bile duct stones.

Look for other signs:
• Previous biliary surgery may indicate possible obstructive jaundice.
• Fever – suspect cholangitis although hepatitis and acute cholecystitis may cause a low-grade fever.
• Personality change or confusion may indicate encephalopathy.
• Constructional apraxia may indicate encephalopathy.
• Asterixis – flapping tremor of outstretched hands, with fingers splayed.
• Dilated abdominal veins are rare – flow radiating away from the umbilicus ("caput medusa") indicates portal hypertension. Flow towards the head only indicates inferior vena cava obstruction.
• Arterial bruit over the liver is rare – this may be due to a hepatoma or acute alcoholic hepatitis.

• Rectal examination for stool color – pale in cholestatic jaundice.

Investigations

Blood tests

The following blood tests should be performed:
• **Liver enzymes** – bilirubin, alkaline phosphatase, transaminases (AST and ALT), gamma-GT, albumin. Typical values that help distinguish different types of jaundice are shown in Table 5.4. An AST >500 is very rare in alcoholic hepatitis and usually indicates coexistent viral infection or drug toxicity (e.g. acetaminophen/paracetamol) or prolonged hypotension. In rare instances, ALT can be seen in biliary obstruction but biliary pain is a feature. Gamma-GT is an unreliable test for alcohol abuse. Gamma-GT will be elevated in liver disease of any cause including

Table 5.2 Differentiating obstructive jaundice from hepatic jaundice (from ref. 1 with permission).

Suggests obstructive jaundice	Suggests hepatic jaundice
History	
Abdominal pain	Anorexia, malaise, myalgias, viral-type illness
Fever, rigors	Known infectious exposure
Prior biliary surgery	Receipt of blood products, use of intravenous drugs
Older age	Exposure to known hepatotoxin
Dark urine and pale stools	Family history of jaundice
Physical examination	
High fever	Ascites
Abdominal tenderness	Stigmata of liver disease (e.g. gynecomastia, spider nevi, Kayser–Fleischer rings)
Palpable abdominal mass	
Abdominal scar	Asterixis, encephalopathy
Urinalysis – large amount of bilirubin with little or no urobilinogen	Urinalysis – mixture of bilirubin and urobilinogen
Laboratory tests	
Predominant elevation of serum bilirubin and alkaline phosphatase	Predominant elevation of serum transaminases
Prothrombin time that is normal or normalises with vitamin K administration	Prothrombin time that does not correct with vitamin K administration
Elevated serum amylase	Blood tests indicative of specifice liver disease, e.g. autoantibodies, positive viral serology

Table 5.3 Drugs which can cause dose-independent hepatotoxicity (from ref. 2).

Liver lesion	Common culprits
Hepatitis	Isoniazid
	Sodium valproate
	Rifampicin
	NSAIDs
	Azathioprine
Cholestasis	Co-amoxiclave
	Chlorpromazine
	Prochlorperazine
	Fusidic acid
	Glibenclamide
Chronic hepatitis	Methyldopa
	Nitrofurantoin
	Dantrolene
Alcoholic hepatitis-like	Verapamil
Granulomas	Hydralazine
	Allopurinol
	Phenylbutazone

nonalcoholic fatty liver disease. A combination of a high gamma-GT and ALP is consistent with cholestasis/obstruction. Albumin is a better marker of liver function although it can be altered by redistribution of body fluids.

• *Prothrombin time* – this is a good marker of liver function.

The following blood tests should be performed depending on the type of jaundice. In *prehepatic jaundice*, the following should be performed:
• peripheral blood film;
• reticulocyte count – raised in hemolysis;
• Coomb test (direct antihuman globulin);
• serum haptoglobins – absent in hemolysis but also low in cirrhosis.

In *hepatic jaundice*, the following should be performed:
• hepatitis A, B, C serology;
• monospot (Paul-Bunnell) for infectious mononucleosis, serum for CMV, mycoplasma. If renal failure is present, check *Leptospira* titers;
• autoantibody screen – mitochondrial, smooth muscle, nuclear; (liver, kidney, microsomal);

Table 5.4 Liver enzymes in different types of jaundice (from ref. 2).

Test	Normal	Prehepatic	Hepatic	Cholestatic/obstructive
Bilirubin (μmol/L)	<17	50–150	50–400	100–900
(mg/dL)	<1	3–9	3–20	6–45
AST (IU/L)	<35	<35	300–10 000	35–400
ALP (IU/L)	<120	<120	<120–300	>300
γ GT (IU/L)	15–40	15–40	15–200	80–1000
Albumin (g/dL)	3.5–5	3.5–5	2–5	3–5
Prothrombin time (s)	13–15	13–15	15–45	15–45

- immunoglobulins;
- iron studies – iron, iron-binding capacity (transferrin saturation) and ferritin to look for hemochromatosis. In hemochromatosis, serum iron is high and transferrin saturation is high, often >80% although values of >55% warrant further investigations. Ferritin is markedly elevated when cirrhosis is present but may be at the upper limit of normal in earlier stages. It is an acute phase protein and is elevated in inflammatory conditions as well as in alcoholics.

The following blood tests should be considered if history or physical examination suggests this:
- alpha-1-antitrypsin – if deficiency is considered;
- copper and ceruloplasmin and 24-hour urinary copper – if Wilson disease is considered, e.g. <40 years old, viral titers and autoantibodies negative;
- alpha fetoprotein – should be checked if a hepatoma is suspected.

Urine

Bilirubin is absent in prehepatic causes. Urobilinogen is absent in complete cholestasis/obstruction.

Ultrasound scan

This is the preferred initial screening test for evaluating biliary obstruction. This determines the calibre of the extrahepatic biliary tree and reveals mass lesions. The sensitivity of abdominal ultrasound for the detection of biliary obstruction in jaundiced patients ranges from 55% to 91% and the specificity from 82% to 95%. It can demonstrate cholelithiasis. Common duct stones may not be seen; the negative predictive value of a dilated duct seen on scan with no stones seen is about 50% for actual common duct stones. The positive predictive value of a dilated duct with

ductal stones seen on scan is about 90%. The variability in sensitivity reflects limitations from overlying bowel gas, site and size of the stones, and presence or absence of duct dilation. Ultrasound is inconsistent in determining the site of obstruction, partly because the distal duct is not well seen in 30–50% of patients. In cases of acute obstruction it may take 4 hours to 4 days for the ducts to dilate. The ducts of some patients with partial or intermittent obstruction may not dilate. Ultrasound can detect space-occupying lesions greater than 1 cm in diameter.

Computed tomography

Computed tomography (CT) is not as accurate as ultrasound in detecting cholelithiasis. It can detect space-occupying lesions as small as 5 mm. It provides technically superior images to ultrasound in obese patients and those in whom the biliary tree is obscured by bowel gas. Its accuracy for detecting biliary obstruction is similar to ultrasound. CT with intravenous contrast material can evaluate the etiology of biliary obstruction such as stone or stricture.

Magnetic resonance imaging

Magnetic resonance cholangiopancreatography (MRCP) can detect bile duct stones or extrahepatic and intrahepatic strictures. MRCP is comparable to ERCP in the detection of bile duct stones (sensitivity and specificity 93% and 100%; 94% and 100% respectively). For the detection of strictures, e.g. in primary sclerosing cholangitis, MRCP is comparable to ERCP (sensitivity and specificity about 90%). MRI is more sensitive and specific than CT with contrast for the detection and evaluation of focal and malignant lesions. In patients with renal impairment, MRI has the advantage over CT in avoiding the potentially nephrotoxic agents used with CT. In patients who may not require therapeutic intervention, MRCP can be performed and if a stone or stricture is identified then a therapeutic intervention can follow. In patients who are likely to require intervention such as stone extraction or stenting, ERCP may be preferable as the initial investigation rather than MRCP.

Endoscopic retrograde cholangiopancreatography

Endoscopic retrograde cholangiopancreatography (ERCP) is highly accurate in the diagnosis of biliary obstruction with a sensitivity of 89–98% and specificity of 89–100%. Biopsy specimens, brushings for cytology can be obtained. If a focal cause for biliary obstruction such as a stone or stricture is detected, then therapeutic maneuvers to relieve the obstruction such as sphincterotomy, stone extraction, dilatation and stent placement can be performed during the same session. However it is invasive with a risk of complications in about 5–10% (pancreatitis, hemorrhage, perforation, cholangitis). See Chapter 11 regarding ERCP complications.

Percutaneous transhepatic cholangiography

Percutaneous transhepatic cholangiography (PTC) visualizes the biliary tree in 90–100% of patients with dilated ducts. PTC requires the passage of a needle through the skin into the hepatic parenchyma and peripheral bile duct. The sensitivity and specificity are comparable to ERCP. PTC may be technically more difficult in the absence of intrahepatic duct dilatation. Therapeutic procedures such as stent placement can be performed. However, bile duct stones cannot be extracted. Minor complications occur in 30% of patients. Major complications, including sepsis, bleeding, biliary leak, pneumothorax, arteriovenous fistula, hematoma, abscess and peritonitis occur in 1–10%. PTC is usually performed for therapeutic indications such as biliary stenting if ERCP is unsuccessful. In patients with bile duct stones where ERCP is unsuccessful in obtaining biliary access, a combined PTC followed by ERCP rendezvous procedure can be performed to allow biliary access with sphincterotomy and stone extraction.

Endoscopic ultrasound

Endoscopic ultrasound (EUS) is superior to ultrasound and CT for diagnosing bile duct stones. Its accuracy is comparable to MRCP and ERCP. EUS may be more accurate than MRCP or ERCP in detecting biliary sludge. It has fewer complications than ERCP. EUS should be considered for diagnosing or excluding bile duct stones when there are contraindications to MRCP or if prior ERCP was unsuccessful.

Liver biopsy

Liver biopsy provides information regarding hepatic lobular architecture and is most helpful in patients with undiagnosed persistent jaundice. It permits the diagnosis of viral hepatitis, nonalcoholic steatohepatitis, alcoholic hepatitis, Wilson disease, hemochromatosis, alpha-1-antitrypsin deficiency, fatty liver of pregnancy, primary biliary cirrhosis, granulomatous hepatitis, and neoplasms. It may provide clues to unsuspected biliary tract obstruction. There is a small complication rate (bleeding and perforation) of about 1.7% (see Chapter 13). Overall this is a safe procedure but the risk to benefit ratio needs to be carefully assessed and explained to the patient.

Management

Gilbert syndrome

Jaundice is rare, as the bilirubin level is usually <70 µmol/L except in concomitant illness with anorexia. Bilirubin increases on fasting. Liver enzymes are normal. The diagnosis is made by a combination of elevated bilirubin, normal liver enzymes and asymptomatic. No treatment other than reassurance is necessary.

Biliary obstruction

Therapy is directed at the mechanical relief of obstruction. The options include ERCP (sphincterotomy, stone extraction, stent insertion), PTC (stent insertion) or surgery. The therapeutic strategy depends on the likely etiology and local expertise.

Hepatic jaundice

The therapy is directed towards the underlying etiology, e.g. stopping alcohol, discontinuation of a drug, antiviral agents, phlebotomy for hemochromatosis, copper chelation for Wilson disease.

Table 5.5 Management of pruritus (from ref. 3).

Topical therapy
Lower bathing water temperature and use fewer or lighter clothing and bed coverings
Minimize dry skin by using moisturizing soaps and applying topical moisturizers

Anion-exchange resins
Cholestyramine or colestipol: start with 4 g (packet or scoop) twice daily, starting before and after breakfast, and increasing to six
    packets or scoops daily, separated from other medications by 2 hours

Bile salts
Ursodeoxycholic acid, 15 mg/kg per day

Doxepin
25–50 mg once daily

Hepatic microsomal enzyme induction
Rifampicin 300–600 mg once daily

Opioid receptor antagonists
Naltrexone, 12.5 mg once daily, increasing slowly to 50–100 mg once daily
Naloxone and nalmefene are only commonly available for parenteral use

Drug-induced jaundice

All possible drugs that can cause jaundice should be stopped. All other possible causes of jaundice should be excluded. Severe acute liver failure is managed as for other causes (see Chapter 25, acute liver failure). Liver biopsy is not necessary if the drug is well known to cause liver dysfunction. Liver biopsy is indicated if the diagnosis is uncertain or if liver enzymes have not returned to normal after 8 weeks as drug reactions may unmask pre-existing liver disease. The liver enzymes should be monitored until they return to normal, usually over several weeks. Most hepatotoxic effects resolve completely after the drug is withdrawn, unless liver dysfunction is unrecognised for several months such as with methotrexate or methyldopa. Very rarely, persistent loss of small intrahepatic bile ducts (ductopenia) can occur and is manifest by persistently elevated ALP.

Pruritus

The pruritogen is thought to be a bile acid, bile acid derivative or some other substance that undergoes enterohepatic circulation. The management of pruritus is outlined in Table 5.5 [3].

Hepatic osteodystrophy

Hepatic osteodystrophy is the metabolic bone disease encompassing osteoporosis and osteomalacia, which occurs in patients with chronic liver disease, particularly cholestatic disease. Osteoporosis is usually dominant. The management of hepatic osteodystrophy involves the early identification through bone mineral density screening by dual energy x-ray absorptiometry of all patients with cholestatic liver disease. If bone density measurement confirms osteoporosis, worsens rapidly or there are symptomatic fractures, antiresorptive medication with bisphosphonates or calcitonin is indicated.

Fat-soluble vitamin deficiency

This condition is common in patients with prolonged cholestasis. Replacement will depend on the extent of deficiency and response to treatment. Table 5.6 outlines the vitamins that can be monitored and replaced if deficient. Evaluation of therapy is monitored by 24-hour urine calcium after 3 months if vitamin D was low, followed by yearly 25-OH vitamin D levels. Annual vitamins A and E levels and prothrombin time can be monitored.

Jaundice in pregnancy

Consider other coincidental causes of jaundice. The following are specific conditions related to pregnancy.

Hyperemesis gravidarum – occurs in the first trimester. Jaundice occurs in 10% especially those with Gilbert syndrome. High serum transaminases are common. This is self limiting and liver failure does not occur.

Table 5.6 Monitoring and replacement of fat-soluble vitamin deficiency in prolonged cholestasis.

Monitoring fat-soluble vitamins	Replacement
25-OH Vitamin D level	Calcium
Vitamin A level	β carotene
Vitamin E level with fasting total lipid profile	D-α-tocopherol
Vitamin K – measure prothrombin time	Vitamin K 10 mg subcutaneously daily for 3 days, then monthly if cholestatic

Intrahepatic cholestasis of pregnancy – occurs in the third trimester. This is preceded by pruritus. The liver enzymes are cholestatic. The condition resolves within 2 weeks after pregnancy. Ursodeoxycholic appears to improve fetal outcome but has not been subject to a randomized controlled trial. It can recur with subsequent pregnancies. It is associated with increased fetal mortality and therefore early delivery may be necessary.

Acute fatty liver of pregnancy – occurs in the third trimester. The features are nausea, abdominal pain and encephalopathy. AST and uric acid are elevated. Coagulopathy and acidosis are seen. There is no hemolysis. As this condition is potentially fatal, early delivery is essential and will result in resolution.

HELLP syndrome – occurs in the third trimester. It is characterized by hemolysis, elevated liver enzymes and low platelets (hence the acronym). It is associated with pre-eclampsia. It has a clinical spectrum of severity up to acute liver failure. Hence early delivery is also needed to resolve the condition.

References

1. Lidofsky S, Scharschmidt BF. Jaundice. Sleisenger and Fordtran's Gastrointestinal and Liver Disease, 6th edition, Feldman M, Scharschmidt BF, Sleisenger MH (eds). WB Saunders & Co., Philadelphia, 1998.
2. Travis SPL, Ahmad T, Collier J, Steinhart AH. Pocket Consultant: Gastroenterology. Blackwell Publishing Ltd, Oxford, 2005.
3. Merriman RB, Peters MG. Approach to the patient with jaundice. Textbook of Gastroenterology, 4th edition, Yamada T, Alpers DH, Kaplowitz N, Laine L, Owyang C, Powell DW (eds). Lippincott Williams & Wilkins, Philadelphia, 2003; 911–28.

6 Acute Severe Lower Gastrointestinal Bleeding

Tonya Kaltenbach, Roy Soetikno

Introduction

Lower gastrointestinal bleeding is common, resulting in approximately 25 hospitalizations per 100 000 adults per year and accounting for an estimated 30% of all major gastrointestinal bleeding. It is more common in the elderly, and its presentation can range from trivial bleeding to massive, life-threatening hemorrhage with a reported mortality rate up to 5%.

The approach to lower gastrointestinal bleeding is controversial and not standardized. Various factors, including the suspected etiology, location and rapidity of bleeding, time of admission, and center experience impact the choices for radiological, surgical or endoscopic diagnosis and treatment approaches.

Definition

The bleeding is of recent limited duration and associated with hemodynamic instability as measured by tachycardia, hypotension and anemia. It also emanates from a source between the ligament of Treitz and the anus.

Presentation and differential diagnosis

Bleeding from colonic diverticula is the most common etiology of acute lower gastrointestinal bleeding (see Table 6.1).

Gastrointestinal Emergencies, 2nd edition. Edited by Tony Tham, John Collins and Roy Soetikno. © 2009 by Blackwell Publishing, ISBN: 978-1-4051-4634-0.

Important historical questions should be asked to help aid in making a correct diagnosis: focusing on age, comorbid conditions, NSAID and antiplatelet agent use, radiation exposure, abdominal surgical history and anorectal trauma. For example, in patients with lower gastrointestinal bleeding over age of 65, diverticular bleeding, arteriovenous malformation or ischemic colitis are most common, while in younger patients, infectious or inflammatory conditions are more likely.

Evaluation

The initial step in management should be stratification of risk. In most cases, lower gastrointestinal bleeding is self-limiting, therefore patients with stable vital signs, no recent bloody effluent and no syncope have a low risk of continued bleeding and elective colonoscopy is appropriate. Urgent interventions should be targeted for patients with severe bleeding.

Independent correlates of severe bleeding
- Bleeding per rectum during the first 4 hours of evaluation
- Vital sign instability
  - Tachycardia (heart rate ≥ 100 bpm)
  - Hypotension (systolic blood pressure ≤ 115 mmHg)
- Syncope
- Non-tender abdominal exam
- Aspirin use
- ≥ 2 comorbid conditions.

Investigations:
- Complete blood count

Table 6.1 Etiology of lower gastrointestinal hemorrhage.

Condition	Cause of hemorrhage
Congenital abnormalities	Meckel diverticulum
	Arteriovenous malformation
	Telangiectasia
	Hemorrhoids
	Rectal/colonic varices
	Vasculitis
	Aortoenteric fistula
Ischemia	ischemic colitis
	Mesenteric ischemia
	Necrotizing enterocolitis
	Marathon runner's colon
Dysentery	Bacterial (salmonellosis, shigellosis, *E. coli* enterocolitis, *Campylobacter* colitis, *Yersinia* enterocolitis)
	Parasitic (amebiasis, giardiasis, schitosomiasis)
Neoplasia	Hemangioma
	Leiomyoma/leiomyosarcoma
	Polyps (adenoma, hyperplastic, hamartoma)
	Colorectal cancer
Inflammation	Ulcerative colitis/Crohn's disease
	Radiation enterocolitis/proctitis
	Henoch–Schönlein purpura
Trauma	Surgery
	Endoscopic polypectomy
Structural abnormality	Diverticulosis
	Pneumatosis coli
	Collagen disorders (Ehlers–Danlos syndrome, pseudoxanthoma elasticum)
	Endometriosis
	Dieufaloy lesion
Pharmacological	Anticoagulants
	Nonsteroidal antiinflammatory drugs
	Cytotoxic chemotherapy

Exclude an upper gastrointestinal source:
- Upper endoscopy
  - patients with a positive nasogastric aspirate;
  - patients where a colonic source is not identified.

Management

Once the patient has been resuscitated, the severity and acuity of bleeding assessed, and an upper gastrointestinal source of bleeding excluded, urgent colonoscopy should be performed (Figure 6.1). In cases of continued bleeding not amenable to endoscopic therapy angiography or surgery should be considered. We emphasize a multidisciplinary team approach with close collaboration between the gastroenterologist, radiologist, surgeon and internist in the successful approach to acute severe lower gastrointestinal bleeding.

Colonoscopy
Preparation – rapid purge with polyethylene glycol based solutions
Administration should be achieved with a nasogastric tube or by drinking 1 L every 30–45 minutes. The median dose should be 5.5 L (range 4–14 L) over 3–4 hours. Metolopramide 10 mg iv can be given immediately prior to administration to control nausea and promote gastric emptying. The stomach should be aspirated before colonoscopy. Purging is contraindicated in the presence of bowel obstruction or suspected gastroparesis.

Equipment and accessory selection
An adult endoscope or therapeutic enteroscope in cases of a suspected small bowel bleeding source should be used. A foot-controlled irrigation device and an additional suction line which is directly locked to the working channel attachment aid visualization and a clear field for therapeutic intervention.

The use of a clear endoscopic mucosal resection cap or a banding cap can improve visualization behind a fold or a turn in the colon. The target bleeding source should be aligned with the axis of the accessory channel with an en face view. Direct pressure can be applied for temporary tamponade.

Techniques
In the treatment of lower gastrointestinal bleeding, various endoscopic techniques (see Table 6.2), such as clipping, looping, banding, argon plasma coagulation (APC) and thermal therapies, used alone and in combination, have been reported to be safe and efficacious. Familiarity with the different techniques is encouraged.

Technetium scan
Literature dating since 1990 suggests that technetium scans are not particularly useful to confirm and localize

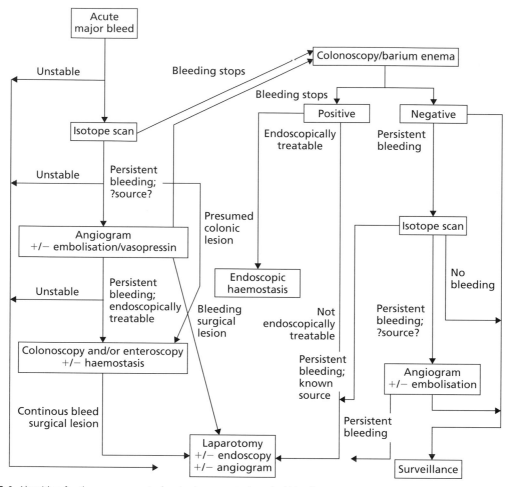

Figure 6.1 Algorithm for the management of major lower gastrointestinal bleeding.

Table 6.2 Therapies for lower gastrointestinal hemorrhage.

Diagnosis	Endoscopic therapy
Diverticular	Clip, thermal
Ischemic colitis	Self-limited
Neoplasm	Clip, loop, thermal
Arteriovenous malformation	Clip, APC, thermal
Radiation proctopathy	APC
Hemorrhoids	Banding

APC, argon plasma coagulation.

the bleeding site in order to direct further angiographic or surgical intervention.

Angiography

Small studies, using the coiling or gel foam embolization technique, have shown high rates of successful primary hemostasis in patients with active bleeding. However, short-term (less than 1 week) rebleeding rates were high at about 25% with a mean of 10–53%; data on long-term rebleeding rates is lacking. Ischemia was notably reported in close to 20% of patients despite using smaller catheters and more directed therapy.

Surgery

Whenever possible, it is preferable to perform surgery on an elective basis rather than emergently. Operative mortality is 10% even with accurate localization and up to 57% with blind subtotal colectomy.

Further reading

Elta GH. Urgent colonoscopy for acute lower-GI bleeding. Gastrointest Endosc 2004; 59:402–8.

Rockey DC. Lower gastrointestinal bleeding. Gastroenterology 2006; 130:165–71.

Strate LL, Syngal S. Predictors of utilization of early colonoscopy vs. radiography for severe lower intestinal bleeding. Gastrointest Endosc 2005; 61:46–52.

Jensen DM, Machicado GA, Jutabha R, Kovacs TO. Urgent colonoscopy for the diagnosis and treatment of severe diverticular hemorrhage. N Engl J Med 2000; 342:78–82.

Soetikno R, Kaltenbach T, Kelsey P, McQuaid K. Endoscopic Interpretation and Therapy of Severe Lower Gastrointestinal Bleeding – Educational DVD. American Society of Gastrointestinal Endoscopy Endoscopic Learning Library 2007.

Juthaba R, Kaltenbach T, Soetikno R. Endoscopic Approach to Hemorrhoids – Educational DVD. American Society of Gastrointestinal Endoscopy Endoscopic Learning Library 2006.

Khanna A, Ognibene SJ, Koniaris LG. Embolization as first-line therapy for diverticulosis-related massive lower gastrointestinal bleeding: evidence from a meta-analysis. J Gastrointest Surg 2005; 9:343–52.

Bender JS, Wiencek RG, Bouwman DL. Morbidity and mortality following total abdominal colectomy for massive lower gastrointestinal bleeding. Am Surg 1991; 57:536–40.

7 Approach to Diarrhea

John S. Collins

Definition

Diarrhea is defined as a decrease in consistency or increased liquidity of the stool. Some definitions of diarrhea also include increased frequency of defecation or increased daily stool weight, but these criteria have been limited by normal variation in a patient population. Chronic diarrhea is usually defined as persistence of symptoms for at least 4 weeks.

Differential diagnosis

The normal gut receives 6–7 L of fluid from ingested food and liquid plus intestinal secretions daily. Most of this fluid is reabsorbed by the small intestine. The colon absorbs 1.5–2.0 L and about 200 mL is excreted in the feces. Thus a fall in small bowel absorption, increased small bowel secretion or a fall in colonic absorptive capacity can lead to diarrhea. Acute diarrhea can be classified according to the deranged underlying physiological mechanisms (see Table 7.1).

Osmotic diarrhea results from the presence of poorly absorbed solutes, usually carbohydrates or peptides, within the gut lumen leading to a net increase in stool water and the passage of large volumes of liquid feces. In disaccharidase enzyme deficiency disorders such as alactasia, ingestion of lactose-rich foods such as milk can precipitate acute diarrhea due to the accumulation of high concentrations of lactose in the small bowel and loss of luminal glucose and galactose which are the substrates for sodium-dependent sugar

Gastrointestinal Emergencies, 2nd edition. Edited by Tony Tham, John Collins and Roy Soetikno. © 2009 by Blackwell Publishing, ISBN: 978-1-4051-4634-0.

Table 7.1 Physiological mechanisms in acute diarrhea.

Mechanism	Disorder
Osmotic	Disaccharide deficiencies
	Magnesium salts
	Short bowel
	Extensive mucosal disease
	Bile salt malabsorption
	Pancreatic insufficiency
Secretory	Stimulant laxatives
	Chemical toxins
	Bacterial toxins
	Drugs
	Allergic response
	Bacterial overgrowth
	Congenital
	Bile acids
	Long chain fatty acids
	Hormone-producing tumors
	Villous adenoma
Dysmotility	Irritable bowel syndrome
	Endocrine disorders
	Autonomic neuropathy
Inflammatory	Infection
	Inflammatory bowel disease
	Ischemic enteritis/colitis

absorption mechanisms. The net result is an increase in stool water leading to diarrhea. The therapeutic use of this mechanism is employed in the use of polyethylene glycol solution or magnesium and sodium salts as bowel preparation agents or laxatives.

Osmotic diarrhea can be classified into two types:
• **Exogenous** – ingested laxatives, bowel preparations; antacids – magnesium hydroxide; dietary sugar ingestion, sorbitol, xylitol; drugs – cholestyramine, lactulose

• **Endogenous** – disaccharidase deficiencies; abetali-poproteinemia; congenital lymphangiectasia; pancreatic insufficiency.

Secretory diarrhea is the result of disturbed transport of water and electrolytes, mainly Na, K, Cl and HCO_3 in the presence of gut mucosal disease, toxins or inflammatory mediators. In these conditions there is usually a stimulation of intestinal Cl and HCO_3 and inhibition of Na and Cl absorption by agents such as enterotoxins, long chain fatty acids or ingested laxatives with a secretogogue effect. Again these can be classified as:

• **exogenous**

laxatives including anthraquinones, bisacodyl, senna

drugs – diuretics, theophylline, prostaglandins

chemical toxins

bacterial toxins – *C. difficile*, *S. aureus*

gut allergy

• **endogenous**

congenital (rare) – microvillus inclusion disease

bacterial enterotoxins

endogenous laxatives due to buildup of dihydroxy bile acids and long chain fatty acids

hormone-producing tumors – vipoma, medullary carcinoma of the thyroid, mastocytosis

Dysmotility diarrhea is caused by increased transit time of luminal contents and may be compounded by bacterial overgrowth due to stasis. **Inflammatory or exudative diarrhea**, as the term suggests, is the result of an acute inflammatory mucosal process which may be idiopathic as in ulcerative colitis or Crohn's disease or more commonly with an infectious microorganism.

Diarrhea is often caused by several coexistent factors. For example, in ulcerative colitis, there is altered colonic permeability to water, increased prostaglandin production and disordered motility with increased loss of blood, mucus and water into the lumen.

The differential diagnosis of acute diarrhea is summarized in Table 7.2.

History

The onset of diarrhea is often acute and the symptoms may be of short duration.

It is important to establish that the patient is complaining of diarrhea as defined above and not frequent, normally formed, stools or the large-volume

Table 7.2 Differential diagnosis of acute onset diarrhea.

Cause	Remarks
Infections:	
Viral	adenovirus, astrovirus, calicivirus, rotavirus
Bacterial	*Salmonella* spp, *Shigella* spp, *B. cereus*
Parasites	*Entamoeba histolytica*, *Giardia lamblia*
Toxins	*C. difficile*, *S. aureus*
Inflammatory bowel disease	Ulcerative colitis
	Crohn's disease
	Collagenous colitis
Drugs	Antibiotics
	ACE inhibitors
	Digoxin
	Chemotherapeutic agents
	Lipid lowering drugs
	Prostaglandin analogues
	Proton pump inhibitors
	All laxatives
Ischemic colitis	
Fecal impaction with overflow	

pale stool associated with steatorrhea. Rapid onset of symptoms with abdominal cramps and sleep disturbance usually suggests an infective or toxic etiology. The patient should be asked about recent food ingestion and its timing in relation to symptom onset. Nausea and vomiting again suggests an enteric infection. Current medications may be a factor and particular inquiry should be made about antibiotics, ACE inhibitors, laxatives, digoxin, proton pump inhibitors, lipid lowering agents, prostaglandin analogues and magnesium-containing antacids.

Recent foreign travel to areas where acute enteric infections are common should raise the suspicion of infection from agents such as *Vibrio cholerae*, *Shigella* or *Entamoeba histolytica*. The passage of bloody diarrhea may indicated an acute infective dysentery but should always raise the suspicion of inflammatory bowel disease.

Examination

In general, the following should be assessed in all cases:
• Signs of dehydration and circulatory collapse due to water and electrolyte depletion. The patient will be pale

with a rapid, low volume pulse. The blood pressure may be low with a postural drop on standing. There will be increased skin turgor and dry mucous membranes.

- Abdominal examination is often normal but in acute onset of inflammatory bowel, the abdomen may be distended with generalized tenderness or an abdominal mass in patients with Crohn's disease.
- Rectal examination may show blood on the glove.

Investigation

Acute diarrhea is very common in the community, often occurring in isolated outbreaks associated with enteric viral infections. Most cases are diagnosed and managed by primary care physicians without resort to further investigations. However a small proportion of cases where the symptoms are associated with dehydration, systemic illness or rectal bleeding are referred for hospital assessment.

The following investigations are most likely to lead to a rapid diagnosis in the majority of cases.

- Fresh stool sample for ova, cysts and parasites, culture and sensitivity as necessary, *C. difficile* enterotoxin and *Giardia* antigen. In the immunocompromised patient, it is essential to rule out the presence of cryptosporidiosis.
- Test stool for occult blood.
- Full blood count.
- Urea and electrolytes.
- ESR, C-reactive protein and alpha-1 antiglobulin as inflammatory markers.
- Tissue transglutaminase assay to rule out celiac disease.
- Blood culture if fever/rigors present.
- Visualization of the colonic mucosa by colonoscopy or flexible sigmoidosopy, and biopsy if inflammatory bowel is suspected.
- Plain abdominal radiographs erect and supine in the presence of abdominal tenderness, decreased bowel sounds and in all cases where acute inflammatory bowel disease is suspected.
- Duodenal aspirates are uncommonly required if giardiasis is suspected.

Management

The management of acute infectious diarrhea and inflammatory bowel disease will be discussed in detail in the respective chapters.

In general the management has three important components:

1. Correction of dehydration, electrolyte disturbance, anaemia and nutritional abnormalities.

2. Oral rehydration solutions which were originally developed for fluid replacement in patients with cholera are useful in the treatment of severe acute diarrhea provided an oral intake is tolerated. **WHO/UNICEF solution** contains Na 90 mmol/L, K 20 mmol/L, Cl 80 mmol/L, HCO_3 30 mmol/L and glucose 111 mmol/L. **Dioralyte** is a commercial preparation which contains Na 35 mmol/L, K 20 mmol/L, Cl 37 mmol/L, HCO_3 18 mmol/L and glucose 200 mmol/L. Both solutions can be administered by nasogastric tube if necessary until the diarrhea has resolved.

3. Consideration of antimicrobial therapy. If an infecting agent is detected in the stool, specific antibacterial therapy is usually not indicated except in certain cases as the enteric infection is commonly self-limiting. If the patient has a severe systemic illness with fever and positive blood cultures, e.g. *Salmonella* bacteremia, then antiobiotic therapy is essential.

It should be noted that infective causes of diarrhea can present with rectal blood loss which can mimic inflammatory bowel disease. Stool cultures should be carried out in these patients to rule out infection before steroid therapy specific for inflammatory bowel disease is commenced.

Further reading

Camilleri M. Chronic diarrhoea: a review of pathophysiology and management for the clinical gastroenterologist. Clin Gastroenterol Hepatol 2004; 2:198–206.

Powell DW. Approach to the patient with diarrhoea. In: Yamada T, ed. *Textbook of Gastroenterology* Vol 1. Philadelphia: Lippincott. 1991; 732–70.

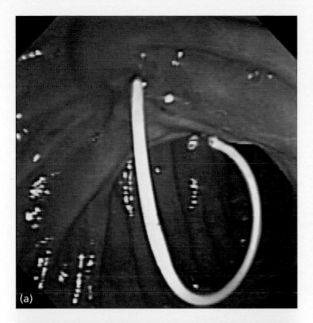

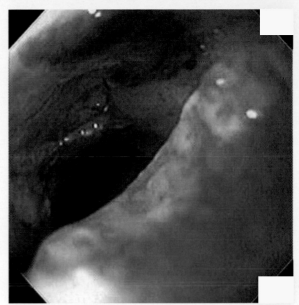

Plate 16.1 Esophageal tear after passage of the echoendoscope.

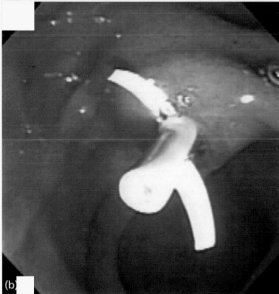

Plate 11.1 Prophylactic pancreatic duct stents. (a) 3-Fr, 4-cm long single-pigtail stent. (b) 5-Fr, 3-cm long flanged stent.

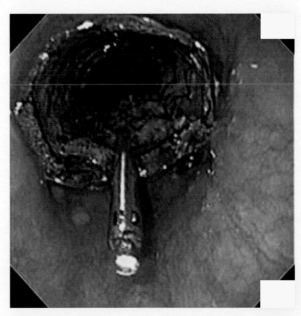

Plate 16.2 Esophageal stent placed over the site of perforation.

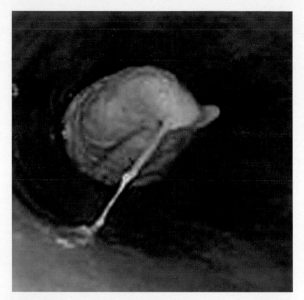

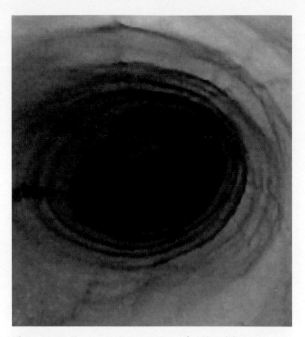

Plate 17.1 A. chicken meat bolus impacted above a distal esophageal mucosal (Schatzki) ring (not shown). The bolus was grasped using the polypectomy snare and lifted off the distal esophageal stenosis before being removed by mouth using the Roth net.

Plate 17.3 Characteristic appearance of eosinophilic esophagitis, a clinical condition that underlies many foreign body impactions today. This endoscopic photograph, depicting multiple rings along the esophageal body, was taken upon introduction of the endoscope in the proximal esophagus and hence provided an endoscopic clue to the etiology of impaction, which occurred more distally in this patient (not shown).

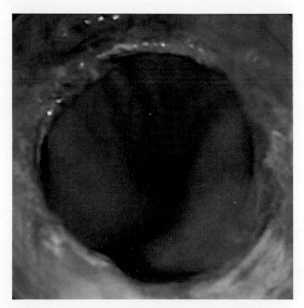

Plate 17.2 Endoscopic appearance of a distal esophageal mucosal (Schatzki) ring severed by the passage of the food bolus into the stomach under direct endoscopic visualization, water and air instillation, and gentle pressure by the endoscope tip. Mucosal rings account for many episodes of acute esophageal impaction, typically with a meat bolus (steakhouse syndrome).

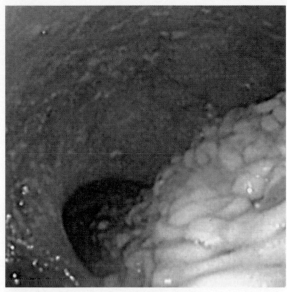

Plate 17.4 Food impaction in a patient with severe scleroderma esophagus and secondary esophageal candidiasis. Note the dilated esophagus and the esophageal mucosal changes consistent with *Candida* infection. Careful water instillation allowed the endoscope to break up the food residue that initially appeared as a cast of the esophageal body. The repeated use of the Roth retrieval net eventually relieved the patient's impaction and associated acute dysphagia.

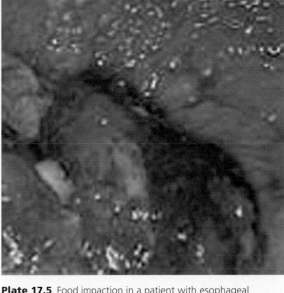

Plate 17.5 Food impaction in a patient with esophageal achalasia. Note the distorted appearance of the distal esophageal mucosa consistent with stasis esophagitis. Because of the associated atony and dilation of the esophageal body, water instillation allowed the endoscope to bypass the impaction and break up the food residue into small particles. Using the endoscope, the food particles were then pushed into the stomach and relieved the patient's dysphagia.

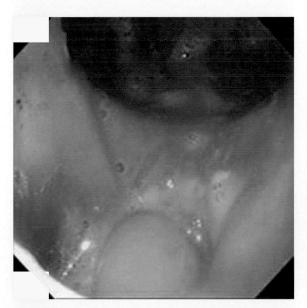

Plate 18.1 Wound dehiscence in the distal esophagus following resection of a diverticulum. The drainage tube in the pleural space is clearly seen.

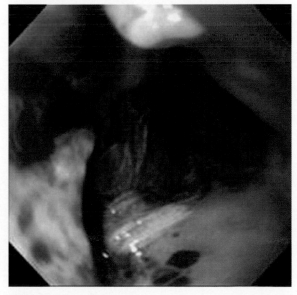

Plate 18.2 Esophageal perforation caused by rigid esophagoscopy.

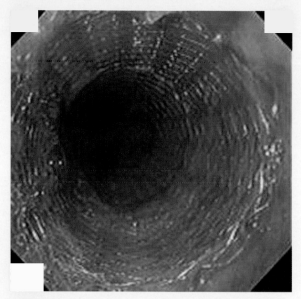

Plate 18.3 Same patient as in Figure 18.1, showing a Flamingo Wallstent in the distal esophagus covering the perforation. The stent was removed after 14 weeks, however a persisting fistula revealed a retained metallic strand which was endoscopically removed (Figure 18.4).

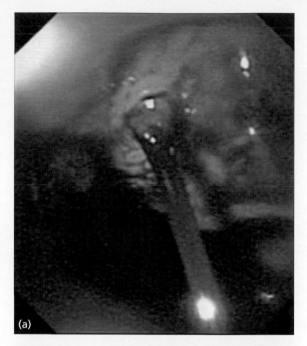

(a)

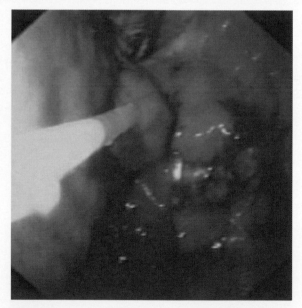

Plate 24.1 Endoscopic picture of huge fundic varices. Venography obtained after complete obliteration therapy using a total of 6 mL Histoacryl-Lipiodol mixture (Figure 24.6).

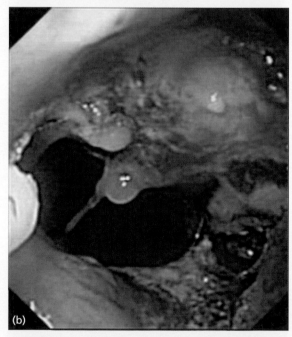

(b)

Plate 24.2 Endoscopic pictures showing an acute bleeding from a sclerotherapy-induced ulcer on a varix at the distal esophagus (a). Immediate control of bleeding by intravariceal injection of 0.5 mL Histoacryl-Lipiodol mixture (b).

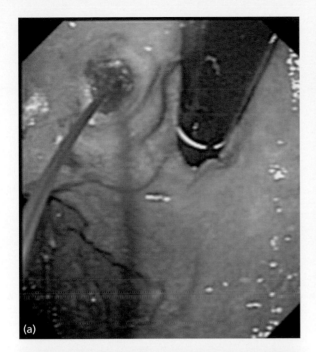

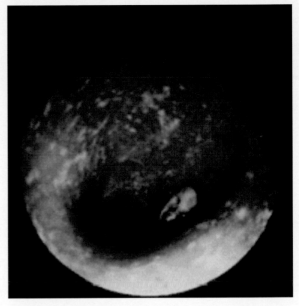

Plate 30.1 Sigmoidoscopic appearance of acute severe ulcerative colitis 6 days after IV steroid therapy.

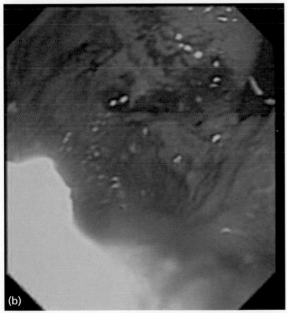

Plate 24.3 Endoscopic pictures showing an acute bleeding from huge fundic varices (a). Immediate control of bleeding is achieved by obliterating the varices using cyanoacrylate glue (b).

2 Complications of Gastrointestinal Procedures

8 Complications of Upper Gastrointestinal Endoscopy

Colm O'Loughlin, Reza Shaker

Complications related to diagnostic upper gastrointestinal endoscopy are rare. The American Society for Gastrointestinal Endoscopy estimated that the overall complication rate of this commonly performed diagnostic procedure was 0.13% with an associated mortality of 0.004% [1]. Estimated average major complication rates for diagnostic and therapeutic upper endoscopic procedures range from 0.2% to 8% with associated mortality rates of 0.01% to 1.5% [2]. Major complications include cardiorespiratory compromise, sedation-related side effects, infectious complications, perforation and hemorrhage.

Late complications may be underestimated primarily due to underreporting. In prospective studies complications have been reported in 2.1% of patients after upper endoscopy with an 18.2% complication rate up to 30 days after the procedure [3]. Oropharyngeal or abdominal discomfort accounted for the majority of these late complications.

Appreciation of potential complications and the frequency of their occurrence by both physicians and patients allows for improved risk benefit analysis. The early recognition of complications permits prompt investigation and treatment, hence minimizing patient morbidity and mortality.

Complications of sedation

Premedications used for moderate sedation in the majority of endoscopy suites include intravenous benzodiazepines, usually midazolam, together with a narcotic such as merperidine (pethidine) or fentanyl. Titrated dosing is administered by an intravenous line during the procedure with continuous monitoring of the patient's hemodynamic stability, cardiac rhythm and oxygen saturation. Continuous clinical assessment is of the foremost importance in cardiopulmonary monitoring.

Cardiorespiratory depression is the most serious adverse effect of sedative and analgesic medications. Cardiorespiratory complications account for approximately half of the morbidity and mortality related to diagnostic endoscopic procedures [4]. Serious cardiorespiratory events may complicate as many as 0.5% of upper endoscopic procedures and more than 50% of deaths are related to cardiorespiratory complications [5,6]. Complications range from minor changes in vital signs to acute myocardial infarction, cardiac arrhythmias, respiratory depression and shock. Hence, full resuscitation equipment should be readily available in the endoscopy area. Use of a combination of medications, such as midazolam and fentanyl, for moderate sedation increases the incidence of respiratory depression significantly [7]. Midazolam or fentanyl alone can be utilized for upper endoscopy.

Management

Naloxone reverses the respiratory depression, sedation and hypotensive effects of narcotics in 1–2 minutes. Flumazenil, a benzodiazepine antagonist, significantly reduces patient recovery time following moderate sedation. Recurrent doses of both may be required in view of the relatively short half-life of these medications. Both naloxone and flumazenil should be readily available in the endoscopy room and familiarity with dosage administration is of the utmost importance.

Gastrointestinal Emergencies, 2nd edition. Edited by Tony Tham, John Collins and Roy Soetikno. © 2009 by Blackwell Publishing, ISBN: 978-1-4051-4634-0.

Cardiorespiratory complications

Oxygen desaturation may occur in up to 70% of patients undergoing various endoscopic evaluations [8]. Factors contributing to oxygen desaturation include difficulty with intubation of the esophagus, advanced patient age and a history of cardiopulmonary disease [7]. Vasovagal reflex secondary to esophageal intubation, overinsufflation of the stomach or small bowel with air and the use of larger diameter endoscopes for upper endoscopy contribute significantly to hypoxemia during the procedure. Cardiac rhythm abnormalities during upper endoscopy are most frequently seen in patients with underlying chronic heart or lung disease [9].

Other adverse events related to perioperative medications include drug allergy, paradoxical excitement with benzodiazepines, and benzocaine-induced methemoglobinemia in genetically predisposed individuals. Sedation, supine positioning and pharyngeal anesthesia utilized for upper endoscopy contribute to the development of pulmonary aspiration. Aspiration may occur in only 0.08% of cases but the mortality rate of this complication may reach 10%. Hence, aspiration precautions and readily available suctioning apparatus are integral to performing upper endoscopic procedures safely.

Infectious complications

Infectious complications may be related to the procedure itself or the equipment used during the procedure. The incidence of bacteremia is low and the rate of subacute bacterial endocarditis (SBE) in patients not at risk for SBE is extremely low and has been estimated to be 1 in 5–10 million [10]. Bacteremia is highest following esophageal dilation and esophageal variceal sclerotherapy with a mean incidence of 45% and 18% respectively and extremely low, less than 5%, in diagnostic upper endoscopy [11,12]. Therapeutic procedures and endoscopic mucosal resection are associated with higher rates of bacteremia than diagnostic endoscopy.

Cardiac conditions at high risk for SBE include prosthetic heart valves, prior history of SBE, and surgically placed systemic pulmonary shunts [13]. SBE prophylaxis is recommended for such patients undergoing procedures with a high risk of bacteremia (esophageal dilation and variceal sclerotherapy). For patients with an intermediate risk for endocarditis (rheumatic valvular disease, mitral valve prolapse, hypertrophic obstructive cardiomyopathy and congenital malformations) antibiotic prophylaxis is a consideration for high-risk procedures but is not recommended for low-risk procedures such as upper endoscopy with biopsy. Prophylactic regimes for gastrointestinal procedures include ampicillin and gentamicin for high-risk cases. Vancomycin may be substituted in penicillin-sensitive patients.

Other infectious complications include retropharyngeal and retroesophageal abscesses. These are related to trauma or unrecognized perforations at the time of the procedure.

Infectious complications related to equipment are very rare and are estimated to be 1 per 1.8 million procedures. Transmission of bacteria such as *H. pylori* and viruses such as HBV and HCV (hepatitis B and C) have been reported and are fortunately very rare. Transmission of HIV (human immunodeficiency virus) has not been reported.

Perforation

(See also Chapter 19.) The rate of perforation in upper endoscopy is relatively low and has been reported in 0.03% to 0.1% of procedures, with a mortality rate of 0.001% [1]. Factors predisposing to perforation include blind passage of the endoscope, anterior cervical osteophytes, presence of a Zenker diverticulum, esophageal strictures and esophageal malignancy. Perforation occurs more frequently in the esophagus than the stomach and is associated with a relatively high mortality rate approximating 25% [14]. Pain is the most common symptom related to perforation. Other symptoms include shortness of breath, pleuritic chest pain, fever and crepitance of the neck (subcutaneous emphysema). Early recognition of this complication, confirmation of perforation radiographically, and collaboration with cardiothoracic surgery are critical in the management of these patients.

Bleeding

Bleeding from diagnostic upper endoscopy is very rare, estimated to occur in 0.03% of cases, and is usually gastric in origin [1]. A Mallory–Weiss tear may occur during upper endoscopy secondary to patient retching. These arise in less than 0.1% of diagnostic endoscopies and are usually not associated with significant bleeding. Overall therapeutic procedures cause bleeding more frequently than diagnostic evaluations. Generally this rare complication occurs primarily in patients with thrombocytopenia and/or coagulopathy. Upper endoscopy without biopsy has been determined to be safe in patients with platelet counts greater than 20000.

Complications of specific endoscopic procedures

Dilation

(See also Chapter 19.) Major complications may occur in 0.5% of esophageal dilations and death in 0.01% [15]. The complication rate for esophageal dilation with mercury dilators has been reported to be 0.4% [1]. There is no evidence that push dilators (balloon versus bougie dilation) result in a higher rate of perforation when dilating benign esophageal strictures [16]. Other complications of esophageal dilation include abdominal pain, bleeding and bacteremia.

Balloon dilation of benign esophageal strictures is complicated by perforation in 0.4% of cases. In pyloric stenosis the risk of perforation is 0.5%, whereas with gastroenterostomy (anastomotic) stricture and gastric staple line dilation, the risk is 2.2% and 0.8% respectively [17]. Caustic strictures are at higher risk of perforation due to the length of the lesion and luminal compromise. Perforation rates up to 17% have been reported [18].

In achalasia the rate of perforation with pneumatic balloon dilation is 5%. There is a reduced risk with gradual dilation and avoidance of inflation pressures of greater than 11 psi [19].

With regard to malignant strictures, the rate of perforation is approximately 10% [2,20]. Post-radiation strictures have the same risk of perforation as malignant stricture, ranging from 2% to 6.5% [21]. It has been established that relatively safe dilation of malignant strictures can be performed up to a diameter of 15 mm. Esophageal malignancies can be treated with thermal, photodynamic or stenting procedures which carry increased risk of complication. The main risk of endoscopic mucosal resection (EMR) is perforation, ranging from 0.7% to 2.5% in esophageal cancer and 0.06% to 2.4% for gastric cancers [22,23].

Dilation of malignant gastric outlet obstruction carries a perforation risk of 0% to 6.7%. Limitation of dilation to less than 15 mm should be considered as perforation rates of 4 to 6.7% are reported with dilation greater than 15 mm [2].

Variceal sclerotherapy and banding

(See also Chapter 10.) The overall complication rate for variceal sclerotherapy (EVS) is between 35% and 78%. Major complications occur in 8.0% of cases and the mortality rate is in the range of 1% to 5% [30,31]. Esophageal ulcers occur in 50% to 78% of cases. Treatment with proton pump inhibitors does not prevent occurrence but may allow healing. Significant bleeding occurs in up to 6% of patients [32,33]. The retreatment interval should be greater than 1 week as the only factor relating to multiple ulcerations is a treatment interval shorter than 1 week. The perforation rate ranges from 2% to 5% [34]. Chest pain after EVS occurs in up to 50% of patients but rarely lasts longer than 48 hours. Strictures can occur weeks to months after variceal sclerotherapy sessions in 2% to 20% of cases. Other complications of this emergent procedure include aspiration (5%), pneumonitis, pleural effusions and bacteremia [35].

Esophageal band ligation (EBL) is fortunately associated with a lower complication rate of 2% to 3%. The overall mortality attributed to an acute complication of EBL is 1%. Hence, EBL is the endoscopic intervention of choice in the management of esophageal varices. Esophageal ulcers are reported in 5% to 15% of patients after EBL with a low tendency for bleeding [35]. Perforation had been reported in 0.7% of cases when band ligation was performed with a facilitating overtube. The introduction of multiple band devices has resulted in the discontinuance of the use of overtubes for this procedure. Formation of strictures has been reported but is rare. Bacterial peritonitis may occur in 4% of cases. Antibiotic prophylaxis is recommended in those patients known to have ascites.

Endoscopic nonvariceal hemostasis

Randomized controlled trials using MPEC (multipolar electrocoagulation) have reported rates of perforation of 0% to 2%. Induction of bleeding by electrocoagulation occurs in up to 5% of cases [36]. Repeated therapy with electrocoagulation within 24 to 48 hours is associated with an up to 4% risk of perforation [37].

Epinephrine, the most commonly used injection agent to achieve initial hemostasis, may cause mucosal ulceration but has not been associated with perforation [38].

Foreign body removal

Complications of endoscopic foreign body removal and meat disimpaction have been reported in up to 8% of cases [39]. The risks of aspiration and perforation may be decreased by the use of an overtube [40]. The use of overtubes has been associated with complications such as bleeding and perforation, and require judicious use by an experienced operator.

Rare complications

These include temporomandibular joint dislocation, teeth injury and parotid enlargement.

Summary

Upper gastrointestinal endoscopy, a very commonly performed procedure, is fortunately relatively safe with few complications and extremely low mortality. Awareness of potential complications and the expected frequency of complications leads to improved risk benefit analysis by both patients and physicians. Early recognition of complications and prompt investigation and treatment minimizes patient morbidity and mortality.

References

1. Silvis SE, Nebel O, Rogers G, Sugawa C, Mandelstam P. Endoscopic complications. Results of the 1974 American Society of Gastrointestinal Endoscopy Survey. JAMA 1976; 235(9):928–30.
2. Newcomer MK, Brazer SR. Complications of upper gastrointestinal endoscopy and their management. Gastrointest Endosc Clin N Am 1994; 4(3):551–70.
3. Zubarik R, Eisen G, Mastropietro C, et al. Prospective analysis of complications 30 days after outpatient upper endoscopy. Am J Gastroenterol 1999; 94(6):1539–45.
4. Hart R, Classen M. Complications of diagnostic gastrointestinal endoscopy. Endoscopy 1990; 22(5):229–33.
5. Arrowsmith JB, Gerstman BB, Fleischer DE, Benjamin SB. Results from the American Society for Gastrointestinal Endoscopy/US Food and Drug Administration collaborative study on complication rates and drug use during gastrointestinal endoscopy. Gastrointest Endosc 1991; 37(4):421–7.
6. Bell GD. Review article: Premedication and intravenous sedation for upper gastrointestinal endoscopy. Aliment Pharmacol Ther 1990; 4(2):103–22.
7. Fleischer D. Monitoring the patient receiving conscious sedation for gastrointestinal endoscopy: issues and guidelines. Gastrointest Endosc 1989; 35(3):262–6.
8. Dark DS, Campbell DR, Wesselius LJ. Arterial oxygen desaturation during gastrointestinal endoscopy. Am J Gastroenterol 1990; 85(10):1317–21.
9. Lee JG, Leung JW, Cotton PB. Acute cardiovascular complications of endoscopy: prevalence and clinical characteristics. Dig Dis 1995; 13(2):130–5.
10. Mogadam M, Malhotra SK, Jackson RA. Pre-endoscopic antibiotics for the prevention of bacterial endocarditis: do we use them appropriately? Am J Gastroenterol 1994; 89(6):832–4.
11. Botoman VA, Surawicz CM. Bacteremia with gastrointestinal endoscopic procedures. Gastrointest Endosc 1986; 32(5):342–6.
12. Neu HC, Fleischer D. Controversies, dilemmas, and dialogues. Recommendations for antibiotic prophyaxis before endoscopy. Am J Gastroenterol 1989; 84(12): 1488–91.
13. Standard of Practice Committee, American Society for Gastrointestinal Endoscopy: Antibiotic prophylaxis for gastrointestinal endoscopy. Gastrointest Endosc 1995; 42(6):630–5.
14. Pettersson G, Larsson S, Gatzinsky P, Sudow G. Differentiated treatment of intrathoracic oesophageal perforations. Scand J Thorac Cardiovasc Surg 1981; 15(3):321–4.
15. Mandelstam P, Sugawa C, Silvis SE et al. Complications associated with esophagogastroduodenoscopy and with esophageal dilation. Gastrointest Endosc 1976; 23(1):16–9.
16. Saeed ZA, Winchester CB, Ferro PS, Michaletz PA, Schwartz JT, Graham DY. Prospective randomized comparison of polyvinyl bougies and through-the-scope balloon for dilation of peptic strictures of the esophagus. Gastrointest Endosc 1995; 41(3):189–95.
17. Kozarek RA. Hydrostatic balloon dilation of gastrointestinal stenoses: a national survey. Gastrointest Endosc 1986; 32(1):15–19.
18. Karnak I, Tanyel FC, Buyukpamukcu N, Hicsonmez A. Esophageal perforations encountered during dilation of caustic esophageal strictures. J Cardiovasc Surg 1998; 39(3):373–7.
19. Nair LA, Reynolds JC, Parkman HP, Ouyang Q, Strom BL, Rosato EF, Cohen S. Complications during pneumatic dilation for achalasia or diffuse esophageal

spasm. Analysis of risk factors, early clinical characteristics, and outcome. Dig Dis Sci 1993; 38(10):1893–904.

20. Neuhaus H, Hoffman W, Dittler HJ, Neidermeyer HP, Classen M. Implantation of self-expanding esophageal metal stents for palliation of malignant dysphagia. Endoscopy 1992; 24(5):405–10.

21. Ng TM, Spencer GM, Sargeant IR, Thorpe SM, Brown SG. Management of strictures after radiotherapy for esophageal cancer. Gastrointest Endosc 1996; 43(6):584–90.

22. Inoue H, Tani M, Nagai K, Kawano T, Takeshita K, Endo M, Iwai T. Treatment of esophageal and gastric tumors. Endoscopy 1999; 31(1):47–55.

23. Makuuchi H, Kise Y, Shimada H, Chino O, Tanaka H. Endoscopic mucosal resection for early gastric cancer. Semin Surg Oncol 1999; 17(2):108–16.

24. Disario JA, Fennerty MB, Tietze CC, Hutson WR, Burt RW. Endoscopic balloon dilation for ulcer-induced gastric outlet obstruction. Am J Gastroenterol 1994; 89(6):868–71.

25. Mathus-Vliegen LM, Koning H. Percutaneous endoscopic gastrostomy and gastrojejunostomy: a critical reappraisal of patient selection, tube function, and the feasibility of nutritional support during extended follow-up. Gastrointest Endosc 1999; 50(6):746–54.

26. Wolfsen HC, Kozarek RA, Ball TJ, Pattterson DJ, Botoman VA, Ryan JA. Long-term survival in patients undergoing percutaneous endoscopic gastrostomy and jejunostomy. Am J Gastroenterol 1990; 85(9):1120–2.

27. Gossner L, Keymling J, Hahn E.G., Ell C. Antibiotic prophylaxis in percutaneous endoscopic gastrostomy (PEG): a prospective randomized clinical trial. Endoscopy 1999; 31(2):119–24.

28. Kulling D, Sonnenberg A, Fried M, Bauerfeind P. Cost analysis of antibiotic prophylaxis for PEG. Gastrointest Endosc 2000; 51(2):152–6.

29. Person JL, Brower RA. Necrotizing fasciitis/myositis following percutaneous endoscopic gastrostomy. Gastrointest Endosc 1986; 32(4):309.

30. Schuman BM, Beckman JW, Tedesco FJ, Griffin JW, Assad RT. Complications of endoscopic injection sclerotherapy: a review. Am J Gastroenterol 1987; 82(9):823–30.

31. Zambelli A, Arcidiacano PG, Arcidiacano R et al. Complications of endoscopic variceal sclerotherapy (EVS): a multicenter study of 1192 patients. Gastroenterology 1993; 104:1023.

32. Piai G, Cipolleta L, Claar M, Marone G, Bianco MA, Forte G, Iodice G, Mattera D, Minieri M, Rocco P, et al. Prophylactic sclerotherapy of high risk esophageal varices: results of a multicentric prospective controlled trial. Hepatology 1988; 8(6):1495–500.

33. Gimson A, Polson R, Westaby D, Williams R. Omeprazole in the management of intractable esophageal ulcerations following injection sclerotherapy. Gastroenterology 1990; 99(6):1829–31.

34. The Copenhagen Esophageal Varices Sclerotherapy Project. Sclerotherapy after first variceal hemorrhage in cirrhosis. N Engl J Med 1984; 311(25):1594–600.

35. Stiegmann GV, Goff JS, Michaletz-Onody PA, Korula J, Lieberman D, Saeed ZA, Reveille RM, Sun JH, Lowenstein SR. Endoscopic sclerotherapy as compared with endoscopic ligation for bleeding esophageal varices. N Engl J Med 1992; 326(23):1527–32.

36. Jensen DM. Endoscopic control of nonvariceal upper gastrintestinal hemorrhage. In Yamada T, Alpers DH, Laine L, Owyang C, Powell DW, eds. Textbook of Gastroenterology. Philadelphia, Lippincott Williams & Wilkins, 1999; 2857–79.

37. Lau JY, Sung JJ, Lam YH, Chan AC, Ng EK, Lee DW, Chan FK, Suen RC, Chung SC. Endoscopic retreatment compared with surgery in patients with recurrent bleeding after initial endoscopic control of bleeding ulcers. N Engl J Med 1999; 340(10):751–6.

38. Lin HJ, Tseng GY, Perng CL, Lee FY, Chang FY, Lee SD. Comparison of adrenaline injection and bipolar electrocoagulation for the arrest of peptic ulcer bleeding. Gut 1999; 44(5):715–19.

39. Berggreen PJ, Harrison E, Sanowski RA, Ingebo K, Noland B, Zierer S. Techniques and complications of esophageal foreign body extraction in children and adults. Gastrointest Endosc 1993; 39(5):626–30.

40. Ginsberg GG. Management of ingested foreign objects and food bolus impactions. Gastrointest Endosc 1995; 41(1):33–8.

9

Complications of Percutaneous Endoscopic Gastrostomy

Freddy Vandenbussche, Jo Vandervoort

Introduction

In 1980 Gauderer et al. introduced percutaneous endoscopic gastrostomy (PEG). Its use has become accepted and widespread [1]. It is considered the safest and easiest method to provide long-term enteral feeding in patients who have a functioning gastrointestinal tract, but for whom the intake of food through the mouth is difficult or impossible.

The most frequent indications for PEG placement are neurological impairment, general debilitating disorders and oropharyngeal or esophageal obstruction by benign or neoplastic lesions [2]. The procedure is easy to perform with a high success rate of 95–98% [3]. The procedure-related mortality is less than 1% [2,4]. Published incidence rates for minor and major complications range from 10% to 13% and 1 to 3% respectively. Minor complications are aspiration, infection of the insertion site, PEG tube dislodgement, gastric ileus, pneumoperitoneum and parastomal leakage and can be treated conservatively. Major complications which require surgical intervention are hemorrhage, fistulization, necrotizing fasciitis and buried bumper syndrome [5].

Minor complications

Aspiration

Procedure-related aspiration is only reported in 0.3–1% of cases [4]. Risk factors are age, supine position,

Gastrointestinal Emergencies, 2nd edition. Edited by Tony Tham, John Collins and Roy Soetikno. © 2009 by Blackwell Publishing, ISBN: 978-1-4051-4634-0.

neurological impairment and sedation. Symptoms are high temperature and respiratory distress. Usually there is oxygen desaturation during the procedure. Shorter procedure times, titrated sedation, controlled air-insufflation and maximal aspiration of gastric juices can prevent this. Treatment with intravenous antibiotics is aimed at the expected microbiology (piperacilline-tazobactam or ceftriaxone + ornidazol) [8].

Pneumoperitoneum

Benign pneumoperitoneum after PEG placement occurs in 40% to 56%. [4]. It originates from air-insufflation at endoscopy and by introducing air via the puncture needle. It can be present for a few days, but may persist up to 4 weeks [9]. In the absence of signs of peritonitis it is of no clinical significance. It is seen on plain abdominal radiograph and a CAT scan rules out other complications [9–11].

Infectious complications

The most common complication is PEG site infection [3]. Incidences differ greatly, but the risk for infection is increased in patients with cancer, AIDS and underlying heart disease [12]. Serious infections are more rare, with an incidence of 1.6%. Prophylactic administration of antibiotics significantly reduces the number of post-PEG infections [3,13]. An important reduction in the number of MRSA infections, which is the most commonly found organism in stomal infections, is seen when using a combination regimen for oro-nasopharyngeal decolonization [14]. Treatment consists of good local wound care and intravenous antibiotic therapy. Evolution to peritonitis is only seen in 0.4–1.6% of cases and should be treated with intravenous antibiotics and surgical exploration [4].

Parastomal leakage

Parastomal leakage is a common problem of PEG. It may be precipitated by the use of corrosive agents such as ascorbic acid or hydrogen peroxide to cleanse the tube, parastomal infection, granulation tissue, sideways traction on the tube, sliding of the tube through absence of the external bolster or by complications such as buried bumper. Diagnosis and subsequent treatment should be directed against the presumed inciting factor. The patient should be treated with proton pump inhibitors, hydrogen peroxide and ascorbic acid should be stopped, and zinc oxide or an antifungal paste should be applied around the PEG site [4].

Major complications

Hemorrhage and perforation

Gastrointestinal hemorrhage following PEG is rare with an incidence of 0.2–2.5% [4,15]. It may be due to direct puncture of a blood vessel in the abdominal wall. This risk is elevated in cirrhotic patients with portal hypertension and dilated venous structures in the wall. More careful transillumination of the abdominal wall should prevent this complication [15]. Unsatisfactory transillumination whatever the cause – obesity, prior surgery or ascites – should always be an absolute contraindication for PEG [2,15].

Bleeding can also occur with ischemic necrosis of the gastric mucosa under a too tightly fixed internal bolster. If the head of the PEG is too mobile, it can erode underlying mucosa, causing bleeding ulcers [15]. Kanie et al. [16] found gastric ulcers in 9.9% of cases after PEG placement. Another mechanism of ulcer formation after PEG insertion is friction of the tip of the PEG against the posterior gastric wall [16]. Treatment should be aimed at loosening of the internal bolster in combination with classical antiulcer therapy based on H2-antagonists or proton pump inhibitor. Only in case of deep ulceration, at risk of perforation, should the PEG tube be removed. [15].

Larson et al. [3] described gastric or esophageal perforation in 4 of the 314 cases during or after PEG placement, often with evolution to peritonitis. It occurs when the mushroom-shaped head of the PEG is pulled through the tighter gastroesophageal junction or, more likely, through a (benign or malignant) stricture. In such cases dilatation of the

stricture to at least 36 F is necessary prior to PEG insertion [3].

Gastroenteric fistula

PEG can also be complicated by formation of gastroenteric fistulae. In a retrospective review in 343 children Patwardhan et al. [17] reported an incidence of 3.5% (12/343). This is confirmed by Khatak et al. [18] with a 2–3% incidence.

During PEG insertion there is a risk of direct puncture of a segment of the jejunum or part of the transverse colon which has been displaced between the anterior gastric wall and the abdominal wall. The cause is overinsufflation of the stomach and air-filling of the duodenum which causes rotation of the greater curvature anteriorly thereby pulling on the gastrocolic omentum and positioning the transverse colon in the puncture trajectory [7]. Abnormal posture of the patient, spinal deformations and previous abdominal surgery with adhesions are risk factors and are considered as contraindications for PEG placement [19]. Pathwardan et al. found that the posterior wall of the stomach was the point of entry in all their patients, suggesting that the insertion of the puncture needle was too deep and thus perforated the stomach. [17].

Gastroenteric fistulae can stay asymptomatic for a long time. The fistulae are discovered when the patient develops watery diarrhea, when they develop intestinal obstruction or fecaloid output through the gastrostomy. Persistent parastomal leakage and inflammation can also be indicative for fistula formation. Sometimes it is only discovered by chance during elective PEG replacement after several months. Patients do not always present with obstructive symptoms because there is usually part of the colonic lumen free for passage [4].

On plain abdominal radiograph, a "side-on" view of the PEG flange as opposed to the normal "end-on" view is seen. There is also an excess length of gastrostomy tubing within the abdomen, suggesting fistula formation [17]. Contrast injection through the PEG tube can show the fistula trajectory to the colon. Endoscopy contributes little to the diagnosis but confirms that the internal bolster of the PEG is no longer visible in the stomach. Occasionally the internal opening of the fistula is visible.

When fistula formation is suspected, it is best to remove the PEG tube immediately. One possible technique would be to pull the PEG tube tightly against the abdomen and to cut the external portion. The remaining piece can be pushed inside either the stomach or the colon and removed endoscopically. Although fistulae close spontaneously, Kim et al. advise closure of the fistula opening with a metal clip to prevent further fecaloid leakage. This also allows for an earlier trial of oral feeds [20]. Nevertheless in patients with a formed fistula, there is an absolute contraindication for a new PEG, as the risk of recurrent fistula formation is elevated. In these patients a surgical gastrostomy is recommended.

As a precaution, Quadri et al. [22] propose elevation of the head end of the bed to 30° during PEG insertion to displace the bowel caudally. Careful transillumination is also very important to assist visualization of the colonic shadow. To outline the puncture site one has to use a syringe with saline solution attached to a needle. As the needle is advanced through the abdominal wall the barrel is retracted. A "safe tract" is determined by simultaneous air return and endoscopic visualization of the needle. Despite these precautions, migration of a gastrostomy or penetration of the small bowel can still occur in rare instances [23].

Necrotizing fasciitis

Necrotizing fasciitis (NF), first described by Wilson in 1952, is a rapid and progressive soft tissue infection leading to necrosis of the fascia, subcutaneous tissue and overlying skin. It is a rare complication which constitutes a surgical emergency with high morbidity and mortality [24,25].

Predisposing factors are diabetes, drug use, alcoholism, obesity, hypertension, old age, malnutrition, neoplasia, deficient immunity and chronic illness, active treatment with corticosteroids or immunosuppressant drugs [25–27].

There are several mechanisms causing NF. When the incision of the skin is too small, it can cause necrosis of the abdominal wall and does not allow sufficient drainage of accumulated fluid. Too much traction on the PEG can cause ischemia of the anterior gastric wall while too little traction can cause leakage of nonsterile feeding solutions intra- or subcutaneously.

Symptoms of NF can be very subtle and a high index of suspicion is necessary. Patients present with pain, redness, edema and sometimes fever. The most important clinical sign is subcutaneous crepitus. Diffuse tissue necrosis can swiftly evolve to infectious septic shock. NF is usually seen within 72 hours after placement, though longer intervals have been described [25–29].

A plain abdominal radiograph shows signs of subcutaneous emphysema, a pathognomonic sign for NF. CAT scan or MRI of the abdomen are useful to evaluate the extension of the infection. It may allow the surgeon to avoid opening the visceral fascia if there is no evidence of peritoneal spread [26].

The treatment of NF requires immediate intervention with a rapid and extensive surgical debridement, broad-spectrum antibiotics and, according to certain authors, hyperbaric oxygen. Mortality varies between 35% and 70% and there is a correlation with the delay to surgical intervention. Repeated surgery until all nonviable tissue has been resected is necessary for the wound to heal and healthy granulation tissue to form [25–29].

The most common organisms are group A hemolytic streptococcus, often together with *Staphylococcus* species, *Enterococcus*, *E. coli*, *Proteus* and *Bacteroides*. In post-traumatic NF *Clostridium* is usually present in association with another aerobic or anaerobic germ [24]. Some authors suggest treatment with hyperbaric oxygen therapy [24].

Supply of sufficient nutrition is an important issue in these patients. Placement of nasoenteric feeding tubes or even surgical gastrostomy or jejunostomy are preferable, given the known limitations of long-term parenteral nutrition. Greif et al. proposed preventive measures such as topical preparation of the oropharyngeal region, the prophylactic administration of antibiotics, restoration of stomach acidity in hypochloremic patients and creation of a more patulous opening at the gastrostomy tube site [29].

Buried bumper

Migration of the internal bolster of the PEG into the gastric mucosa is a rare complication, referred to as the "buried bumper syndrome." It was first described by Klein et al. [31] in 1988. In a series of 115 patients, Gençosmanoglu et al. [32] found two cases of buried bumper (1.7%), which corresponds with the incidence of 1.5–1.9% reported in the literature [4].

Intramucosal migration of the more rigid bumper of a PEG tube is caused by ischemic pressure necrosis from the underlying gastric mucosa. It is followed by re-epithelialization so the bumper gets completely imbedded in the gastric wall. Pressure necrosis is a result of either excessive tension on the bolster causing hypoperfusion of the stomach wall, or because patients exert too much traction on the external portion of the tube. This is a long-term complication after PEG. Often, it is only noticed at endoscopy during PEG replacement [31].

The depth of the intramucosal migration defines the clinical presentation. Symptoms may vary from pain at the insertion place with edema and erythema, more difficult tube mobilization, or difficulties in the infusion of feeding solution.

Patients can also present with melena from bleeding ischemic ulcers at the site of the buried bumper [33]. Most often, patients complain of sudden pain at infusion or have abdominal bloating, indicative of gastric dysmotility [31]. Although the clinical presentation of buried bumper is frequently asymptomatic, it may evolve to gastric perforation, diffuse peritonitis with acute abdomen and even death of the patient.

Diagnosis can be made based on clinical examination which shows immobilization of the PEG at a point where it can no longer be pushed inward. Gastroscopy is the most accurate way of diagnosing a buried bumper. Supplementary diagnostic work-up often comprises a plain abdominal radiograph, contrast radiography through the PEG and a abdominal CAT scan or MRI. These imaging techniques allow differentiation between other causes of PEG immobilization such as gastroenteric fistula. Whatever the presentation, it is imperative that the PEG tube be removed to prevent further migration through the stomach wall and gastric perforation.

Treatment consists of removal of the PEG, leaving behind a replacement tube with a balloon at the tip. One technique uses the needle knife to cut the overlying mucosa, so the bumper can be pushed into the stomach and endoscopically removed. In case of doubtful position, the bumper can be safely localized using endoscopic ultrasound [33]. In another technique a guide wire is pushed through the PEG tube. Next a skin incision is made up to the imbedded bumper, which can then be removed without opening the peritoneum thereby reducing infectious complications. As a precaution it is recommended leaving a space of 1.5 cm free between the external bolster and the skin to prevent pressure necrosis. Nursing staff are best advised to push the tube inward 1 cm and rotating it a few times every time they clean the tube, thus preventing intramucosal migration [33,34].

References

1. Gauderer MWL, Ponsky JL, Izant RJ Jr. Gastrostomy without laparotomy: a percutaneous endoscopic technique. J Ped Surg 1980; 15(6):872–5.
2. Nicholson FB, Korman MG, Richardson MA. Percutaneous endoscopic gastrostomy: a review of indications, complications and outcome. J Gastroenterol Hepatol 2000; 15:21–5.
3. Larson DE, Burton DD, Schroeder KW, DiMagno EP. Percutaneous endoscopic gastrostomy: indications, success, complications and mortality in 314 consecutive patients. Gastroenterology 1987; 93:48–52.
4. McClave A, Chang W-K. Complications of enteral access. Gastrointest Endosc 2003; 58(5):739–51.
5. Mathus-Vliegen EMH, Koning H, Taminiau JAJM, Moorman-Voestermans CGM. Percutaneous endoscopic gastrostomy and gastrojejunostomy in psychomotor retarded subjects: a follow-up covering 106 patient years. J Pediatr Gastroenterol Nutr 2001; 33:488–94.
6. Löser C, Wolters S, Fölsch UR. Enteral long-term nutrition via percutaneous endoscopic gastrostomy (PEG) in 210 patients: a four-year prospective study. Dig Dis Sci 1998; 43(11):2549–57.
7. Gauderer MWL. Percutaneous endoscopic gastrostomy: a 10 year experience with 220 children. J Ped Surg 1991; 26(3):288–94.
8. Kadakia S, O'Sullivan H, Starnes E. Percutaneous endoscopic gastrostomy or jejunostomy and the incidence of aspiration in 79 patients. Am J Surg 1992; 164:114–18.
9. Dulabon GR, Abrams JE, Rutherford EJ. The incidence and significance of free air after percutaneous endoscopic gastrostomy. Am Surg 2002; 68(6):590–3.
10. Roberts PA, Wrenn K, Lundquist S. Pneumoperitoneum after percutaneous endoscopic gastrostomy: a case report and review. J Em Med 2005; 28(1):45–8.
11. Faias S, Buck G, DeLegge M. Peritonitis after percutaneous endoscopic gastrostomy and jejunostomy: where there is smoke, there may not be fire. Endoscopy 2006; 38(7):745–8.
12. Fox VL, Abel SD, Malas S, Duggan C, Leichtner AM. Complications following percutaneous endoscopic gastrostomy and subsequent catheter replacement in children and young adults. Gastrointest Endosc 1997; 45(1):64–71.
13. Miller RE, Castlemain B, Lacqua FJ, Kotler DP. Percutaneous endoscopic gastrostomy: results in 316 patients and review of the literature. Surg Endosc 1989; 3:186–90.

14. Horiuchi A, Nakayama Y, Kajiyama M, Fujii H, Tanaka N. Nasopharyngeal decolonization of methicillin-resistant *Staphylococcus aureus* can reduce PEG peristomal wound infection. Am J Gastroenterol 2006; 101:274–7.

15. Cappell MS, Abdullah M. Management of gastrointestinal bleeding induced by gastrointestinal endoscopy. Gastroenterol Clin North Am 2000;29(1):125–67.

16. Kanie J, Akatsu H, Suzuki Y, Shimokata H, Iguchi A. Mechanism of the development of gastric ulcer after percutaneous endoscopic gastrostomy. Endoscopy 2002; 34(6):480–482.

17. Patwardhan N, McHugh K, Drake D, Spitz L. Gastroenteric fistula complicating percutaneous endoscopic gastrostomy. J Pediatr Surg 2004; 39:561–4.

18. Khatak IU, Kimber C, Kiely EM, et al. Percutaneous endoscopic gastrostomy in paediatric practice: complications and outcome. J Pediatr Surg 1998; 33: 67–72.

19. Yamazaki T, Sakai Y, Hatakeyama K, Hoshiyama Y. Colocutaneous fistula after percutaneous endoscopic gastrostomy in a remnant stomach. Surg Endosc 1999; 13:280–2.

20. Kim HS, Lee DK, Baik SK et al. Endoscopic management of colocutaneous fistula after percutaneous endoscopic gastrostomy. Endoscopy 2002; 34:430.

21. Gyökeres T, Burai M, Hamvas J et al. Conservative vs. endoscopic closure of colocutaneous fistulas after percutaneous endoscopic gastrostomy complications. Endoscopy 2003; 35:246–7.

22. Quadri AHA, Puetz TR, Dindzans V, Canga C, Sincaban M. Enterocutaneous fistula: a rare complication of PEG tube placement. Gastrointest Endosc 2001; 53(4): 529–31.

23. Beasley SW, Catto-Smith AG, Davidson PM. How to avoid complications during percutaneous endoscopic gastrostomy. J Pediatr Surg 1995; 30(5):671–3.

24. Catena F, La Donna M, Ansaloni L, Agrusti S, Taffurelli M. Necrotizing fasciitis: a dramatical surgical emergency. Eur J Emerg Med 2004; 11(1):44–8.

25. Haas D, Dharmaraja P, Morrison JG, Pots III Jr. Necrotizing fasciitis following percutaneous endoscopic gastrostomy. Gastrointest Endosc 1988; 34(6):487–8.

26. Maclean AA, Miller G, Bamboat ZM, Hiotis K. Abdominal wall necrotizing fasciitis from dislodged percutaneous endoscopic gastrostomy tubes: a case series. Am Surg 2004; 70(9):827–31.

27. Martindale R, Witte M, Hodges G, Kelley J, Harris S, Andersen C. Necrotizing fasciitis as a complication of percutaneous endoscopic gastrostomy. J Parenter Enteral Nutr 1987; 11(6):583–5.

28. Cave DR, Robinson WR, Brotschi EA. Necrotizing fasciitis following percutaneous endoscopic gastrostomy. Gastrointest Endosc 1986; 32(4):294–6.

29. Greif JM, Ragland JJ, Ochsner MG, Riding R. Fatal necrotizing fasciitis complicating percutaneous endoscopic gastrostomy. Gastrointest Endosc 1986; 32(4):292–4.

30. Shupak A, Shoshani O, Goldenberg I. Necrotizing fasciitis: an indication for hyperbaric oxygen therapy? Surgery 1995; 118:873–8.

31. Klein S, Heare BR, Soloway RD. The "buried bumper syndrome": a complication of percutaneous endoscopic gastrostomy. Am J Gastroenterol 1990; 85(4): 448–51.

32. Gençosmanoglu R, Koç D, Tözün N. The buried bumper syndrome: migration of internal bumper of percutaneous endoscopic gastrostomy tube into the abdominal wall. J Gastroenterol 2003; 38:1077–80.

33. Anagnostopoulos GK, Kostopoulos P, Arvanitidis DM. Buried bumper syndrome with a fatal outcome, presenting early as gastrointestinal bleeding after percutaneous endoscopic gastrostomy placement. J Postgrad Med 2003; 49:325–7.

34. Rino Y, Tokunaga M, Morinaga S, Onodera S, Tomiyama I, Imada T, Takanashi Y. The buried bumper syndrome: an early complication of percutaneous endoscopic gastrostomy. Hepato-Gastroenterology 2002; 49:1183–4.

10

Complications of Variceal Sclerotherapy, Ligation and Balloon Tamponade

Yan Zhong, Stefan Seewald, Nib Soehendra

The use of sclerotherapy, band ligation and balloon tamponade in acute variceal hemorrhage is described in Chapter 24. Endoscopic sclerotherapy and band ligation are also performed for primary and secondary prophylaxis to prevent esophageal variceal bleeding, whereas balloon tamponade is used only for controlling acute esophagogastric variceal hemorrhage.

This chapter will deal with the recognition, management and prevention of complications related to sclerotherapy, band ligation and balloon tamponade. Prevention is as usual the best treatment, since the majority of the patients are critically ill, and complications of these procedures are frequently serious. Complications of these three treatment modalities used for acute bleeding will include general and specific aspects.

General aspects

Endoscopic treatment and balloon tamponade in acute variceal hemorrhage should be considered as a relatively invasive procedure that may trigger some adverse events related to the general conditions of patients. The underlying liver disease has a profound influence on the course of complications. The risk of aspiration and subsequent pneumonia high in patients with massive bleeding. It may even be higher during the introduction of the instrument when the stomach is filled with blood or food, particularly in

Gastrointestinal Emergencies, 2nd edition. Edited by Tony Tham, John Collins and Roy Soetikno. © 2009 by Blackwell Publishing, ISBN: 978-1-4051-4634-0.

patients with altered consciousness. In such circumstances, endoscopy should best be performed under general anesthesia after securing the circulatory and respiratory status. In conscious patients, endoscopy may be carried out without any sedation or pharyngeal anesthesia. The use of a therapeutic upper gastrointestinal endoscope with a working channel of 6.0 mm is strongly recommended, because it enables rapid evacuation of the gastric contents and simultaneously compresses the bleeding site at the esophagus. An additional suction pump is needed to clear the oropharyngeal cavity [1].

Specific complications

Balloon tamponade

Today, balloon tamponade is mainly used when variceal bleeding cannot be controlled endoscopically or if immediate endoscopy is not available. The Sengstaken–Blakemore double-balloon tube is used for esophageal variceal bleeding and the single-balloon Linton–Nachlas tube for both fundic and esophageal variceal hemorrhages. Transient hemostasis can be achieved in 50–90% of cases with a complication rate of around 15% [2]. In endoscopically uncontrolled variceal hemorrhage, the rate of hemostasis may be lower, and the complication rate subsequently higher. Following failed endoscopic hemostatic attempts, placement of a balloon tube may be cumbersome or even impossible due to swelling of the esophageal wall. A recently modified covered self-expandable metallic stent seems to be a good alternative to balloon tamponade (see Chapter 24). Complications of balloon tamponade include aspiration pneumonia, pressure-induced ulceration, esophageal perforation, migration causing acute airway obstruction, and bleeding.

Aspiration pneumonia

Aspiration may occur during insertion of the balloon tube and when the patient is not intubated. The risk of aspiration is higher when balloon tamponade is used in an unconscious patient without endotracheal intubation. Regular clearance of the oropharyngeal cavity is therefore mandatory. Patients treated with balloon tamponade should be kept in an intensive or intermediate care unit.

Pressure-induced ulceration

This complication is mainly caused by the overinflation and prolonged use of the esophageal balloon. Inflation of the esophageal balloon with 80 mL air or water exerts a pressure of around 40 mmHg which is sufficient to control the bleeding. The use of balloon tamponade should not exceed 24 hours, in order to prevent pressure necrosis of the esophageal wall. Within this time span, endoscopy should be performed to achieve definitive hemostasis.

Esophageal perforation

Perforation is in most cases secondary to pressure-induced wall necrosis which may occur particularly if prolonged balloon tamponade is applied for controlling bleeding following failed extensive sclerotherapy. Perforation may also occur if a gastric balloon is misplaced and inflated in the esophagus. To avoid this, the correct position of the gastric balloon must be checked radiologically before inflating the balloons.

Proximal migration causing acute airway blockage

Proximal migration of the balloon tube occurs if the gastric balloon is underinflated, particularly in the presence of a hiatal hernia, and if the tube is held under traction. In such acute life-threatening situations, the tube is cut using scissors to immediately deflate the balloons allowing for rapid removal of the tube.

Bleeding

Bleeding should be regarded as a complication of balloon tamponade. The rebleeding rate following balloon deflation amounts to 46% [3]. The high rebleeding rate may be explained by the fact that balloon tamponade is mainly used in cases with massive hemorrhage that is refractory to endoscopic treatment. Such variceal bleeding usually occurs in patients with advanced liver disease associated with coagulopathy and other comorbidities.

Sclerotherapy

Endoscopic sclerotherapy is playing a less important role in the management of acute variceal hemorrhage due to the relatively high complication rate despite having a reported immediate hemostasis rate ranging from 70% to 90%. Procedure-related complications are bleeding, stricture formation and perforation. The most common complication is early rebleeding, which occurs in about 35% [4,5]. Most of these adverse effects are related to extensive necrosis of the esophageal wall that occurs when an inappropriate injection needle and/or too much and too concentrated a sclerosant is used.

Post-sclerotherapy bleeding

Acute esophageal variceal bleeding may be transiently controlled by para- or perivariceal injections of sclerosant around the bleeding site creating compressing cushions. However, varices may not be thombosed after the initial session. Severe bleeding may therefore occur due to sclerosant-induced ulcers eroding the still patent varices 2–3 days after sclerotherapy [6,7]. Furthermore, a relatively high volume of sclerosant is usually required to control severe variceal hemorrhage, leading to more extensive and deep wall necrosis, thus causing other secondary complications, such as mediastinitis, perforations and fistulae

Apart from avoiding the use of high-volume sclerotherapy, proper injection is decisive for preventing complications. Injection should not be done intravariceally, since some sclerosants (e.g. sodium morrhuate, ethanolamine oleate) may cause systemic side effects, such as respiratory or renal failure. Injection must be restricted to the submucosal layer. This can only be controlled endoscopically which may not be possible in acute hemorrhage due to poor visibility. Correct submucosal injection is identified by the immediate appearance of a whitish mucosal bulge. If this bulge is not seen, the injection was either too deep or intravascular.

The most effective treatment modality for controlling this kind of bleeding is obliteration therapy using cyanoacrylate tissue glue (see Chapter 24).

Dysphagia, retrosternal discomfort, fever, pleural effusion

Transient dysphagia may occur after sclerotherapy due to swelling and chemical irritation of the esophageal wall. It is therefore advisable to keep the patient on a soft diet during the treatment period. Transmural injection of sclerosant often causes localized mediastinitis that is usually associated with transient retrosternal or chest pain and fever with no further significant sequelae and therefore requires no specific treatment. Pleural and mediastinal changes following sclerotherapy in the form of minor pleural effusion and atelectasis are frequently seen radiologically; such changes usually resolve spontaneously within 2–3 days [8].

Fever may also result from bacteremia, which has been found in up to 50% of patients receiving sclerotherapy [9]. If fever does not subside within 2–3 days and massive pleural effusion occurs, a perforation should be considered.

Perforation, esophageal fistula

Esophageal perforation is mainly a result of deep wall necrosis following excess sclerotherapy or repeated injections at short intervals which happens in patients with massive variceal hemorrhage or early rebleeding. It may also be attributed to the use of balloon tamponade following sclerotherapy [7].

Treatment of this severe complication is generally conservative since patients are usually unfit for surgery. Apart from parenteral nutrition and administration of broad-spectrum antibiotics, thoracic drainage is the mainstay of therapy.

Chylothorax due to perforation of the thoracic duct and bronchoesophageal fistula are very rare complications of sclerotherapy that may be related to the use of excess amounts of sclerosant and a long injection needle [10].

Stricture

Strictures are the most common significant complications of endoscopic sclerotherapy, occurring mainly in the lower part of the esophagus. This may be explained by the excessive use of sclerosant in the most common site of variceal hemorrhage causing deep necrosis and subsequent fibrosis of the lower esophageal sphincter. The more persistent and enthusiastic the performance of sclerotherapy in order to achieve good long-term results, the more likely is the development of strictures. Most sclerotherapy-induced strictures respond to bougienage. As soon as dysphagia occurs, bougienage should be performed, and repeated at weekly intervals as required. In patients with gastroesophageal reflux, additional administration of a proton pump inhibitor is advisable.

Band ligation

Endoscopic band ligation has widely replaced sclerotherapy, especially in the secondary prophylaxis of bleeding esophageal varices. Its principle is similar to that of hemorrhoidal ligation. Band ligation of esophageal varices results in safe and effective obliteration of the vessels by a process of inflammation and scar formation. The bands are displaced after 3–7 days due to ischemic mucosal necrosis and sloughing of the thombosed varix [11]. In several clinical trials, band ligation has shown a significantly lower complication rate as compared to sclerotherapy. Bleeding, perforation, stricture, bacteremia and other infectious sequelae are significantly less frequent following band ligation.

Compared to sclerotherapy, recurrence of varices after initial variceal eradication has been found to be more common [12–14]. Close follow-up and repeated ligation is therefore advisable until complete variceal eradication is achieved by producing sufficient fibrosis of the inner wall of the esophagus similar to sclerotherapy [15].

Bleeding

Bleeding may rarely occur during a banding procedure if the varix ruptures while being sucked into the barrel of the ligator. However, this kind of bleeding is easily stopped by immediately releasing the band. Early rebleeding may occur after initial band ligation sessions as long as varices are not completely thrombosed. Since thrombosis of the varices is the key to the success of band ligation, the rate of early rebleeding may be higher in patients with advanced liver disease and coagulopathy in whom ligation is less likely to lead to thrombosis of the varices. In such cases, obliteration therapy using cyanoacrylate currently represents the most effective treatment modality (see Chapter 24).

Perforation

Since the invention of the multiband ligator, perforation has become a very rare complication. Tears or perforations occurring in the upper esophagus are related to the placement of an overtube when a single-band ligator was used [16,17].

Stricture

Esophageal stricture following band ligation is a very rare complication [18]. It may occur if multiple band ligations are applied to a small area of the esophageal wall, which may happen when controlling massive variceal hemorrhage from an unidentifiable bleeding site.

Retrosternal pain, dysphagia, bacteremia

Post-banding retrosternal discomfort and dysphagia are quite common, especially if more than six bands have been placed too closely. They occur immediately after the procedure and usually last for a few days. Food bolus impaction after band ligation has been reported and is preventable by keeping patients on a soft diet for at least 3 days [19]. Transient bacteremia and other infectious sequelae after band ligation are significantly less frequent as compared to sclerotherapy [20].

References

1. Soehendra N. Treatment of esophagogastric varices. In: Soehendra N, Binmoeller KF, Seifert H, et al., eds. Theraputic Endoscopy. Stuttgart, Thieme, 2005; 74–86.

2. Chojkier M, Conn HO. Esophageal tamponade in the treatment of bleeding varices: a decadel progress report. Dig Dis Sci 1980; 25:267–72.

3. Conn HO. A plethora of therapies. In: Westaby D, MacDougall BR, Williams R, eds. Variceal Bleeding. London, Pitman, 1982; 221–51.

4. Soehendra N, de Heer K, Kempeneers I, et al. Sclerotherapy of esophageal varices: acute arrest of gastrointestinal hemorrhage or long-term therapy? Endoscopy 1983; 15(Suppl 1):136–40.

5. Bernuau J, Rueff B. Treatment of acute variceal bleeding. In: Benhamou JP, Lebrec D, eds. Clinics in Gastroenterology: Portal Hypertension. Philadelphia, Saunders, 1985; 185–207.

6. MacDougall BR, Westaby D, Theodossi A, et al. Increased long-term survival in variceal haemorrhage using injection sclerotherapy: results of a controlled trial. Lancet 1982; 1:124–7.

7. Terblanche J, Bornman PC, Kahn D, et al. Failure of repeated injection sclerotherapy to improve long-term survival after oesophageal variceal bleeding: a five-year prospective controlled clinical trial. Lancet 1983; 2:1328–32.

8. Saks BJ, Kilby AE, Dietrich PA, et al. Pleural and mediastinal changes following endoscopic injection sclerotherapy of esophageal varices. Radiology 1983; 149:639–42.

9. Sontheimer J, Salm R, Friedrich G, et al. Bacteremia following operative endoscopy of the upper gastrointestinal tract. Endoscopy 1991; 23:67–72.

10. Barsoum MS, Bolous FI, El-Rooby AA, et al. Tamponade and injection sclerotherapy in the management of bleeding oesophageal varices. Br J Surg 1982; 69:76–8.

11. Stiegmann GV, Sun JH, Hammond WS. Results of experimental endoscopic esophageal varix ligation. Am Surg 1988; 54:105–8.

12. Hou MC, Lin HC, Kuo BI, et al. Comparison of endoscopic variceal injection sclerotherapy and ligation for the treatment of esophageal variceal hemorrhage: a prospective randomized trial. Hepatology 1995; 21:1517–22.

13. Baroncini D, Milandri GL, Borioni D, et al. A prospective randomized trial of sclerotherapy versus ligation in the elective treatment of bleeding esophageal varices. Endoscopy 1997; 29:235–40.

14. Sarin SK, Govil A, Jain AK, et al. Prospective randomized trial of endoscopic sclerotherapy versus variceal band ligation for esophageal varices: influence on gastropathy, gastric varices and variceal recurrence. J Hepatol 1997; 26:826–32.

15. Soehendra N, Grimm H, Maydeo A, et al. Endoscopic sclerotherapy: personal experience. Hepatogastroenterology 1991; 38:220–3.

16. Goldschmiedt M, Haber G, Kandel G, et al. A safety maneuver for placing overtubes during endoscopic variceal ligation. Gastrointest Endosc 1992; 38:399–400.

17. Berkelhammer C, Madhav G, Lyon S, et al. "Pinch" injury during overtube placement in upper endoscopy. Gastrointest Endosc 1993; 39:186–8.

18. Laine L, Cook D. Endoscopic ligation compared with sclerotherapy for treatment of esophageal variceal bleeding: a meta-analysis. Ann Intern Med 1995; 123:280–7.

19. Saltzman JR, Arora S. Complications of esophageal variceal band ligation. Gastrointest Endosc 1993; 39:185–6.

20. Lo GH, Lai KH, Shen MT, et al. A comparison of the incidence of transient bacteremia and infectious sequelae after sclerotherapy and rubber band ligation of bleeding esophageal varices. Gastrointest Endosc 1994; 40:675–9.

11 Complications of Endoscopic Retrograde Cholangiopancreatography

Victor K. Chen, Richard C.K. Wong

Introduction

Endoscopic retrograde cholangiopancreatography (ERCP) involves the passage of a specially designed side-viewing duodenoscope through the mouth into the duodenum with visualization of major papilla (ampulla of Vater) and injection of contrast to examine the biliary and pancreatic ducts. A wide variety of accessories (catheters, sphincterotomes, guidewires, balloons, wire baskets, stents, etc.) can be used to cannulate the desired system and for therapeutic interventions. Since the advent of ERCP in the 1960s, competing noninvasive imaging modalities (magnetic resonance cholangiopancreatography, high-resolution CT, and endoscopic ultrasonography) have significantly shifted the indications for ERCP from diagnostic imaging towards therapeutic intervention.

Definition

A complication is an unplanned adverse event occurring as a direct result of the procedure of interest. Prospective studies more accurately reflect true complication rates while retrospective studies tend to underestimate complications. Post-ERCP pancreatitis is the most common ERCP-related complication. From a well-established consensus statement published in 1991, all three of the following are needed for the diagnosis of ERCP-induced pancreatitis: (1) new

Gastrointestinal Emergencies, 2nd edition. Edited by Tony Tham, John Collins and Roy Soetikno. © 2009 by Blackwell Publishing, ISBN: 978-1-4051-4634-0.

or worsening abdominal pain; (2) serum amylase elevation 3 or more times the upper limits of normal at 24 hours after the ERCP; (3) requiring at least 2 days of hospitalization. The severity of post-ERCP pancreatitis was also defined in this consensus statement by the length of hospitalization: 'mild' − 2 to 3 days, 'moderate' = 4 to 10 days, and 'severe' = more than 10 days or with pseudocyst formation or requiring intervention. Other major complications of ERCP include bleeding, perforation and cholangitis [1].

Overview of potential complications

Prior to performing ERCP, the endoscopist should review the procedural indications and carefully consider whether other less invasive tests would be preferred. For example, if diagnostic imaging of the pancreatobiliary system is the main goal, would an MRCP (magnetic resonance cholangiopancreatography) suffice? Alternatively, if the ERCP is being performed for a suspected pancreatic malignancy without symptomatic obstructive jaundice, would an endoscopic ultrasound-guided fine-needle aspiration (EUS-FNA) be preferred for staging and tissue diagnosis? Moreover, if there is a low clinical suspicion of a retained bile duct stone in a patient with acute gallstone pancreatitis, would proceeding directly to laparoscopic cholecystectomy with an intraoperative cholangiogram (IOC) be the preferred management? If a stone is found at IOC, then a postoperative ERCP can be performed for stone extraction. These are all preferred alternative strategies depending on local expertise and availability as ERCP remains technically demanding and has the highest associated complication rate of any procedure performed by gastroenterologists.

Although not traditionally considered a complication, failure to accomplish anticipated goals of ERCP (e.g. failed cannulation of desired ductal system, inability to extract stones, etc.) are undesired outcomes, since further testing and/or invasive procedures such as percutaneous transhepatic cholangiography (PTC) may be required that would otherwise be unnecessary after a successful procedure. Guidelines from the American Society for Gastrointestinal Endoscopy (ASGE) suggest an appropriate target cannulation rate of ≥90%, with most endoscopists being able to achieve a rate of ≥85% for successful cannulation, excluding failed ERCPs because of gastrointestinal tract-altering surgeries (e.g. Whipple pancreaticoduodenectomy, Billroth II, etc.) [2].

Case volume is an important factor in successful bile duct cannulation, and endoscopists performing on average more than two ERCPs per week have significantly greater success than those performing fewer (96.5% versus 91.5%, $p = 0.0001$) [3]. Precut access sphincterotomy improves cannulation rates, but complication rates vary markedly (2% to 34%) depending on the endoscopist's skill level [4].

The overall short-term complication rate for ERCP (see Table 11.1) is 5% to 10%. Post-ERCP pancreatitis is the most common complication and typically occurs in around 5% of patients. Post-sphincterotomy bleeding, cholangitis and cholecystitis are other major complications unique to ERCP [5–7]. Other risks associated with general endoscopy (e.g. upper endoscopy and colonoscopy) such as medication-related or cardiopulmonary adverse outcomes (e.g. "oversedation"), aspiration and perforation can also occur with ERCP. Rare systemic contrast related adverse reactions have been reported [8]. Water-soluble iodine-based contrast media is used to opacify the biliary and/or pancreatic ducts during ERCP.

Emergency ERCP

There are essentially two indications that may necessitate emergency ERCP: (1) acute suppurative cholangitis; (2) severe gallstone pancreatitis (not responding to medical management).

Acute suppurative cholangitis, even with the administration of appropriate antibiotics, is life threatening without prompt biliary decompression. ERCP is performed in acute cholangitis to decompress the bile ducts of pressurized bacteria-ridden bile. Emergency ERCP is preferred over surgery since endoscopic biliary drainage has a significantly lower associated mortality rate [9–11].

There are no studies specifically comparing the complication rates of emergency versus non-emergency ERCP. However, prior studies of emergency ERCP for the treatment of acute cholangitis report complication rates of 34% and mortality rates of 5% to 10%, which are higher than the expected ERCP complication and mortality rates in non-emergency settings [9–11]. Emergency ERCP for acute gallstone pancreatitis has similarly higher overall complications (10–46%) and mortality (0.08–0.1%) rates than non-emergency ERCP [12–14].

Post-ERCP pancreatitis

There are many important risk factors for post-ERCP pancreatitis, which can be divided into patient-related risk factors and endoscopist-related risk factors. Importantly, the presence of multiple risk factors is more than simply additive as post-ERCP pancreatitis rates can range from 1% to 40%. Therapeutic ERCP may result in higher rates of post-ERCP pancreatitis than diagnostic ERCP, but more recent multivariate analysis studies have failed to confirm this except for specific interventions such as pancreatic sphincterotomy and biliary sphincter balloon dilation. In addition, purely diagnostic ERCP has been largely replaced by less-invasive imaging technologies such as MRCP and EUS.

Table 11.1 Complications of endoscopic retrograde cholangiopancreatography [5–7].

ERCP-related complication	Estimated complication rate (%)
Overall	5–10
Pancreatitis	5
Post-sphincterotomy bleeding	1–2
Cholangitis	<1
Cardiopulmonary complications	<1
Perforation	0.3–0.6
Cholecystitis	0.2–0.5
Mortality	0.2
Contrast-related reaction	Rare

Patient selection is an important consideration when performing ERCP, as certain patient populations are at significantly higher risk for ERCP-related pancreatitis. A prospective multi-center study examined risk factors (OR = odds ratio) for post-ERCP pancreatitis and, in multivariate analysis, found the following patient factors to be significantly associated with risk of post-ERCP pancreatitis: (1) prior history of post-ERCP pancreatitis (OR 5.35); (2) suspected sphincter of Oddi dysfunction (OR 2.60); (3) female gender (OR 2.51); (4) normal serum bilirubin (OR 1.89); (5) absence of chronic pancreatitis (OR 1.87) [3]. Thus an older male patient presenting with obstructive jaundice from pancreatic cancer has a relatively lower risk (around 1%) for post-ERCP pancreatitis. In contrast, a young female with normal liver tests presenting for suspected sphincter of Oddi dysfunction has a very high risk (30% or more) for post-ERCP pancreatitis.

Endoscopist skill and procedural techniques are important determinants of post-ERCP pancreatitis. Papillary edema from trauma induced during difficult cannulation is an etiology of ERCP-related pancreatitis. Difficult cannulation (OR 3.07), multiple pancreatic duct injections (OR 2.72), pancreatic sphincterotomy (OR 3.07) and biliary sphincter balloon dilation (OR 4.51) are all significant risk factors for post-ERCP pancreatitis [3]. Low procedural case volume is associated with higher risks of complications. Pancreas divisum appears to be a risk factor for ERCP-related pancreatitis only if minor papilla cannulation is attempted. Biliary sphincterotomy and sphincter of Oddi manometry (with the use of aspirating catheters) do not appear to be risks factors for pancreatitis. Post-ERCP pancreatitis and overall complication rates may be reduced with using pure cut current versus blended current for biliary sphincterotomy [15]. Monopolar current may cause less pancreatitis after biliary sphincterotomy as opposed to bipolar current. It has been suggested that cannulation using a soft-tip hydrophilic guidewire may reduce the incidence of post-ERCP pancreatitis, but this is more likely related to experience of the endoscopist. The risk of pancreatitis from precut access papillotomy is highly dependent on the technique of the endoscopist [4,6]. Balloon dilation of the native biliary sphincter should be avoided since it is associated with increased morbidity and death due to severe pancreatitis [16].

Prevention of post-ERCP pancreatitis

The best way to prevent post-ERCP pancreatitis is to avoid unnecessary ERCPs, especially in high-risk patients. Endoscopists who perform ERCP should be skilled at performing both diagnostic and therapeutic procedures. Less experienced endoscopists should consider referral to high-volume centers.

Data are conflicting as to whether the use of low-osmolality contrast media (e.g. Omnipaque, Isovue, Optiray, Ultravist or Oxilan) versus high-osmolality contrast media (e.g. Hypaque, Renograffin, RenoCal, Urografin or Conray) reduces the incidence of post-ERCP pancreatitis. However, most studies show no benefit of one contrast media over another [8].

Several pharmacological agents have been studied to evaluate their effects in reducing post-ERCP pancreatitis. Allopurinol, antibiotics, calcium channel blockers, corticosteroids, heparin derivatives, interleukin-10, gabexate mesylate, nitrates, nonsteroidal antiinflammatory drugs (NSAIDs), octreotide, platelet activating factor (PAF) inhibitors, and somatostatin are examples of medications that have been studied in post-ERCP pancreatitis, all of which show negative or conflicting results [17]. Thus, none of these pharmacological agents are commonly utilized in clinical practice.

Prophylactic temporary pancreatic duct stent placement is the one intervention that convincingly reduces the risk of post-ERCP pancreatitis [17]. Impaired drainage of the pancreatic duct from papillary edema during cannulation and contrast injection is one of the possible triggers for post-ERCP pancreatitis. Pancreatic stent placement facilitates drainage of the pancreatic duct. A meta-analysis showed that high-risk patients without pancreatic stent placement had 3-fold higher odds (OR 3.2) of developing pancreatitis when compared with those with pancreatic stents (15.5% vs. 5.8%). The number needed-to-treat analysis showed that one in every 10 patients (95% CI, 6–18) at high risk for post-ERCP pancreatitis could be expected to benefit from pancreatic duct placement [18]. Endoscopists attempting to place pancreatic duct stents should be familiar with performing therapy in the pancreatic duct.

Prophylactic pancreatic stent placement should be considered in high-risk patients or 'difficult' cannulations. Small caliber (less than 5 Fr) plastic pancreatic stents can be inserted into the main pancreatic duct over a guidewire for prophylaxis against post-ERCP pancreatitis. Depending on the type of pancreatic stent, a single pigtail or plastic flanges in the duodenum keeps the stent from migrating proximally into the pancreatic duct (Plate 11.1). Short (less than 5 cm in length) 4 Fr or 5 Fr plastic pancreatic stents can be inserted into the head of the pancreas to prevent occlusion of the pancreatic orifice from edema. Short stents facilitate anticipated dislodgement after resolution of papillary edema. However, other endoscopists prefer long (10 to 12 cm in length) 3 Fr plastic pancreatic stents inserted into the body or tail of the pancreas to avoid the possibility of stent-induced ductal changes in the head. 5 Fr pancreatic stents fit over a 0.035-inch guidewire, while 4 Fr stents require a 0.025-inch or smaller guidewire, and 3 Fr stents only fit over a 0.018-inch guidewire. All prophylactic pancreatic duct stents should be removed within a week by esophagogastroduodenoscopy if they have not spontaneously dislodged into the gastrointestinal tract, which can be assessed by plain radiograph of the abdomen.

Post-sphincterotomy bleeding

Hemorrhage after sphincterotomy occurs in 0.76–2% of cases. Immediate bleeding can occur at the time of sphincterotomy in 10–30%, but most are not clinically significant and can be controlled at the initial ERCP. Delayed post-sphincterotomy bleeding can occur up to 2 weeks in about half the cases. The risk of clinically significant, severe hemorrhage requiring blood transfusions and/or surgical or angiographic intervention is uncommon at 0.1–0.5%.

In multivariate analyses, significant risk factors for post-sphincterotomy hemorrhage are: (1) coagulopathy; (2) anticoagulation less than 3 days after endoscopic sphincterotomy; (3) cholangitis; (4) observed bleeding during endoscopic sphincterotomy; (5) endoscopists with lower ERCP case volumes (less than one ERCP per week). Precut access sphincterotomy may be a risk factor for hemorrhage depending on technique. Cirrhosis in the absence of coagulopathy is probably not a risk factor for post-sphincterotomy bleeding. Newer electrosurgical units with microprocessor software-controlled feedback may decrease the incidence of immediate hemorrhage, but do not appear to affect delayed bleeding rates. The following were not found to be significant risk factors for hemorrhage after endoscopic

sphincterotomy: (1) use of aspirin or NSAIDs; (2) ampullary tumor; (3) larger sphincterotomy; (4) extension of prior endoscopic sphincterotomy [6,7].

Post-sphincterotomy bleeding can often be prevented with careful pre-procedural preparation and assessment of the patient, their medication list and laboratory studies. The endoscopist should know the results of a complete blood count, platelet count and basic coagulation studies prior to a planned sphincterotomy and any abnormalities should be corrected. For anticoagulant medications, the patient's risks of thromboembolism should be weighed against the risks of post-sphincterotomy bleeding. In such cases, the endoscopist should consult with the physician who prescribed the anticoagulant medication as to the patient's risk of a thromboembolic event. In complicated cases, the endoscopist might wish to consult with a hematologist before performing an elective ERCP with sphincterotomy. It is also important that the endoscopist carefully review, on a case-by-case basis, the indications for endoscopic sphincterotomy and whether it is essential. This is especially critical in high-risk patients. For example, in a critically ill patient with ascending cholangitis and coagulopathy from sepsis, decompressing an obstructed bile duct by placement of a temporary plastic biliary stent is typically preferred. Delayed biliary sphincterotomy and stone extraction can then be performed after the patient's clinical status has improved and coagulopathy resolved.

The vast majority of post-sphincterotomy bleeding can be controlled with endoscopic interventions. Injection of dilute epinephrine, thermal-coaptive coagulation (heat probe or bipolar electrocoagulation) and endoclips are commonly used methods of endoscopic hemostasis for post-sphincterotomy bleeding. Some endoscopists believe that bleeding may occur with partial severing of blood vessels and recommend extending the biliary sphincterotomy in order to completely sever the artery and cause vasospasm. Another potentially useful technique is large volume (e.g. 15–20 mL) submucosal injection with dilute epinephrine or normal (0.9%) saline just proximal to the apex of the biliary sphincterotomy.

Medical management of post-sphincterotomy bleeding includes resuscitation and hemodynamic support with intravenous crystalloid fluids, blood transfusions and correction of any coagulopathy. Patients with thrombocytopenia or platelet dysfunction (e.g. from aspirin) and severe, ongoing bleeding should be considered for transfusion of fresh platelets. Those who continue to bleed should be urgently referred to the interventional radiologist for visceral angiography with super-selective coil embolization of the bleeding artery. A few preliminary case reports have suggested that recombinant factor VII (rFVIIa) may be a useful adjunctive measure to massive or refractory bleeding. Nowadays, surgery is rarely necessary to stop post-sphincterotomy bleeding.

Infectious complications

The risk of cholangitis and cholecystitis after ERCP is less than 1%. Possible risk factors for ERCP-related biliary infections include jaundice, stent placement for malignant strictures, and low endoscopist case volume. The most important risk factors for infectious complications after ERCP are inadequate biliary drainage and combined percutaneous transhepatic cholangiography and ERCP (i.e, "rendezvous technique") [6,7]. Retained bile duct stones were thought to be a risk factor for cholangitis but increased rates of infection may be related to inadequate biliary drainage rather than the retained stones. Primary sclerosing cholangitis is a risk factor for cholangitis after ERCP and is thought to be secondary to contrast injection into an obstructed biliary tree with intra- and/or extrahepatic biliary strictures that drain poorly. In patients with primary sclerosing cholangitis and jaundice, therapeutic interventions (e.g., biliary stent placement), and history of recurrent cholangitis may increase the risk of infectious complications after ERCP. Performing ERCP in patients with pancreatic pseudocysts may result in infection of the pseudocyst. Liver abscess, endocarditis and endovasculitis are rare but reported infectious complications of ERCP. Antibiotic prophylaxis is recommended in patients undergoing ERCP who have communicating pancreatic cysts or pseudocysts. Antibiotic prophylaxis is also recommended in patients undergoing transpapillary or transmural drainage of pseudocysts.

Guidelines for antibiotic prophylaxis for ERCP have recently changed [19]. In patients with bile duct obstruction without cholangitis, ASGE guidelines now recommend antibiotic prophylaxis only in cases where there is known or suspected incomplete biliary drainage, for example, in patients with primary sclerosing cholangitis or hilar bifurcation strictures. In such cases,

antibiotic prophylaxis should be administered together with continuation of antibiotics after the procedure. Conversely, antibiotic prophylaxis is not recommended in cases where it is likely that complete biliary drainage will be achieved, for example, in patients with common bile duct obstruction without cholangitis. An exception would be for patients with obstructive jaundice from post-transplant biliary strictures where antibiotic prophylaxis is recommended together with continuation of antibiotics after the procedure.

ASGE guidelines for antibiotic prophylaxis have also changed regarding the prevention of infective endocarditis [19]. Antibiotic prophylaxis is no longer recommended for the sole purpose of preventing infective endocarditis even if the patient has a preexisting high-risk cardiac lesion (e.g., prosthetic cardiac valve, history of infective endocarditis, valvular abnormalities in cardiac transplant recipients, certain types of congenital heart disease). An exception would be in patients with preexisting high-risk cardiac lesions who are undergoing emergent ERCP as treatment for ascending cholangitis. In this instance, antibiotic prophylaxis is recommended because of concern for infective endocarditis caused by enterococci from the infected bile. It is thus important that the choice of antibiotic should cover biliary flora including enteric gram-negative organisms and enterococci with consideration of local antibiotic resistance and susceptibility.

Failure to drain the biliary system after injection of contrast by ERCP can result in ascending cholangitis. Common diseases at risk for cholangitis with inadequate biliary drainage include: (1) primary sclerosing cholangitis; (2) cholangiocarcinoma; (3) pancreatic cancer; (4) incomplete clearance of bile duct stones; (5) postoperative ischemic biliary strictures. The basic principle behind cholangitis occurring in these situations is the injection of contrast medium which, together with inadequate biliary drainage, can become a nidus for subsequent infection. Biliary stents inserted for strictures should ideally be large (10 Fr), being placed using a therapeutic duodenoscope: smaller-diameter stents can easily become occluded with biliary sludge or debris. Great care should be taken when placing the stent to ensure that it completely bridges the entire length of the stricture with adequate overlap at both ends. With incomplete clearance of choledocholithiasis, a temporary plastic biliary stent should be placed until complete stone clearance can be achieved at a second procedure.

Similarly, if there is marked ampullary edema at the end of ERCP, drainage of the bile duct should be observed on fluoroscopy: if drainage is inadequate, a temporary plastic biliary stent (or a nasobiliary drainage catheter) should be placed. Caution should be taken when inserting covered self-expanding metallic biliary stents as this may result in cholangitis from blockage of smaller intrahepatic bile ducts, or acute cholecystitis if the cystic duct becomes blocked. Prevention is always the best treatment against post-ERCP cholangitis: prophylactic antibiotics should be administered in certain situations as described above. Most importantly, ERCP should never be attempted if an endoscopist is not proficient in therapeutic ERCP. If biliary drainage is unsuccessful, the patient should be continued on broad-spectrum intravenous antibiotics, and urgent plans must be made to secure adequate biliary drainage in order to prevent potentially life-threatening cholangitis. In such situations, possible therapeutic options include urgent referral to a more experienced endoscopist for repeat attempt at ERCP versus referral to interventional radiology for emergency percutaneous transhepatic cholangiography. Management of post-ERCP cholangitis is based upon heightened clinical awareness of the diagnosis, which results in rapid diagnosis and treatment. Broad spectrum intravenous antibiotics, supportive care, sufficient fluid resuscitation, and most importantly, securing prompt and adequate biliary drainage are key elements to the treatment of infectious complications resulting from ERCP.

Cardiopulmonary complications

In general, ERCP requires higher doses of sedatives than colonoscopy or upper endoscopy. Patients with severe suppurative cholangitis are very ill and, in addition to jaundice, fever and abdominal pain (Charcot's triad), they may also be hypotensive and delirious (Reynold's pentad). In such patients, it is paramount that the anesthesiologist be involved in providing monitored anesthesia care during ERCP, which is often performed in the operating room. Furthermore, patients who undergo ERCP for suspected pancreatic malignancy tend to be older and have more comorbidities. One should be careful when performing ERCP in all of these patients, as the combination of these factors may be associated with higher rates of cardiopulmonary complications. Overall, cardiopulmonary complications occur in less than 1% of ERCP but are the leading cause of death from ERCP. Cardiac arrhythmias, hypoventilation or aspiration can occur [7]. "Oversedation" in the setting of acute illness and preexisting comorbidities contributes to most cardiopulmonary complications from ERCP, many of which respond rapidly to intravenous reversal agents (flumazenil and/or naloxone), close monitoring and supportive care.

Bowel perforation

Although uncommon, perforation is a potential complication that occurs in fewer than 0.6% of therapeutic ERCPs. Perforation can result from endoscope trauma, sphincterotomy or guidewire puncture. By univariate analysis, significant risk factors for perforation include sphincterotomy, sphincter of Oddi dysfunction and dilated common bile duct. Increased risks associated with sphincter of Oddi dysfunction and dilated common bile duct likely reflect perforation risks of therapeutic intervention (e.g. sphincterotomy, biliary dilation, etc.) and "overly aggressive" cannulation rather than inherent perforation risks of these disease processes. By multivariate analysis, significant risk factors for perforation include duration of procedure and biliary stricture dilation [20].

The "side-viewing" duodenoscope used to perform ERCPs facilitates visualization of the major papilla in the duodenum, but has quite different dynamics than the "forward-viewing" endoscopes used for general endoscopy (e.g. upper endoscopy and colonoscopy). Intubation of the esophagus with a duodenoscope is essentially "blind" with advancement through minimal resistance felt at the upper esophageal sphincter. A Zenker diverticulum and cricopharyngeal bar can increase the risk of perforation and care must be taken with esophageal intubation to prevent inadvertent hypopharyngeal perforation into the mediastinum. Pulsion diverticulum, esophageal strictures and hiatal hernias may increase risks of perforation within the esophagus. Commonly found in the elderly, periampullary diverticulum may increase the risk of perforation by making cannulation more difficult. Biliary sphincterotomy in this setting may carry higher risks of perforation as the periampullary diverticulum can distort typical anatomic landmarks that aid the endoscopist in knowing how far to extend the sphincterotomy. Gastrointestinal tract-altering surgeries such as a Billroth II partial gastrectomy may also increase perforation risks and the endoscopist should consider using a forward-viewing endoscope to first identify the afferent limb. Gastroduodenal outlet obstruction, which occurs in many patients with advanced pancreatic cancer, may make duodenal intubation more difficult and risky. Inadvertent retroperitoneal contrast injection and perforation through a "false tract" is a concern with ulcerated ampullary tumors that distort the major papilla and make identification of the biliary and pancreatic orifices more difficult.

Perforation can also result from extending a sphincterotomy incision beyond the intraduodenal portion of the bile duct. Precut needle-knife access techniques are highly operator-dependent and may increase risks of perforation. Bowel wall perforation can result from inadvertent guidewire puncture. Intrahepatic guidewire puncture and injury also have been reported.

Small or "contained" retroperitoneal perforations resulting from sphincterotomy and/or guidewire injury can frequently be managed conservatively without surgical intervention. Broad-spectrum intravenous antibiotics are recommended to prevent intraabdominal sepsis. The patient should be kept nil per os and placed on intravenous proton pump inhibitor to suppress gastric acid production. Decompression with nasogastric and nasobiliary drainage tubes can be helpful. Esophageal, gastric and duodenal perforations usually require surgery [20] (See chapters 18 and 19 on esophageal and gastrointestinal perforations respectively).

Contrast media-related reactions

As part of the pre-procedural assessment before ERCP, all patients should be asked whether they are allergic to intravenous contrast media used in computed tomography (CT) studies or are allergic to shellfish. Such patients are at increased risk for adverse reactions from the contrast used in ERCP and should receive nonionic contrast agents as well as an appropriate prophylactic allergy preparation, beginning at 12 to 13 hours before the ERCP (see below).

Water-soluble iodine-based contrast media are used to opacify the biliary and/or pancreatic ducts during ERCP. Practice standards are based primarily on radiological recommendations for intravenous contrast. The actual risk of systemic contrast-related reactions from ERCP is much less than with intravenous contrast administration because of limited systemic absorption. Nonetheless, idiosyncratic non-IgE mediated anaphylactic reactions can occur immediately and nonidiosyncratic reactions can occur from 1 hour to 7 days after contrast injection, but are usually mild and self-limited.

Patients at increased risk for adverse reactions, such as those with prior history of allergy to contrast media or shellfish, should receive nonionic contrast agents. For such patients, corticosteroid prophylaxis should be administered at several time points before the ERCP, as a single dose of corticosteroid given before the procedure is inadequate. Recommendations from the American College of Radiology are for intravenous contrast-related reactions, but gastrointestinal endoscopists extrapolate them for use in ERCP [8]. Possible regimens for prophylaxis against contrast-related systemic reactions include:

(1) prednisone 50 mg by mouth at 13 hours, 7 hours and 1 hour before ERCP, plus diphenhydramine 50 mg intravenously 1 hour before ERCP; or

(2) methylprednisolone 32 mg by mouth 12 hours and 2 hours before, plus diphenhydramine 50 mg intravenously 1 hour before ERCP.

Adverse reactions to contrast media used in ERCP can be serious and potentially life-threatening. Mild symptoms include sensation of warmth, metallic taste in mouth, pruritus, nausea, brief vomiting, diaphoresis, coughing, rhinorrhea and dizziness. Moderate symptoms include diffuse urticaria or rash, persistent vomiting, headache, facial edema, laryngeal edema, mild bronchospasm, dyspnea, vasovagal reaction, palpitations, tachycardia or bradycardia, hypertension and abdominal cramps. Severe reactions include life-threatening arrhythmias, hypotension, shock, severe bronchospasm, laryngeal edema, pulmonary edema, seizures, syncope, and death.

Mild to moderate urticaria can be treated with diphenhydramine 50 mg intravenously. The addition of cimetidine 300 mg or ranitidine 50 mg intravenously can also be considered. Bronchospasm and laryngeal edema should be taken extremely seriously: treatment includes supplemental oxygen, hemodynamic monitoring and support, and immediate transport to the nearest emergency department. For more severe cases of bronchospasm and laryngeal edema, epinephrine 1:10,000 can be administered 0.3–0.5 mg intramuscularly (0.3–0.5 mL) every 3–5 minutes as needed. Patients with poor response to intramuscular epinephrine can be given intravenous epinephrine 0.1 mg. Of note, patients taking beta blockers may not respond optimally to epinephrine and, in these patients, glucagon 1 mg can also be given intravenously every 1 minute up to a maximum of 5 mg. Hypotension and vasovagal reactions can be treated by elevating the patient's legs in the Trendelenburg position, oxygen supplementation and intravenous isotonic fluid administration. In severe vasovagal reactions, intravenous atropine 0.6–1 mg, repeated every 3–5 minutes as needed until a total of 3 mg is administered, should be considered. In unresponsive patients, an immediate 'code blue' should be called with strict adherence to ACLS (advanced cardiac life support) protocols, as appropriate. It is important that all patients with moderate to severe allergic reactions (or those with uncertain severity) should be immediately referred and transported by ambulance to the nearest emergency department for evaluation and continuing treatment [21,22].

Conclusions

Of all gastrointestinal endoscopic procedures, ERCP has the greatest potential for complications, yet can be truly life-saving in certain disease states. For each patient, the risks and benefits of ERCP should be carefully considered by the endoscopist. In some circumstances, less invasive imaging modalities may be preferred. Physicians performing ERCP should be skilled at performing both diagnostic and therapeutic interventions, and be adept at recognizing and treating any complications as soon as they arise.

References

1. Cotton PB, Lehman G, Vennes J, Geenen JE, Russell RC, Meyers WC, et al. Endoscopic sphincterotomy complications and their management: an attempt at consensus. Gastrointest Endosc 1991; 37(3):383–93.
2. Baron TH, Petersen BT, Mergener K, Chak A, Cohen J, Deal SE, et al. Quality indicators for endoscopic retrograde cholangiopancreatography. Gastrointest Endosc 2006; 63(4 Suppl):S29–34.
3. Freeman ML, DiSario JA, Nelson DB, Fennerty MB, Lee JG, Bjorkman DJ, et al. Risk factors for post-ERCP pancreatitis: a prospective, multicenter study. Gastrointest Endosc 2001; 54(4):425 34.
4. Freeman ML, Guda NM. ERCP cannulation: a review of reported techniques. Gastrointest Endosc 2005; 61(1):112–25.
5. Freeman ML, Nelson DB, Sherman S, Haber GB, Herman ME, Dorsher PJ, et al. Complications of endoscopic biliary sphincterotomy. N Engl J Med 1996; 335(13):909–18.
6. Freeman ML. Adverse outcomes of ERCP. Gastrointest Endosc 2002; 56(6 Suppl):S273–82.
7. Mallery JS, Baron TH, Dominitz JA, Goldstein JL, Hirota WK, Jacobson BC, et al. Complications of ERCP. Gastrointest Endosc 2003; 57(6):633–8.
8. Mishkin D, Carpenter S, Croffie J, Chuttani R, DiSario J, Hussain N, et al. ASGE Technology Status Evaluation Report: radiographic contrast media used in ERCP. Gastrointest Endosc 2005; 62(4):480–4.
9. Leese T, Neoptolemos JP, Baker AR, Carr-Locke DL. Management of acute cholangitis and the impact of endoscopic sphincterotomy. Br J Surg 1986; 73(12):988–92.
10. Leung JW, Chung SC, Sung JJ, Banez VP, Li AK. Urgent endoscopic drainage for acute suppurative cholangitis. Lancet 1989; 1(8650):1307–9.
11. Lai EC, Mok FP, Tan ES, Lo CM, Fan ST, You KT, et al. Endoscopic biliary drainage for severe acute cholangitis. N Engl J Med 1992; 326(24):1582–6.
12. Neoptolemos JP, Carr-Locke DL, London NJ, Bailey IA, James D, Fossard DP. Controlled trial of urgent endoscopic retrograde cholangiopancreatography and endoscopic sphincterotomy versus conservative treatment for acute pancreatitis due to gallstones. Lancet 1988; 2(8618):979–83.
13. Fan ST, Lai EC, Mok FP, Lo CM, Zheng SS, Wong J. Early treatment of acute biliary pancreatitis by endoscopic papillotomy. N Engl J Med 1993; 328(4):228–32.
14. Folsch UR, Nitsche R, Ludtke R, Hilgers RA, Creutzfeldt W. Early ERCP and papillotomy compared with conservative treatment for acute biliary pancreatitis. The German Study Group on Acute Biliary Pancreatitis. N Engl J Med 1997; 336(4):237–42.
15. Elta GH, Barnett JL, Wille RT, Brown KA, Chey WD, Scheiman JM. Pure cut electrocautery current for sphincterotomy causes less post-procedure pancreatitis than blended current. Gastrointest Endosc 1998; 47(2):149–53.
16. Disario JA, Freeman ML, Bjorkman DJ, Macmathuna P, Petersen BT, Jaffe PE, et al. Endoscopic balloon dilation

compared with sphincterotomy for extraction of bile duct stones. Gastroenterology 2004; 127(5):1291–9.

17. Freeman ML, Guda NM. Prevention of post-ERCP pancreatitis: a comprehensive review. Gastrointest Endosc 2004; 59(7):845–64.

18. Singh P, Das A, Isenberg G, Wong RC, Sivak MV, Jr., Agrawal D, et al. Does prophylactic pancreatic stent placement reduce the risk of post-ERCP acute pancreatitis? A meta-analysis of controlled trials. Gastrointest Endosc 2004; 60(4):544–50.

19. Banerjee S, Shen B, Baron TH, Nelson DB, Anderson MA, Cash BD, et al. Antibiotic prophylaxis for GI endoscopy. Gastrointest Endosc 2008; 67(6):791–8.

20. Enns R, Eloubeidi MA, Mergener K, Jowell PS, Branch MS, Pappas TM, et al. ERCP-related perforations: risk factors and management. Endoscopy 2002; 34(4):293–8.

21. Cochran ST. Anaphylactoid reactions to radiocontrast media. Curr Allergy Asthma Rep. 2005; 5(1):28–31.

22. Grammer LC, Greenberger PA. Drug Allergy in Patterson's Allergic Diseases, 6th edition. Philadelphia, Lipincott Williams & Wilkins, 2002: 354–35.

12 Complications of Laparoscopic Surgery

Stephen Attwood

Introduction

The advantages of laparoscopy are numerous and it is important to emphasize at the beginning of this chapter on complications that the advantages of laparoscopy outweigh the disadvantages and potential complications.

In general, compared to the equivalent open surgical procedure, laparoscopy results in reduced pain, early mobility, reduced incidence of chest infections, deep venous thrombosis and pulmonary embolus, early return to normal gut function (less ileus), reduced wound infections, early discharge from hospital and early return to work and sporting activity. Long-term outcomes show that with laparoscopy there is a reduced rate of incisional hernia, reduced rate of peritoneal adhesions, and improved cosmetic appearance. Laparoscopy often allows for a more accurate diagnosis especially in acute abdominal pain and malignancy. It also allows a useful alternative access, for example in recurrent inguinal hernia where the previous scar tissue from open surgery can be avoided, and it allows multiple operations through the same access – e.g. bilateral inguinal hernia.

While bleeding can be a difficult problem to control if it occurs during laparoscopy, in general there is reduced blood loss, less transfusion and less cost of blood replacement. Laparoscopy allows an improved opportunity for teaching, an operative field visible to all personnel and facilitates telemedicine or even telepresence operating.

Gastrointestinal Emergencies, 2nd edition. Edited by Tony Tham, John Collins and Roy Soetikno. © 2009 by Blackwell Publishing, ISBN: 978-1-4051-4634-0.

The best way of avoiding complications is to know about them. This chapter will highlight as many of the known complications of laparoscopic surgery as possible.

Many will be the same as for the equivalent open operation. Some will be unique and some will be commoner because of the laparoscopic approach (see Table 12.1). An interesting feature of complications after laparoscopy is that the skin incisions may give little clue as to what has been done internally. From a periumbilical access point the laparoscopist may have been operating anywhere from the mid mediastinum down to the lowest part of the pelvis. Therefore accurate, contemporaneous notes are an essential part of laparoscopic practice and reading these is an essential part of assessing a patient with complications after laparoscopic surgery.

Many of the complications of laparoscopy have been associated with the learning curve of taking a new approach to an old problem. Despite the large number of potential pitfalls the balance of benefit (by avoiding other complications from open surgery, or improving overall outcomes) is still in favor of laparoscopy.

Assessment, investigation and management of laparoscopic complications

Assessment
- Understand the underlying operation: read the operation notes.
- Look for method of access to peritoneum (Veress needle/open cutdown).

Table 12.1 Categorization of specific risks of complications in laparoscopic versus open operations.

Operations which have a specific risk of complication when done laparoscopically

Gastric bypass for obesity: anastomotic leaks

Resection of the stomach or esophagus: anastomotic leaks

Pancreatic resection: anastomotic leaks

Colectomy: anastomotic leaks

Nissen fundoplication: bougie perforation of the cardia

Incisional hernia repair: enterotomy, seroma

Adrenalectomy: renal arterial injury

Operations where there is significant debate on the relative risks of open versus laparoscopic approach

Appendicectomy: deep pelvic abscess

Cholecystectomy: relative risk of common bile duct injury

Operations where the complications of laparoscopic surgery seem little different in nature, and no more frequent than open surgery

Inguinal hernia repair

Heller's myotomy

Splenectomy

Rectopexy

Nephrectomy (live related donor)

Liver resection (for disease)

Ovarian tubal surgery

• Consider the underlying primary pathology.

• Consider any secondary pathology in the operative field (adhesions).

• Does the patient have comorbidity (obesity, cardiac failure, respiratory failure)?

• Use a multidisciplinary approach (radiology, gastro-enterology, anesthesiology and surgical teams)

• Examine the patient comprehensively:
   – area of surgery – abdomen or chest;
   – outside the area – head, neck, limbs, and cardio-respiratory system.

Investigation

• Radiography – within 24 hours note that the free air may be due to pneumoperitoneum.

• Ultrasound not often helpful initially because of gas.

• Blood tests: check for anemia, blood gases, and after cholecystectomy liver function tests.

Management

• Discuss the case with the operating surgeon and anesthetist.

• Inform the patient of the concerns.

• Do not delay with reoperation if the need arises.

• Reoperation usually is by laparoscopy.

• There is no gain in laparoscopy if open surgery is safer in the hands of the local team.

• Involve specialist referral for specific complications such as bile duct injury.

• Collect data for subsequent audit.

Types of complication

Cardiorespiratory system
Gas in the wrong cavity

Extraperitoneal insufflation may result in surgical emphysema, palpable anywhere on neck, chest or abdomen.

Pneumothorax or carbothorax (since the gas is CO_2) occurs by accidental pleural puncture, when dissecting the mediastinum or diaphragm. As long as positive pressure ventilation is maintained, an underwater seal drain is not required at the end of the procedure. Gas can also escape through a congenital foramen such as Morgagni or Bochdalek into the chest without any instrumental injury. A needle placed into the suspected chest cavity and CO_2 analysis may reveal a 100% concentration and confirm the diagnosis. This is treated by leaving in a wide-bore needle during the operation to allow gas to escape and remove the needle after ceasing the insufflation of CO_2 at the end of the procedure.

Gas embolism is a possibility but is rarely reported. It results in acute hypotension, cyanosis, hypoxia and a characteristic "millwheel" murmur on cardiac auscultation. Treat by releasing the pneumoperitoneum, place the patient in a steep Trendelenburg, left lateral decubitus position and aspirate gas using a central line.

Hypercarbia may occur with underlying lung disease such as emphysema and chronic obstructive airway disease causing premature ventricular contraction and arrhythmias. The anesthetist should be aware of the risk and monitor the exhaled CO_2 concentration. Increasing ventilation volume and frequency at an early stage will prevent this becoming a substantial problem.

Postoperative shoulder tip pain (Kehr sign) is common and may be due to carbonic acid irritating the diaphragm, overstretch of the diaphragm muscle fibers, or chemical irritating effects of blood in the peritoneal cavity. This is treated with reassurance, simple analgesia and mobilization of the patient. It almost always resolves within 24 hours.

Complications in the systemic circulation

Reduced venous return due to compression of the IVC is a theoretical risk that is rarely a clinical problem. In obese patients the upright position actually makes ventilation easier and venous return is usually good.in practice. Bradycardia can occur with vasovagal activity induced by the rapid insufflation of CO_2 during the establishment of the pneumoperitoneum. Treat by reduction of the CO_2 insufflation and administration of intravenous atropine. Respiratory gas exchange increases during laparoscopy and core temperature rises but there is no scientific evidence that this effect is beneficial or detrimental [1].

Deep venous thrombosis is relatively rare after laparoscopic surgery due to the improved mobilization postoperatively and the often shorter operative time than open surgery for cholecystectomy and hernia repair.

Complications of access
Enterotomy, vascular injury and bladder injury

When a vascular injury occurs during laparoscopic access it is usually after the use of a Veress needle (spring-mounted ball on the tip of a safety needle) to introduce the CO_2 into the peritoneum and may occur from the needle itself or the blind introduction of a sharp port. When it occurs it is catastrophic and so it has received much attention but it is rare, at 1 in 1333 cases, and the associated mortality is 1 in 33333 [2]. All of the complications of access are reduced by the use of a direct cutdown technique. While some experienced operators continue to safely use a Veress needle, particularly among gynecologists, it is easier and safer to teach the open cutdown method.

A new alternative is a translucent plastic port with a 0° lens to allow direct view of the inserted port, useful for obese patients, for bariatric surgery, or for placing the first port laterally when starting a laparoscopic incisional hernia repair.

No method of port insertion is perfectly safe in the presence of dense adhesions but being aware of the possibility, taking specific steps to avoid the problem and carefully assessing any areas of potential damage will limit these events to a minimum [2,3].

Port site hernia

It is rare for a port site hernia to occur (1%) and much less common than incisional hernias for midline laparotomy (10%). They usually occur within 3–6 weeks of the operation, may be associated with wound infection and obesity, and occur at 10–12 mm port sites, often one that has been extended to remove a large gallbladder. They are best repaired with a polypropylene mesh.

Complications of operative injury during laparoscopy
Enterotomy

Inadvertent injury of an abdominal organ can occur during the removal and replacement of surgical instruments. If this happens out of view of the camera then the injury may go unnoticed until there is a significant leakage of intestinal content and possible established peritoneal sepsis.

Enterotomy may occur during the dissection of adhesions of intestinal loops. In many circumstances adhesions may be left alone but in patients with adhesion obstruction, or patients with incisional hernia, there is a need to clear the operative field of adhesions. During laparoscopy the detection of such an injury may be hampered by limitations of the field of view of the laparoscopic camera. Recognition is critically important because immediate repair is simple either laparoscopically or by externalizing the bowel through a small incision.

Diathermy

Diathermy injury may occur as in open surgery, with the additional risk of capacitance coupling, which occurs if a conductor is placed inside an insulator (such as a plastic sheath around a metal port) and this can randomly discharge electricity out of view of the operator.

Adhesions

Laparoscopy greatly reduces the incidence of adhesions compared to equivalent open operations, resulting in fewer early and late postoperative complications of pain and obstruction. The long-term comparative figures are not well reported but clinical experience indicates a dramatic reduction in scar tissue compared to the effects of open intraabdominal surgery.

Hemorrhage

The problem of bleeding during laparoscopy has required the design of special tools. The Harmonic scalpel, a vibrating blunt blade device that coagulates with minimal heat and can seal arteries up to 7 mm in diameter, is useful for Nissen fundoplication. The Ligasure™ is a form of mulipolar electrocoagulation, useful for large arteries and popular in colectomy or splenectomy. For liver resection compression collars, microwave application and argon beam plasma coagulation (a form of spray diathermy) all have a role to play in dealing with potential major hemorrhage.

Conversion to open surgery

Whether conversion to open surgery can be defined as a complication is debatable. From the perspective of consent and education, the patient must be aware of the possibility but it may not be appropriate to term it a complication. When applied to large numbers conversion rates do give an indication of the quality of outcome from laparoscopic surgery and they may be audited in departments of surgery. For some operations such as Nissen fundoplication conversion to open surgery is so rare (<1% in expert institutions) that a high rate signifies potential problems with surgical standards. In contrast, for colectomy, conversion rates still vary from 11% to 29% and it will take some time before we understand whether such conversion is required to achieve adequate cancer clearance or whether the underlying issue is a lack of appropriate laparoscopic technique to achieve the same result [3,5].

Complications specific to procedures
Cholecystectomy, exploration of common bile duct

The complications of bile duct injury were frequent during the introduction of laparoscopy cholecystectomy (see Table 12.2) but are now much less frequent due to improved training. The risk of a major duct injury (incision, transaction, ischemic stricture) of a major bile duct is now less than 1 : 500 [6]. Cholecystectomy is relatively common and in a unit such as ours where we perform up to 1,000 cholecystectomies per annum

Table 12.2 Complications of laparoscopic cholecystectomy.

Injury to common bile duct or other biliary anatomy
Strictures, bile leaks, obstructive jaundice
Injury to duodenum
Leak from closure of cholecystoduodenal fistula
Retained gallstones in peritoneum
Retained common bile duct stones
Postoperative hemorrhage

such a risk may produce two injuries each year. The risk of minor injuries (bile leaks requiring stenting or suture) is approximately 1 : 200 (see also chapter on 23 – biliary emergencies). All of these are reduced by careful technique with good exposure of the Calot triangle and assurance of the anatomy of the cystic duct and cystic artery before clipping or division. The mobilization of the Hartmann pouch and extending this along the body of the gallbladder can greatly help in defining any potential aberrant anatomy. In patients with very inflamed thickened tissues it is safer to steer clear of the Calot triangle and perform a fundus first dissection. This requires the ability to deal with oozy hemorrhage from the liver bed, and having an argon beam plasma coagulator is a great asset in this circumstance.

When in doubt about the anatomy an intraoperative cholangiogram is useful. Referral centers seeing common bile duct injuries tend to advise routine cholangiography. This is a subject about which there has been controversy since before the days of laparoscopy.

Spilt gallstones may cause the rare complication of infection from actinomycosis and reports of this are unique to laparoscopy. To reduce the risk of stones being left behind use a tissue retrieval bag whenever the gallbladder wall is opened and place any loose stones in the bag before attempts are made to remove it from the abdomen.

Hernia repair, inguinal, femoral, incisional

Retention of urine after hernia repair is common (10% after bilateral repair). Bruising in the scrotum is common but significant hematoma in the scrotum is rare. Small bowel obstruction may occur due to adhesion or internal hernia through peritoneal repair. Nerve entrapment from a staple or tack can cause significant groin pain, but overall chronic groin pain is less common after laparoscopy than open surgery. After incisional hernia repair the sac may fill with blood-stained fluid (seroma) and be palpable as a persistent lump. These nearly always resolve after 6 months.

Enterotomy is likely when extensive adhesions require division during incisional hernia repair. This occurs in 2–5% of complex incisional hernias. Enough postoperative observation (2–3 days) is needed to ensure that peritonitis is not developing. In our experience we have seen delayed perforation at 7–10 days postoperatively and patients need to be educated to return and given easy access to the surgical team if significant postoperative symptoms develop.

Nissen fundoplication

The only complication of fundoplication that is specific to the laparoscopic approach is perforation of the esophagogastric junction. It is related to the use of a bougie. The incidence is 1–2%. Most observers advise careful use of the bougie with the anesthesiologist in direct view of the laparoscopic image during its introduction. The author believes that there is no need to subject the patient to the risk of a bougie perforation and the wrap can be calibrated using instruments that are 10mm in diameter (such as a 10mm Babcock introduced between the completed wrap and the esophagus.

Wrap migration may occur into the chest but is reduced by closing the diaphragmatic hiatus even when a hernia is not present. A slipped Nissen occurs when the fundoplication moves down onto the proximal stomach and is prevented by fixing the wrap to the esophagus and retaining the hepatic branch of the vagus nerve. Dysphagia may occur regardless of the approach. There is no difference between preserving, or dividing, the short gastric arteries, in randomized trials. These trials compare one blanket policy versus another. In some patients a tight fundus might benefit from mobilization of the short gastric arteries, whereas some loose fundi, especially after mobilizing a large hiatus hernia, become excessively mobile (and therefore liable to tort) if the short gastric arteries are mobilized as well. Therefore the author believes that the right technique is to be selective and choose mobilization of the short gastric arteries when there is an operative feeling of tension in the wrap (20%).

Splenectomy

Residual splenunculi may be more common after laparoscopic splenectomy as they occur along the surface of the pancreas, within and behind the greater omentum, areas not easily seen at laparoscopy.

Major operative hemorrhage is a worry during laparoscopic splenectomy but measures to handle it are well established. Having a swab available to place laparoscopically directly on arterial bleeding while suction, irrigation and proximal control is achieved allows laparoscopic control of such a surgical mishap.

Operations for morbid obesity: gastric bands/stapling/bypass

These are frequently performed laparoscopically. For laparascopic bands, slippage may occur in 0.7–3% [7,8], erosion in 0.7% and band obstruction in 1.5%. All these require revisional surgery. For bypass operations anastomotic leaks are the gravest of problems and the incidence of these after laparoscopic operations may be higher than after open ones (2.3% vs 4.2%) [7,9].

Colectomy

Conversion to open surgery is frequent (11–29% in recent series) [10] and current thinking accepts the need to convert to achieve cancer clearance. Complications are equivalent between open and laparoscopic approaches but the long-term outcomes are not clearly defined. Specific early fears about the high incidence of metastatic deposits along the track of the ports used for laparoscopic access, especially among UK observers, have not proved to be a real issue. Randomized trials show comparative figures for port site or incisional metastases (0.5–0.9% vs 0.2% laparascopy vs open) [4,5] and these differences are not clinically significant in the overall context of survival.

During colectomy, swelling and dependent edema of head, neck and upper limbs may occur from prolonged positioning in steep Trendelenburg. A sensible precaution is to provide the patient and the surgeons some respite from the positional effects by reversing the head-down position after each hour. These can be very long procedures – median operating times 275 minutes.

Appendicectomy

Specific complications after appendicectomy performed by the laparoscopic route are rare but pelvic abscesses are commoner in some series. A thorough cleansing by irrigation and aspiration and the use of drains for patients with significant peritoneal soiling after perforation will minimize this problem. A very rare event is the reinfection of the stump of appendix and this will be minimized by careful dissection of the appendix down onto the cecum at the time of the first operation.

Upper gastrointestinal cancer resections

Pancreatic, esophageal and gastric resection are probably not done in sufficient numbers to be regarded as routine and the risks of complication are not well described. Anastomotic leak rates for esophageal resections are 12% but, so far, only small series have been reported [11].

Adrenalectomy

For laparoscopic adrenalectomy there is the potential for rare complications such as renal arterial injury, not reported with open adrenalectomy [12].

Solid organ resection

Nephrectomy, common for live related donor, or for disease, and liver resection have a greater challenge for the surgeon in control of major blood vessels and techniques are evolving to deal with these issues using specific new technologies. Radical prostatectomy performed laparoscopically has the same range of operative complications as the open operation.

Gynecology

Tubal surgery, ectopic pregnancy, ovarian cyst and endometriosis treatment are all achievable by laparoscopy and the main issue in dealing with operative complications is the potential lack of the necessary skills of the gynecologist to deal with them. For instance, bowel injury may occur from dissection or from laser/argon beam and so it is good practice to ensure that there is a suitably qualified general surgeon available to handle these (or prevent them) by laparoscopic techniques.

References

1. McHoney MC, Corizia L, Eaton S et al. Laparoscopic surgery in children is associated with an intraoperative hypermetabolic response. Surg Endosc 2006; 20: 452–7.

2. Bonjer HJ, Hazebrook EJ, Kezemier G, Giuffrida MC, Meijer WS, Lange JF Open versus closed establishment of pneumoperitoneum in laparoscopic surgery. Br J Surg 1997; 84:599–602.

3. Pickersgill A, Slade RJ, Falconer GF, Attwood S. Open laparoscopy: the way forward. Br J Obs Gynae 1999; 106:1116–19.

4. Clinical Outcomes of Surgical Therapy Study Group. A comparison of laparoscopically assisted and open colectomy for colon cancer. N Engl J Med 2004; 350:2050–9.

5. Lacy Am, Garcia-Valdecasas JC, Delgado S, Castells A, Taura P. Pique JM et al. Laparosopcially assisted colon resection for treatment of non-metastatic colon cancer: a randomised trial. Lancet 2002; 359:2224–9.

6. Gentileschi P, DiPaola M, Catarci M et al. Bile duct injuries during laparoscopic cholecystectomy: a 1994–2001 audit on 13,718 operations in the Rome area. Surg Endosc 2004; 18:232–6.

7. Nguyen NT, Morton JM, Wolfe BM, Schirmer B, Ali M, Traverson LW. The Sages Bariatric Surgery Outcome Initiative. Surg Endosc 2005; 19:1429–38.

8. Parikh MS, Fielding GA, Ren CJ. US experience with 749 laparoscopic adjustable gastric bands: intermediate outcomes. Surg Endosc 2005; 19:1631–5.

9. Fernandez AZ, DeMaria EJ, Tichansky DS, Kellum JM, Wolfe LG, Meador J, Sugerman HJ. Experience with over 3,000 open and laparoscopic bariatric procedures: multivariate analysis of factors related to leak and resultant mortality. Surg Endosc 2004; 18:193–7.

10. Reza MM, Blasco JA, Andradas E, Cantero R, Mayol J. Systematic review of laparoscopic versus open surgery for colorectal cancer. Br J Surg 2006; 93:921–8.

11. Collins G, Johnson E, Korshus T et al. Experience with minimally invasive esophagectomy. Surg Endosc 2006; 20:298–301.

12. Brunt LM. Minimal access adrenal surgery. Surg Endosc 2006; 20:351–61.

13 Complications of Liver Biopsy

Ramsey C. Cheung

Introduction

Liver biopsy is performed using percutaneous, transjugular or laparoscopic techniques.

This chapter focuses on percutaneous biopsy (blind or under ultrasound guidance), which is the most common technique and hence used in all large published series. Depending on the definition of complications, the reported complication rate ranges from 0.56–3.7%, and mortality rate from 0.01–0.3%. In a pooled analysis of 189 085 liver biopsies, the overall complication rate from 0.28% and mortality rate was 0.03%.

Over 90% of complications are encountered within the first 24 hours, and 60% within 2 hours of the procedure. However, it is important to recognize complications such as hemorrhage which may be delayed for up to 3 weeks. Less than 5% of patients who undergo percutaneous liver biopsy require hospitalization as a result of a complication, with the main indications for admission being pain or hypotension. The complication rate increases with factors such as number of passes, presence of hepatic malignancy and advanced liver disease. Some studies also found the complication rate to be related to the type of biopsy needle and operator experience.

Transjugular liver biopsy is preferred if there are contraindications to percutaneous biopsy (Table 13.1), such as severe coagulopathy (especially if not corrected with transfusion), massive ascites, or suspected vascular lesion. The risk of bleeding is reduced since the biopsy is performed through the vessel. Other indications for a transjugular approach include morbid obesity, failure of percutaneous liver biopsy, or as part of another procedure such as portal pressure measurement and placement of a transjugular intrahepatic portosystemic shunt.

Table 13.1 Contraindications for percutaneous liver biopsy.[a]

Absolute
Uncooperative patient
Echinococcal cysts
Suspected hemangioma
Absence of a safe unobstructed access route for biopsy
History of unexplained bleeding
Coagulopathy[b]
Bleeding time >10 min
Platelet count <60 000/mm^3
INR ≥ 1.5
Relative
Biliary obstruction or cholangitis
Right-sided pleural disease (e.g. empyema) or subdiaphragmatic infection
Significant ascites
Severe uncontrolled anemia
Uremia[c]

[a]Consider transjugular approach in uncooperative patients, and patients with coagulopathy or ascites.
[b]Unless corrected with transfusion of fresh frozen plasma or platelets.
[c]Dialysis should be performed the day before liver biopsy, and deamino-8-D-arginine vasopressin (DDAVP) can also be given to reduce risk of hemorrhage.

Complications

See Table 13.2.

Pain
Clinical features

Up to one-third of patients will have at least some degree of pain in the right upper quadrant and/or right

Gastrointestinal Emergencies, 2nd edition. Edited by Tony Tham, John Collins and Roy Soetikno. © 2009 by Blackwell Publishing, ISBN: 978-1-4051-4634-0.

shoulder. Moderate pain occurs in approximately 20% and severe pain in <5%.

Investigation

Severe pain that responds poorly to analgesics, especially if accompanied by hypotension, should prompt work-up for hemorrhage or bile peritonitis.

Management

• Pain should be treated with analgesics, depending on the severity. For moderately severe pain, an opiate analgesic should be given intravenously for rapid onset of action.

• Monitor vital signs every 4–6 hours for hypotension (vasovagal or otherwise), and serial hematocrit or hemoglobin if bleeding is suspected.

Hemorrhage

Hemorrhage may be intraperitoneal, intrahepatic, subcapsular, or into the biliary tract (hemobilia). Mortality is usually related to intraperitoneal hemorrhage which is the most serious bleeding complication. Intrahepatic or even subcapsular hemorrhage may evolve into intraperitoneal hemorrhage. As a result, management will be similar if the patient is symptomatic. However, asymptomatic or minimally symptomatic intrahepatic or subcapsular hematoma is found in up to 23% if ultrasound is performed on all patients after liver biopsy. Large hematomas may be symptomatic and respond well to conservative therapy.

Clinical features

Risk of hemorrhage is higher in the presence of cirrhosis, intrahepatic malignancy, use of True-cut needle and multiple passes. There is also an increased risk in the presence of coagulopathy, but the safe threshold is not clear. Aspirin or other antiplatelet agents should be avoided for 5–7 days and NSAIDs for 1–3 days prior to biopsy to reduce risk of hemorrhage. Patients on oral anticoagulant should cease the medication for at least 3 days prior to the procedure. Risk of fatal hemorrhage is 10-fold higher in patients with malignancy as compared to those without malignancy.

Bleeding can occur immediately, and intraperitoneal hemorrhage usually becomes clinically obvious within the first 2–3 hours. However, other types of bleeding can be delayed (>24 h post-biopsy) in up to 70%. Delayed hemorrhage from pseudoaneurysms or rupture of intrahepatic hematoma can occur up to 18 days after liver biopsy.

Delayed hemorrhage has a high mortality since the correct diagnosis may not be made in a timely fashion or the bleeding may occur at home.

Hemorrhage should be considered in a patient with severe abdominal pain who responses poorly to analgesics, accompanied by a drop in serum hemoglobin, tachycardia and hypotension.

Investigation

• Hemoglobin/hematocrit every 6 h.

• Abdominal ultrasound or CT scan to look for intrahepatic or subcapsular hematoma.

• CT scan is preferred to determine intraperitoneal hemorrhage.

• Pseudoaneurysms and arteriovenous fistulae, which are the causes of delayed hemorrhage following liver biopsy, are detected by ultrasound with Doppler and biphasic CT scan.

Management

• Admit to hospital for observation.

• Type and cross packed red blood cells.

• Intravenous fluid and transfusion to support blood pressure and/or hematocrit.

• Correct any preexisting coagulopathy with transfusion of platelets and/or fresh frozen plasma.

• If patient is in shock, consult a surgeon or interventional radiologist depending on local expertise, for immediate intervention after the patient is stabilized.

• Pseudoaneurysms should be managed initially with angiographic embolization, and if it fails then surgery will be required (hepatic lobectomy or debridement followed by ligation of the pseudoaneurysm).

• Selective arteriography is both diagnostic and therapeutic in the patient with high clinical suspicion but negative CT scan.

• Surgical exploration if angiographic intervention failed.

Hemobilia
Clinical features

• Up to 90% present as upper gastrointestinal bleeding.

• Others present as gastrointestinal hemorrhage with a drop in hemoglobin and guaiac positive stool.

• Abdominal pain, usually in the right upper quadrant, is a finding in 70%.

• Jaundice is a presenting feature in 60% of cases.
• The mean interval of onset of hemobilia is 5 days after percutaneous liver biopsy but rarely can occur on the day of biopsy or as long as 21 days later. One-third can present with biliary colic, jaundice and gastrointestinal hemorrhage (Quincke triad).
• The bleeding is usually arterial in origin.

Investigation
• Upper endoscopy and/or ERCP. Upper endoscopy to rule out other etiology of upper gastrointestinal bleeding. Bleeding and clot from the ampulla of Vater can be seen on upper endoscopy. ERCP is recommended to establish the diagnosis and also for therapeutic intervention.
• Abdominal CT scan or ultrasound to rule out other causes of biliary obstruction. Ultrasound frequently shows the clot as an echogenic shadow in the biliary tree.

Management
• Stop bleeding by correcting any coagulopathy with vitamin K and/or fresh frozen plasma.
• ERCP to decompress and remove clots if there is evidence of obstruction. This could be achieved simply with sphincterotomy, balloon extraction of the clot, or placing a nasobiliary tube or biliary stent for drainage.
• Type-and-cross packed red blood cells. Transfuse if evidence of active bleeding at endoscopy and/or development of anemia.
• Angiography with embolization of the pseudoaneurysm by an interventional radiologist should be performed if significant bleeding persists after all attempts at conservative intervention. This will include superselective transcather embolization with gelfoam or metallic coils.

Bile peritonitis with or without gallbladder perforation
Clinical features
• Aspiration of bile in the suction syringe at the time of biopsy.
• Sudden onset of severe abdominal pain and right shoulder pain within minutes of the biopsy.
• Right upper quadrant tenderness, peritoneal signs, ileus and shock if accompanied by biliary peritonititis. Bile leak could be delayed for up to 10 days.
• Fever and leukocytosis.

Bile peritonitis is more common in the presence of biliary obstruction. In the absence of a dilated biliary tree, bile peritonitis is usually due to a gallbladder perforation.

Symptoms may be mild even with development of bile ascites.

Investigation
• Abdominal ultrasound or CT scan to detect bile collections.
• Technetium-99m dimethyl iminodiacetic acid (HIDA) scan to detect any ongoing bile (radionucleotide) leaks.

Management
• Nothing by mouth, intravenous fluid resuscitation and broad-spectrum antibiotics to cover biliary tract pathogens. Conservative medical treatment if patient is stable and no peritoneal findings. Surgical consult if peritoneal signs are present.
• Percutaneous drainage and cholecystostomy for the leak to seal in unstable patient.
• Biliary drainage in the presence of biliary obstruction.
• Laparotomy or laparoscopy in patients with signs of biliary peritonitis. Cholecytectomy is a definitive treatment.

Pulmonary complications
Clinical features
• Right-sided chest wall pain at the site of needle entry.
• Right-sided pleuritic chest pain immediately or 2–3 hours post-biopsy.
• Rarely dysnpea, cough or hemoptysis.

Investigation
• Chest radiography (posteroanterior and lateral) to rule out hemothorax and pleural effusion.
• Complete blood count if hemoptysis occurs or hemothorax is suspected.

Management
• Transfuse packed red blood cells if anemia developed as a result of hemothorax.
• Chest tube if pnemothorax is large, tension pneumothorax, or patient is symptomatic.
• Remove pleural effusion if large or symptomatic.

Other complications
Some rare complications are listed in Table 13.2. Bacteremia is usually transient and asymptomatic.

Table 13.2 Complications of percutaneous liver biopsy.

Complication	Incidence (%)
Pain	0.06–33
Intraperitoneal hemorrhage	0.03–0.7
Intra-/extrahepatic hematoma	0.06–2.7[a]
Biliary	
Perforation of gallbladder	0.012
Hemobilia	0.06–1
Bile peritonitis	0.03–0.22
Pulmonary complications	0.01–0.35
Pneumothorax	0.08–0.8
Hemothorax	0.18–0.49
Sepsis	0.09
Seeding of malignant lesion	0.003–0.009
Biopsy of other organs	0.004–0.12
Rare complications	
Subphrenic abscess	
Bile embolism	
Air embolism	
Biloma from bile leak	
Hemobilia-related obstructive jaundice, acute cholecystitis, acute pancreatitis	

[a]Up to 23% if post-biopsy ultrasound is performed on all patients.

Penetration of other organs such as the colon is infrequent and usually benign with rare cases of peritonititis. Another rare complication when biopsy is performed for intrahepatic malignancy, primary or metastatic, is seeding of the needle tract.

Further reading

Bravo AA, Sheth SG, Chopra S. Liver biopsy. N Engl J Med 2001; 344:495–500.

Campbell MS, Jeffers LJ, Reddy KR. Liver biopsy and laparoscopy. In: Schiff ER, Sorrell MF, Maddrey WC, eds. Diseases of the Liver, 10th edition. 2007: 61–81.

Piccino T, Sagnelli E, Pasquale G, Giusti G. Complications following percutaneous liver biopsy: a multicenter retrospective study on 68,276 biopsies. J Hepatol 1986; 2:165–73.

Sheela H, Seela S, Caldwell C, Boyer JL, Jain D. Liver biopsy: evolving role in the new millennium. J Clin Gastroenterol 2005; 39:603–10.

14 Complications of Colonoscopy

Sybile Van Lierde, Jo Vandervoort

Introduction

Since the introduction of colonoscopy in the late 1960s, the therapeutic and diagnostic applications of the technique have increased dramatically. Colonoscopy is now recommended for primary colorectal cancer screening in average-risk persons [1]. Colorectal cancer screening targets healthy people, therefore the magnitude of the risk and severity of complications from screening are important issues to consider when selecting a screening strategy.

Up to 1.9% of more than 500000 colonoscopies performed in the US each year result in significant complications. Complications of colonoscopy include bleeding from biopsy and polypectomy site, colonic perforation and postpolypectomy syndrome (a transmural colonic burn, marked by localized abdominal pain without evidence of frank perforation) [2]. Diverticulitis, which is caused by a microscopic perforation of the colon, can also theoretically be caused by colonoscopy in persons with preexisting diverticulosis.

Furthermore, there is a 9-fold increased risk of serious complications with polypectomy or when biopsies are taken.

Complications

Haemorrhage

Hemorrhage is the most common polypectomy complication, occurring in 0.3–6.0% of cases in various reports [2–4]. Bleeding can occur immediately

Gastrointestinal Emergencies, 2nd edition. Edited by Tony Tham, John Collins and Roy Soetikno. © 2009 by Blackwell Publishing, ISBN: 978-1-4051-4634-0.

following or be delayed up to 29 days. The severity of bleeding ranges from arterial pumping to slight ooze.

The risk is related to the type and size of the polyp, the technique of polypectomy, and the coagulation status of the patient [2,3]. The risk of immediate bleeding is increased when blended current (rather than pure coagulation current) is used or when the snare is pulled through the polyp without the use of cautery "cheese wiring." Bleeding is more frequent in patients with coagulation disorders, in patients with large (>2.5 cm) polyps, those with a thick stalk and sessile lesions [5].

Colonoscopy is commonly performed in patients on medication that can affect their coagulation status. Guidelines have been issued by the American Society for Gastrointestinal Endoscopy (ASGE) based upon the available evidence and consensus opinion [6]. It is recommended that nonaspirin antiplatelet agents should be discontinued 7–10 days before the procedure. Low molecular weight heparin should be discontinued 8 hours before the procedure. Warfarin should be discontinued 3–5 days before the procedure. Aspirin and nonsteroidal anti-inflammatory drugs need not be discontinued.

Management of immediate hemorrhage

Most bleeding that occurs immediately after resection can be controlled by the endoscopist [5]. The technique for controlling bleeding depends upon the severity of bleeding, the type of polyp, and individual preference. A combination of techniques is frequently required.

Immediate bleeding after resection of a pedunculated polyp can usually be stopped by regrasping the pedicle with a snare and holding pressure on the pedicle to stop blood flow, permitting the hemostatic cascade to occur. Retransection of the pedicle can be performed but is not the preferred approach since there may be too little of the pedicle remaining to regrasp if bleeding recommences.

If the above technique fails, epinephrine (a dilution of 1:10000) can be directly injected into the bleeding site.

A thermal probe, BICAP or heater probe can be used, but because the colon wall is very thin, the current delivered should be decreased by approximately 50%.

Argon plasma beam coagulation is effective for oozing from a superficial vessel.

Bleeding can be controlled by placement of hemoclips. The clips are especially useful for bleeding from flat polypectomy sites, but have also been used successfully to stop arterial pulsatile bleeding from the severed stalk of pedunculated polyps.

If bleeding persists, a mesenteric angiogram will help to localize the bleeding vessel(s) followed by embolization of this vessel. Also vasopressin can be infused locally to vasoconstrict the mucosal feeding arterioles.

Endoloops can be used to ligate the stalk to stop bleeding. In polyps with thick stalks and/or with a visible pulsation, an endoloop can be applied to the stalk prior to a polypectomy to prevent bleeding.

Management of delayed hemorrhage

Delayed bleeding occurs in up to 2% of patients who have polyps removed [5]. The risk is increased in the elderly, in patients with hypertension, when large sessile polyps are removed from the right colon and when pure coagulation current was used for polypectomy. The risk also rises with the size of polyps.

Although use of NSAIDs and/or aspirin is commonly believed to increase the risk of delayed bleeding, there are no studies that corroborate this impression. In contrast, patients who are recommenced on anticoagulant therapy do have an increased risk for delayed post-polypectomy bleeding [6,7].

Colonoscopy should be performed immediately in patients who appear to be actively bleeding. If the bleeding site is seen, haemostasis should be attempted using the modalities described above.

Postpolypectomy electrocoagulation syndrome

This syndrome refers to the development of abdominal pain, fever, leukocytosis, and peritoneal inflammation in the absence of frank perforation that occurs after polypectomy with electrocoagulation. It usually presents within 12 hours, but symptoms may occur up to 5 days after the procedure. Recognition is important to avoid unnecessary exploratory laparatomy since it resolves with conservative treatment in the majority of patients. It is the second most common complication (after bleeding) occurring in 0.5% of polypectomies. There are no cases of post-polypectomy electrocoagulation syndrome described following the use of submucosal saline elevation of large polyps prior to transection, possibly because it prevents transmural thermal injury. It occurs also most often after the removal of large (>2cm) sessile polyps, which usually require large amounts and long duration of thermal energy [2,5,8].

Management

Radiographic evaluation with a plain abdominal radiograph or an abdominal CT scan is important to distinguish this syndrome from frank perforation. Treatment is conservative, consisting of intravenous fluids, nil by mouth, bed rest and antibiotics until symptoms improve. In most cases, the pain settles with simple analgesia and there are no long-term sequelae.

Colonic perforation

Colonic perforation occurs rarely during colonoscopy but it is still a major complication. A recent large series has reported an incidence of nearly 1 in every 1000 colonoscopies [4,9,10].

The sigmoid colon and the rectosigmoid junction is the area at greatest risk for perforation. The presence of intestinal pathology, such as severe diverticular disease, inflammatory bowel disease, colonic stricture, radiation colitis or previous abdominal surgery predisposes the colon to perforation during endoscopy.

The clinical presentation is quite variable. The most common symptom of perforation is abdominal pain. The onset of pain usually occurs during or soon after completion of the procedure, but it may be delayed or even nonexistent in some instances [11]. Signs can be masked for hours or days by omental plugging. Persistent abdominal pain, distension and tenderness with fever, tachycardia, absent bowel sounds and subcutaneous emphysema indicate colonic perforation. In the most severe cases of perforation, spilling of bowel contents leads to peritonitis, sepsis and circulatory collapse.

Plain radiography of the chest and abdomen often reveals pneumoperitoneum but lack of this finding does not exclude peritonitis. In these patients, computed tomography can be helpful in establishing the size and extent of injury with more precision [11–12].

Management

The management of colon perforation secondary to colonoscopy remains controversial. It can be effectively managed by operative or nonoperative measures. The choice between nonoperative and surgical treatment depends on the patient's general medical condition, the completeness of bowel preparation and the type of colonoscopic procedure that had been performed [12,13]. Perforation from diagnostic colonoscopy requires surgical intervention more frequently than that from therapeutic colonoscopy [14]. The reason is that perforations during diagnostic colonoscopy result from mechanical forces during insertion or from barotraumas, forcible instrument insertion, endoscopic torquing with alpha maneuver and the "slide-by" technique in which the colonoscope is advanced along the mucosal surface without direct visualization. These manipulations cause undue stretching of the bowel with resultant linear tears of the mucosa on the antimesenteric side of the colon, resulting in transmural rupture [15]. Perforations after therapeutic procedures are more frequent. The mechanisms include the direct injury caused by biopsy forceps, brushes, dilators and more commonly the thermal or electrical injury when using laser or electrocautery.

Several large studies have reported that many patients with colonic perforations may be successfully treated without surgery [12]. Nonoperative treatment involves hospitalization, intestinal rest and intravenous fluids and antibiotics to contain peritonitis and allow the perforation to seal. If the perforation is immediately seen after polypectomy and it is small and localized, it can be managed endoscopically. At that time the colon is clean and hemoclips can be placed. Close observation is mandatory and surgical intervention is needed if the patient's condition deteriorates or there is no improvement in 72 hours. On the other hand, operative treatment is indicated for patients with diffuse peritonitis, failure of medical treatment, large colonic injuries, ongoing sepsis and those with underlying pathology (i.e. cancer, unremitting colitis and distal obstruction). Surgical procedures range from primary repair, resection and anastomosis or defunctioning colostomy.

Rare complications of colonoscopy

These include subcutaneous emphysema, pneumatosis coli, pneumoscrotum, pneumopericardium and pneumothorax [16,17].

Insufflated gas can pass into the retroperitoneum, bowel wall (pneumotosis coli), or subcutaneous tissues leading to abdominal discomfort and signs of subcutaneous emphysema.

Management

In these situations, a perforation into the peritoneal cavity with septic risk must be excluded as described above. If the patient has no signs of peritoneal inflammation or no systemic sepsis, a conservative approach can safely be employed although it is advisable to monitor the patient in hospital and obtain an urgent surgical consult.

Even less common but serious complications include acute colonic (pseudo)obstruction [18], splenic trauma [19], cecal volvulus, vasovagal reactions and endocarditis. Sepsis and other infections following colonoscopy are rare.

References

1. Winawer S, Fletcher R, Rex D, Bond J, Burt R, Ferrucci J, et al. Colorectal cancer screening and surveillance: clinical guidelines and rationale. Update based on new evidence. Gastroenterology 2003; 124:544–60.
2. Waye JD, Kahn O, Auerbach ME. Complications of colonoscopy and flexible sigmoidoscopy. Gastrointest Endosc Clin N Am 1996; 6:343–77.
3. Gibbs DH, Opelka FG, Beck DE, Hicks TC. Post-polypectomy colonic hemorrhage. Dis Colon Rectum 1996; 39:806.
4. Levin TR, Zhao W, Conell C, et al. Complications of colonoscopy in an integrated health care delivery system. Ann Intern Med 2006; 145:880.
5. Waye JD, Lewis BS, Yessayan S. Colonoscopy: a prospective report of complications. J Clin Gastroenterol 1992; 15:347.
6. Zuckerman MJ, Hirota WK, Adler DG, et al. ASGE guideline: the management of low-molecular-weight heparin and nonaspirin antiplatelet agents for endoscopic procedures. Gastrointest Endosc 2005; 61:189.
7. Hui AJ, Wong RM, Ching JY, et al. Risk of colonoscopic polypectomy bleeding with anticoagulants and antiplatelet agents: analysis of 1657 cases. Gastrointest Endosc 2004; 59:44.
8. Nelson DB, McQuaid KR, Bond JH, et al. Procedural success and complications of large-scale screening colonoscopy. Gastrointest Endosc 2002; 55:307.
9. Muhldorfer SM, Kekos G, Hahn E.G., Ell C. Complications of therapeutic gastrointestinal endoscopy. Endoscopy 1992; 24:276–83.

10. Anderson ML, Pasha TM, Leighton JA. Endoscopic perforation of the colon: lessons from a 10-year study. Am J Gastroenterol 2000; 95:3418–22.

11. Hall C, Dorricott NJ, Donovan IA, Neoptolomos JP. Colon perforation during colonoscopy: surgical versus conservative management. Br J Surg 1991; 78:542–4.

12. Araghizadeh FY, Timmcke AE, Opelka FG, Hichs TC, Beck DE. Colonoscopic perforations. Dis Colon Rectum 2001; 44(5):713–16.

13. Cobb WS, Heniford BT, Sigmon LB, Hasan R. Colonic perforations: incidence, management and outcomes. Am Surg 2004; 70(9):750–9.

14. Ker TS, Wasserberg N, Beart Jr RW. Colonoscopic perforation and bleeding of the colon can be treated safely without surgery. Am Surg 2004; 70(10):992–4.

15. Orsoni P, Berdah S, Verrier C, Caamano A, Sastre B, Boutboul R, Grimaud JC, Picaud R. Colonic perforation due to colonoscopy: a retrospective study of 48 cases. Endoscopy 1997; 29:160–4.

16. Ho HC, Burchell S, Morris P, Yu M. Colon perforation, bilateral pneumothoraces, pneumopericardium, pneumomediastinum, and subcutaneous emphysema complicating endoscopic polypecto my: anatomic and management considerations. Am Surg 1996; 62:770–4.

17. Lovisetto F, Zonta S, Rota E, Mazzilli M, Faillace G, Bianca A, Fantini A, Longoni M. Left pneumothorax secondary to colonoscopic perforation of the sigmoid colon: a case report. Surg Laparosc Endosc Percutan Tech 2007; 17(1):62–4.

18. Saunders MD. Acute colonic pseudo-obstruction. Gastrointest Endosc Clin N Am 2007; 17(2):341–60.

19. Ahmed A, Eller PM, Schiffman FJ. Splenic rupture: an unusual complication of colonoscopy. Am J Gastroenterol 1997; 92:1201–4.

15 Complications of Capsule Endoscopy

Cecilia Sison, Andres Sanchez Yagüe, Roy Soetikno,
Kenneth Binmoeller

Introduction

Endoscopic evaluation of the small intestines has been severely limited because of its significant length and distance from the oral or rectal orifices. Capsule endoscopy is a noninvasive technology developed to allow diagnostic imaging of the entire length of the small bowel [1]. Images obtained approximate the physiological state of the small bowel since the capsule moves passively, does not inflate the bowel and visualizes the mucosa in its collapsed state. It has become the gold standard in evaluating suspected disease of the small intestines [2].

Capsule endoscopy is a safe procedure. A major risk associated with capsule endoscopy is capsule retention [2]. Clinically significant retention was seen in less than 1% of patients. Other complications include potential interference between the transmitted capsule wavelengths and other implanted electronic devices, most notably cardiac pacemakers and defibrillators. Rare complications include impaction and fracture of the capsule endoscope device and intestinal perforation secondary to a retained capsule endoscope device. The aim of this chapter is to provide a review of the complications of capsule endoscopy.

Contraindications

Capsule endoscopy is contraindicated for the following [1]:
• patients with known or suspected gastrointestinal obstruction, strictures or fistulas based on the clinical picture or preprocedure testing;

Gastrointestinal Emergencies, 2nd edition. Edited by Tony Tham, John Collins and Roy Soetikno. © 2009 by Blackwell Publishing, ISBN: 978-1-4051-4634-0.

• patients with cardiac pacemakers or other implanted electro-medical devices;
• patients with swallowing disorders;
• pregnancy.

Capsule retention

The ICCE 2005 Consensus for Capsule Retention [2] defined capsule retention as having a capsule endoscope remain in the digestive tract for a minimum of 2 weeks. Capsule retention was further defined as the capsule remaining in the bowel lumen unless directed medical, endoscopic or surgical intervention was instituted. Clinically significant retention is different from regional transit abnormalities wherein the capsule remains for at least 60 minutes in a single segment of bowel that may or may not have evidence of visible mucosal abnormality. In a series by Barkin [3], consisting of 937 patients being evaluated for obscure gastrointestinal bleeding, seven cases (0.75%) of capsule retention were reported. A series published by Pennazio et al. [4] reported a capsule retention rate of five (5%) out of 100 patients undergoing capsule endoscopy for obscure bleeding.

Causes of capsule retention include Crohn's disease, NSAID strictures, small bowel tumors, radiation enteritis and surgical anastomotic strictures. Retention has not been reported in patients with a "normal" anatomy or those with anatomical variants such as small bowel diverticulosis and appendiceal orifices [1]. In a retrospective case series by Baichi et al. [5] five cases of retention were reported out of 245 capsule studies. Causes of capsule retention included adenocarcinoma in a patient with hereditary nonpolyposis colorectal cancer (1), idiopathic stenosis (1), stricturing Crohn's disease (2), and adhesions (1). In Pennazio's [4] series, of the five patients with capsule retention, two had Crohn's disease, two had anastomotic strictures and one had a small bowel tumor. A case study conducted by Sears et al. [6] showed NSAID-induced strictures to be the major cause of retention.

Management

• Patients with capsule retention are often asymptomatic [5,6]. The development of pain usually heralds passage through a tight stricture.

• Retention can be suspected from the interpretation of capsule images. A clear image of the obstructing lesion may be seen. Repetitive views of the same mucosal areas may be visualized. Failure to see the colon during the examination is also an indication, although this is not diagnostic since 25% of capsule examinations fail to enter the colon during the 8-hour procedure time.

• If capsule retention is suspected or if the colon is not entered during the acquisition time, an abdominal or kidney, ureter and bladder radiograph should be obtained after 2 weeks [2].

• Endoscopic or surgical intervention has been shown to be effective for capsule removal [2]. Aside from removal of the retained capsule, surgical intervention has the added advantage of treatment and/or resection of the offending pathology that caused the capsule retention (e.g. strictures).

• Studies have shown that initiation of medical therapies such as a course of steroids or infliximab, discontinuing NSAIDs, are not successful in managing capsule retention.

Prevention

There is no guaranteed screening method to completely prevent capsule retention. Obtaining a good medical history with identification of risk factors remains to be the single best method [2]. Risk factors include known Crohn's disease, history of chronic NSAID use, history of previous small bowel obstruction as well as small bowel resection, previous abdominal surgery, and history of abdominal radiation. Patients with abdominal pain, distention and nausea should be suspected of having a potential for capsule retention.

Another attempt to avoid capsule retention has been the development of the "patency capsule" [1,2]. This is a self-dissolving capsule developed by Given Imaging that has the same dimensions as the capsule endoscopy device but which contains lactose. When retained

in a fluid-filled environment, the core of the capsule dissolves after approximately 40 hours, allowing the insoluble outer membrane to collapse and pass. It also carries a radiofrequency identification (RFID) tag that is activated and detected by a hand-held RFID scanner. Detection of a signal by the hand-held scanner indicates that the capsule is still retained in the gastrointestinal tract.

Electromagnetic interference with implanted electro-medical devices

The capsule endoscope device uses a frequency of 440 MHz to transmit images. Theoretically, this system may interfere with the normal operation of cardiac pacemakers. The manufacturers have included a written warning that the capsule should not be used in patients with pacemakers. Electromagnetic interference may alter the operation of pacemakers, potentially causing problems in several ways: (1) interference with the ventricular channel includes oversensing, which may result in ventricular pacing inhibition, resulting in bradycardia with dizziness and syncope; undersensing, which may lead to competition with the native QRS complexes possibly resulting in induction of tachyarrhythmias; and induction of asynchronous ventricular (noise mode) function; (2) interference with the atrial channel resulting in oversensing of electromagnetic signals, with a subsequent increase in ventricular pacing rate [7].

However, there have been studies showing that the capsule is safe to use in patients with implanted cardiac pacemakers and defibrillators. In a small case series [8] of five patients with cardiac pacemakers who underwent capsule endoscopy for obscure gastrointestinal bleeding, no arrhythmia or other adverse cardiac event was noted during capsule transmission. In addition, no pacemaker-induced interference on the capsule endoscopy images was observed. In a study by Dubner et al. [7] a test device, that reproduces the effect of a capsule endoscope device by transmitting at exactly the same frequency, was used to determine the safety of capsule endoscopy in patients with implanted cardiac pacemakers. Electromagnetic interference was observed but this was not clinically significant. No potentially dangerous pacemaker inhibition was observed.

Impaction and fracture of the capsule endoscopy device

Impaction and subsequent fracture of the capsule endoscopy device in the small bowel is a rare complication. In fact, only one case has been reported at this time. Fry et al. [9] published a case of a patient who underwent capsule endoscopy for a 2.5-year history of unexplained abdominal pain. Pertinent in his history was intake of aspirin for atherosclerotic coronary artery disease. Wireless capsule endoscopy revealed multiple ring-like strictures in the mid and distal small bowel resulting in luminal narrowing, as well as ulcerated areas with stricture formation. A diagnosis of NSAID-induced diaphragm disease was established. Aspirin was discontinued and the patient was symptom-free for 6 months. However, he experienced recurrent abdominal pain. Radiographic images showed a metallic-density foreign body in the right lower quadrant. CT enterography identified four capsule fragments in the distal small bowel. Exploratory laparotomy was performed with resection of 40 cm of small bowel. Gross inspection of the resected specimen revealed diaphragm disease and the fragmented video capsule. The patient's postoperative course was uneventful and 4 months later, on follow-up, the patient was doing extremely well with no recurrence of abdominal pain.

Intestinal perforation

Only one case of intestinal perforation due to a retained capsule endoscope device has been published. Gonzales Carro et al. [10] reported a case of an elderly gentleman with a history of a previous cholecystectomy 10 years ago, who underwent capsule endoscopy for anemia. Capsule endoscopy revealed multiple angiodysplastic lesions in the distal jejunum and proximal ileum. The patient had not eliminated the capsule after a month but he remained asymptomatic. Two months later, the patient presented with symptoms suggestive of peritonitis and was found to have diffuse peritonitis secondary to a distal ileum perforation. A large number of adhesions was seen in the area, which were likely due to the previous surgery. The capsule was found in the area of the perforated ileum. The ileal segment was resected. The postoperative course was unremarkable and the patient was discharged.

References

1. Mishkin D, Chuttani R, Croffie J, DiSario J, Liu J, Shah R, Somogyi L, Tierney W, Wong Kee Song LM, Petersen B. ASGE Technology Status Evaluation Report: wireless capsule endoscopy. Gastrointest Endosc 2006; 63(4):539–45.
2. Cave D, Legnani P, de Franchis R, Lewis BS. ICCE Consensus for Capsule Retention. Endoscopy 2005; 37(10):1065–7.
3. Barkin JS, Friedman S. Wireless capsule endoscopy requiring surgical intervention: the world's experience. Am J Gastroenterol 2002; 97:A83.
4. Pennazio M, Santucci R, Rondonotti E, Abbiati C, Beccari G, Rossini FP, de Franchis R. Outcome of patients with obscure gastrointestinal bleeding after capsule endoscopy: report of 100 consecutive cases. Gastroenterology 2004; 126:643–53.
5. Baichi M, Arifuddin R, Mantry PS. What we have learned from 5 cases of permanent capsule retention. Gastrointest Endosc 2006; 64(2):283–7.
6. Sears DM, Avots-Avotins A, Culp K, Gavin MW. Frequency and clinical outcome of capsule retention during capsule endoscopy for GI bleeding of obscure origin. Gastrointest Endosc 2004; 60(5):822–7.
7. Dubner S, Dubner Y, Gallino S, Spallone L, Zagalsky D, Rubio H, Zimmerman J, Goldin E. Electromagnetic interference with implantable cardiac pacemakers by video capsule. Gastrointest Endosc 2005; 61(2):250–4.
8. Leighton JA, Sharma VK, Srivathsan K, Heigh R, McWane TL, Post JK, Robinson SR, Bazzell JL, Fleischer DE. Gastrointest Endosc 2004; 59(4):567–9.
9. Fry LC, De Petris G, Swain JM, Fleischer DE. Impaction and fracture of a video capsule in the small bowel requiring laparotomy for removal of the capsule fragments. Endoscopy 2005; 37(7):674–6.
10. Gonzalez Carro P, Picazo Yuste J, Fernandez Diez S, Perez Roldan F, Roncero Garcia-Escribano O. Intestinal perforation due to a retained wireless capsule endoscope. Endoscopy 2005; 37:684.

16 Complications of Endoscopic Ultrasound

Cecilia Sison, Andres Sanchez Yagüe, Roy Soetikno, Kenneth Binmoeller

Introduction

From its conceptualization more than 20 years ago, endoscopic ultrasonography (EUS) has evolved from a novel diagnostic imaging tool to a standard diagnostic and therapeutic modality. It has made a significant impact on the diagnosis and management of gastrointestinal and nongastrointestinal diseases. These advances are due to the development of the linear array echoendoscope, which allows the placement of devices into the ultrasound plane of view, permitting various interventions to be accomplished. Among these interventions is the endoscopic ultrasound-guided fine-needle aspiration of lesions that are too small to be visualized by CT scan or MRI, or lesions that are well encased by surrounding vascular structures.

EUS as well as EUS-guided fine-needle aspiration (FNA) biopsy have been proven to be safe. Reported complications are related to biopsy of cystic and solid lesions [1]. In a large multicenter trial involving 554 consecutive mass or lymph node biopsies, only five (0.9%) complications were reported, all of which were nonfatal [2]. These complications were endoscope-induced perforation, superimposed infection of aspirated cystic lesions, and hemorrhage. Major complications were observed in 2.5% of 355 patients who underwent EUS-FNA for solid pancreatic masses in another series [3] including infection and acute pancreatitis. There were no deaths reported. The purpose of this chapter is to provide a review of the complications of diagnostic and therapeutic endoscopic ultrasonography.

Complications

Hemorrhage

Hemorrhagic complications including intracystic hemorrhage are uncommon in EUS-FNA procedures. The mechanism for post-EUS-guided FNA bleeding probably relates to injuring the blood supply to the aspirated lesion [7]. In a series of 50 patients who underwent EUS-guided FNA of pancreatic cystic lesions, three (6%) developed acute intracystic hemorrhage. Bleeding in all three cases stopped spontaneously after several minutes [4]. In another study of 208 patients who underwent EUS-guided FNA, two (~1%) patients developed hemorrhage [5]. Only one (0.18%) patient developed hemorrhage in a trial of 554 patients who underwent EUS-guided FNA [2].

Endosonographic appearance

Extraluminal hemorrhage is recognized by the development of an expanding echopoor zone surrounding the site of needle puncture of the targeted lesion [6]. The appearance is compatible with that of a hematoma. This is supported by the aspiration of blood-tinged fluid [6] in the aspirating syringe. In a study conducted by Varadarajulu et al. [4], intracystic hemorrhage was readily recognized during EUS-FNA as an expanding hyperechoic area around the site of needle puncture within the targeted cyst. This is again supported by aspiration of blood-tinged fluid (Figure 16.1).

Gastrointestinal Emergencies, 2nd edition. Edited by Tony Tham, John Collins and Roy Soetikno. © 2009 by Blackwell Publishing, ISBN: 978-1-4051-4634-0.

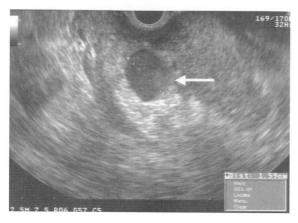

Figure 16.1 Intracystic hemorrhage after fine needle aspiration using a 22 gauge needle of a pancreatic cyst.

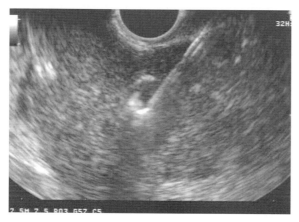

Figure 16.2 Injection of fibrin glue into the cyst cavity after an arterial bleeding occurred and did not stop spontaneously 20 minutes after EUS FNA of a pancreatic cyst. The bleeding stopped instantaneously after injection of fibrin glue.

Management

• Immediate recognition of this complication is important because it permits immediate termination of the procedure.

• The lesion should be observed endosonographically for cessation of bleeding.

• If bleeding does not cease after a short period of time, pressure may be applied for 15–25 minutes at the needle puncture site by inflation of the balloon and by tip deflection of the echoendoscope [6].

• EUS-guided injection of epinephrine at the bleeding site may be performed [4].

• Another option is to inject fibrin glue into the cyst cavity in the region of the bleeding vessel, which can be identified by a pulsating vascular flow (Figure 16.2).

Pancreatitis

Pancreatitis may result from needle passage through healthy pancreatic tissue or inflammation as a result of intracystic hemorrhage [7]. Pancreatitis was noted to occur more commonly after EUS-FNA of pancreatic cystic lesions located in the pancreatic head or uncinate process [7]. In a pooled analysis of 19 centers involving 4909 EUS-guided FNAs of solid pancreatic lesions, pancreatitis occurred in 14 cases (0.29%) [8]. In another trial of 355 patients who underwent EUS-FNA for a solid pancreatic mass, three patients developed pancreatitis [3].

Clinical features

• Presents within the first 24 hours after the procedure.

• Epigastric abdominal pain.

• Abdominal tenderness and guarding are also common.

• Nausea and vomiting.

• Elevated pancreatic enzymes at least 3 times the upper limit of normal.

Management

The management of patients with pancreatitis after EUS-FNA of the pancreas [11] is similar to the management of patients with pancreatitis due to other causes (see Chapter 22).

Perforation

(See also Chapter 18.) Cases of perforation have been described after EUS-FNA [2,5]. This is thought to be related to the passage of the echoendoscope rather than the FNA itself [7], and this may be due to the oblique-viewing optics of the scope [1]. The esophagus is the most common site for perforation (Figure 16.3; Plates 16.1 & 16.2).

Superimposed infection

The possible risk of superimposed infection after aspiration of cystic lesions has led to the suggestion that antibiotics should be administered prophylactically before EUS-FNA [2]. However, the risk of infection in such cases has not been studied prospectively in a

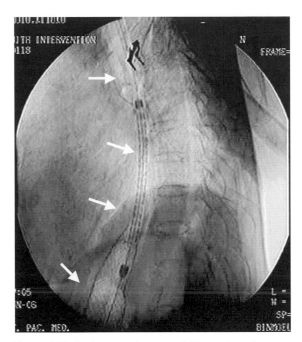

Figure 16.3 Deployment of an expandable esophageal metal stent over the sight of a perforation.

controlled manner. A randomized prospective study is required to address this issue. Although prophylactic use of antibiotics appears logical prior to aspiration of necrotic lesions the risk of infection has not been quantified. In a series of 114 pancreatic cystic lesions, antibiotic prophylaxis was given prior to EUS-FNA in 66% of patients. No cases of infection were observed in patients with or without prophylaxis. Additionally, case reports of infection after EUS-FNA of submucosal lesions have been published.

Management
• Broad-spectrum antibiotics for 7–14 days.

Aspiration
Aspiration of food or fluid into the lungs is an uncommon complication.

Prevention
• No food or drink for at least 6 hours before the procedure.
• Suction oral secretions.
• If possible, keep patient on his or her left side throughout the entire procedure.
• When filling the lumen of the gastrointestinal tract with water, elevate the head of the bed to about 30°.

Management
Management is as follows [12]:
• Terminate the procedure.
• Perform aggressive chest physiotherapy.
• Oxygen support through a nasal cannula or a face mask. If the patient, remains hypoxic, consider ventilatory support.
• Request a chest radiograph.
• Broad-spectrum antibiotics.
• Other laboratory tests: hemoglobin, metabolic panel, sputum culture and sensitivity.

Oversedation
Providing adequate sedation and analgesia is a vital part in the practice of gastrointestinal endoscopy. Most endoscopic procedures are performed under "conscious sedation." At this level of sedation, the patient is able to make a purposeful response to tactile and verbal stimulation. At the same time, pulmonary and cardiovascular function are maintained [13]. This type of sedation is accomplished with the use of a benzodiazepine alone or in combination with an opiate. The most commonly used benzodiazepines are midazolam and diazepam. Midazolam is favored by most endoscopists for its fast onset of action, high amnestic properties and shorter duration of action [13]. Opiates such as fentanyl and meperidine provide both sedation and analgesia. Fentanyl has a faster onset of action and clearance as well as a reduced incidence of nausea compared to meperidine. Combination of these agents are frequently utilized, especially during longer procedures. However, such combinations increase the risk of oversedation, oxygen desaturation and cardiorespiratory complications.

Management
Management is by use of reversal agents [12].
• Flumazenil (Romazicon, Anexate), an imidazobenzodiazepine derivative, is a competitive benzodiazepine antagonist. It has been shown to effectively antagonize benzodiazepine-induced sedation and ventilatory depression, as well as psychomotor impairment and retrograde amnesia. Doses of 0.1 mg to 0.2 mg produce partial antagonism, whereas higher doses of 0.4 mg to 1.0 mg usually produce complete antagonism in patients who have received the usual amount of sedation. Reversal effect is evident within 1–2 minutes after

administration, and the peak effect is seen in 6–10 minutes after injection.

• Naloxone (Narcan) is a competitive opioid antagonist. It reverses opioid-induced respiratory depression, sedation and hypotension. When administered intravenously, the onset of action is apparent within 2 minutes. The usual initial dose is 0.4 mg to 2 mg intravenously. If there is no apparent response or if response is inadequate, doses may be repeated at 2–3 minute intervals. The maximum dosage is 10 mg.

Prevention

Guidelines for conscious sedation and monitoring during endoscopy [13] were formulated by the American Society for Gastrointestinal Endoscopy to minimize complications associated with oversedation. A summary of these guidelines include:

• A focused history and physical is required prior to the administration of moderate sedation.

• Routine monitoring of patients' pulse rate, blood pressure and oxygen saturation are useful in identifying early problems.

• The use of benzodiazepines and/or opiates will result in a satisfactory outcome in nearly all patients.

• Specific antagonists of opiates (naloxone) and benzodiazepines (flumazenil) are available and should be present in every endoscopy unit to treat oversedated patients.

References

1. Gress F, Bhattacharya I. Endoscopic Ultrasonography. Oxford, Blackwell Science, 2001.
2. Wiersema MJ, Villmann P, Giovannini M, et al. Endosonography-guided fine-needle aspiration biopsy: Diagnostic accuracy and complication assessment. Gastroenterology 1997; 112:1087.
3. Eloubeidi MA, Tamhane A, Varadarajulu S, Wilcox CM. Frequency of major complications after EUS-guided FNA of solid pancreatic masses: A prospective evaluation. Gastrointest Endosc 2006; 63:622.
4. Varadarajulu S, Eloubeidi MA. Frequency and significance of acute intracystic hemorrhage during EUS-FNA of cystic lesions of the pancreas. Gastrointest Endosc 2004; 60(4):631–5.
5. Gress FG, Hawes RH, Savides TJ, Ikenberry SO, Lehman GO. Endoscopic ultrasound-guided fine-needle aspiration using linear array and radial scanning endosonography. Gastrointest Endosc 1997; 45:243–50.
6. Affi A, Vasquez-Sequeiros E, Norton I, Clain J, Wiersema M. Acute extraluminal hemorrhage associated with EUS-guided fine needle aspiration: Frequency and clinical significance. Gastrointest Endosc 2001; 53(2):221–5.
7. O'Toole D, Palazzo L, Arotcarena R, Dancour A, Aubert A, Hammel P, Amaris J, Ruszniewski P. Assessment of complications of EUS-guided fine-needle aspiration. Gastrointest Endosc 2001; 53(4):470.
8. Eloubeidi MA, Gress FG, Savides TJ, Wiersema MJ. Acute pancreatitis after EUS-guided FNA of solid pancreatic masses: A pooled analysis from EUS centers in the United States. Gastrointest Endosc 2004; 60:385.
9. Johnsson E, Lundell L, Liedman B. Sealing of esophageal perforation or rupture with expandable metal stents: a prospective controlled study on treatment efficacy and limitations. Dis Esophagus 2005; 18(4):262–6.
10. White RE, Munqatana C, Topazian M. Expandable metal stent for iatrogenic perforation of esophageal malignancies. Gastrointest Surg 2003; 7(6):715–19.
11. Feldman: Sleisenger & Fordtran's Gastrointestinal and Liver Disease, 7th edition. Philadelphia, WB Saunders & Co, 2002.
12. Tham TCK, Collins JSA. Gastrointestinal Emergencies. London, BMJ Books, 2000.
13. Guidelines for conscious sedation and monitoring during gastrointestinal endoscopy. Gastrointest Endosc 2003; 53(3):317–22.

3 Specific Conditions

Foreign Body Impaction in the Esophagus

George Triadafilopoulos

Introduction

Foreign body impaction in the esophagus is associated with significant morbidity and, rarely, mortality due to perforation and sepsis. This emergency is encountered in both children and adults. The most common cause of esophageal foreign body obstruction in adults is meat bolus impaction above a preexisting peptic or malignant esophageal stricture, distal esophageal (mucosal) ring, or eosinophilic esophagitis (Plates 17.1–17.3). In contrast, more than 75% of esophageal foreign body obstructions in children are from coin ingestion. Mentally impaired, edentulous or elderly subjects may also present with accidental foreign body, pill, or large food bolus impaction. Intentional ingestion of foreign bodies by psychiatric patients or prison inmates may also lead to esophageal foreign body impaction. Although the esophagus has three areas of "physiological" narrowing (cricopharyngeus, aortic arch, diaphragmatic hiatus), underlying, clinically silent, structural or functional esophageal diseases (e.g. esophageal achalasia or scleroderma esophagus) (Plate 17.4 & 17.5) are frequently responsible for esophageal foreign body impaction (Figure 17.1).

History and examination

Most adults with esophageal foreign body obstruction present with symptoms, but infants, children,

Gastrointestinal Emergencies, 2nd edition. Edited by Tony Tham, John Collins and Roy Soetikno. © 2009 by Blackwell Publishing, ISBN: 978-1-4051-4634-0.

or mentally impaired adults may not give a history of foreign body ingestion or complain of dysphagia. Typically, acute onset of dysphagia and inability to swallow saliva are the key symptoms of esophageal obstruction. Inability to swallow saliva indicates complete esophageal obstruction and requires urgent attention. Hypersalivation, retrosternal fullness and pain, regurgitation, hiccups and retching may also occur. Odynophagia, or painful swallowing, raises the possibility of esophageal laceration or perforation. In contrast, respiratory symptoms, such as stridor, dyspnea, asthma, or cough, all resulting from tracheal compression, may predominate in young children. If drug smuggling with cocaine body stuffing is suspected, particular attention needs to be taken not to rupture the bag to avoid acute drug overdose.

Treatment

The management of this emergency is summarized in Figure 17.2 [1, 2, 3]. The main steps in management are:
1. Immediate evaluation of the airway.
2. Radiological evaluation to localize the object.
3. Endoscopic retrieval.

Airway assessment

Stridor, choking, or dyspnea suggest a compromised airway. If there is impending asphyxiation, emergency endotracheal intubation is needed. Even in the absence of respiratory symptoms, airway protection and continuous oropharyngeal suction are important to avoid pulmonary aspiration. Airway obstruction can occur during the removal of the foreign body and a laryngoscope should be immediately available.

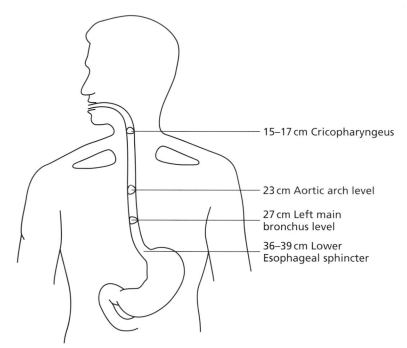

15–17 cm Cricopharyngeus

23 cm Aortic arch level

27 cm Left main bronchus level

36–39 cm Lower Esophageal sphincter

Figure 17.1 Anatomical areas associated with esophageal bolus impaction.

Radiological evaluation

Depending on the reliability of the clinical history and the clinical presentation, plain neck, chest and abdominal radiographs are required and they may reveal a radiopaque foreign body, or mediastinal, subdiaphragmatic, or subcutaneous air or pleural effusion, all suggestive of esophageal perforation. If possible, radiographic localization and identification of esophageal foreign bodies is important prior to any attempt at extraction. In particular, identification of airway landmarks on postero-anterior and lateral chest radiographs is important to differentiate between tracheo-bronchial and esophageal foreign bodies. Flat objects, such as coins, usually orient themselves in the coronal plane when lodged in the esophagus, and are best seen on anteroposterior projections. Tracheal foreign bodies align in the sagittal plane and are best seen on a lateral projection. Disc batteries may be seen as a double shadow or a stack of coins. Toothpicks or fish bones may not be seen on radiographs; thus, failure to locate an object on radiographic examination does not preclude its presence. Food or meat bolus impaction will not be evident radiologically unless bony tissue is present. Barium swallow should not be performed since it may impair subsequent endoscopic visualization and increase aspiration risk.

Endoscopic retrieval [4,5]

No treatment is needed if a patient with a history of foreign body ingestion is asymptomatic and has negative plain radiographs, since the foreign body may have passed out of the esophagus. Sharp objects impacted above the cricopharyngeus should be removed with a laryngoscope. With food boluses, 1 mg of intravenous glucagon may relax the esophagus and allow spontaneous bolus passage into the stomach. If endoscopic visualization distal to the impaction is feasible, gentle pushing of the bolus into the stomach using the tip of the endoscope may be attempted (Plates 17.2 & 17.5).

The appropriate timing for endoscopic retrieval varies with the type of object as well as the site and completeness of obstruction (Tables 17.1 and 17.2). Retained esophageal foreign bodies should be promptly removed to avoid esophageal perforation or pulmonary aspiration and under no circumstances should they be allowed to remain in the esophagus beyond 24 hours after ingestion. Endoscopy should be performed immediately in patients who are unable to handle oral secretions or who have ingested sharp objects (pins, partial dentures, fish bones, toothpicks) that are likely to perforate the esophagus, and in patients with impacted disc or button batteries in

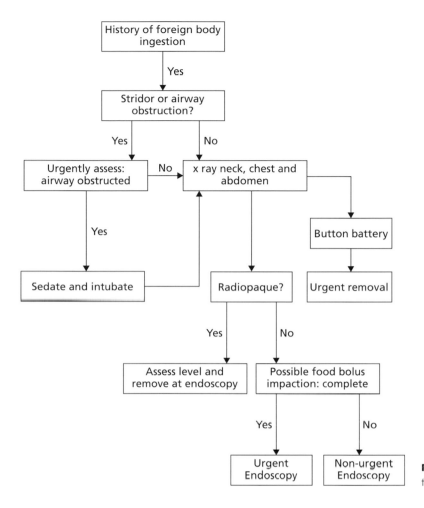

Figure 17.2 Management of esophageal foreign body impaction.

order to avoid caustic injury and perforation. If an esophageal stricture or ring is identified after clearing a food bolus, dilation should be performed during the same session. Esophageal biopsy and esophageal motility should be considered in order to rule out underlying esophageal structural or motor abnormality, such as eosinophilic esophagitis or achalasia (Plates 17.3 and 17.5). If eosinophilic esophagitis is suspected, dilation should be performed with extreme caution because of the risk of perforation (Plate 17.3)[6].

Endoscopy, using a flexible forward-viewing endoscope under conscious sedation, is the procedure of choice and is successful in >90% of cases with <5% complication rate. Rigid esophagoscopy requires general anesthesia and carries a 10% complication rate but it is preferable in children with impacted sharp foreign bodies.

The endoscopic tools used to remove obstructing esophageal bodies vary and a full range of retrieval accessories should always be readily available (Table 17.1). Coins are best retrieved with a rat-tooth or alligator forceps, or the retrieval net. Round objects such as disc or button batteries are best captured using the retrieval net. If there is no distal obstruction, blunt objects (e.g. meat bolus) <2 cm in diameter may be gently pushed into the stomach. Sometimes breaking a food bolus into smaller particles facilitates either its endoscopic retrieval using a retrieval net or its gentle advancement into the stomach using the endoscope. For removal of sharp objects (e.g. safety pins), a protector hood should be placed at the tip of the endoscope or an overtube should be inserted. The protector hood maintains its bell portion inverted during insertion of the endoscope; the bell portion then flips back to its

Table 17.1 Endoscopic accessories needed for esophageal foreign body removal.

Alligator forceps
Rat-tooth forceps
Shark-tooth forceps
Stent removal forceps
V-shaped grasping forceps
Tripod
Stone (Dormia) baskets
Roth retrieval net
Polyp retrieval snare
Nakao snare system
Overtube
Latex protector hood

Table 17.2 Timing for endoscopic retrieval of esophageal foreign body.

Foreign body	Location	Time endoscopy (h)
Coin	Upper	4–6
Coin	Lower	12–18
Meat	Any/complete obs	Urgent
Meat	Any/incomplete obs	8–10
Sharps	Any	4–6

After Webb, 1997.

original shape as it crosses the gastroesophageal junction during withdrawal, thereby protecting the esophageal and pharyngeal walls from injury. It is important to grasp the object so that its sharp end is trailing upon withdrawal. The overtube is also useful in the removal of objects that are difficult to grasp securely or when multiple passes of the endoscope are needed.

Blunt objects <2 cm that have already entered the stomach can usually be managed conservatively since most of them will pass within several days. Surgical removal should be considered if the object remains in the same location for more than 1 week, or in patients who develop fever, vomiting, or abdominal pain, suggestive of perforation. Long objects (>5 cm), such as toothbrushes and spoons, are unlikely to pass and should be removed. Such objects may be grasped with a snare or basket and drawn into an overtube and withdrawn.

Sharp objects (e.g. chicken or fish bones, paper clips, toothpicks, needles, and dental bridges) should be urgently removed endoscopically to avoid perforation. Using a retrieval basket or net, disc batteries should be removed promptly, since their contact with the esophageal wall may rapidly result in necrosis and perforation. Drug packets should not be removed endoscopically because of the risk of rupture. Urgent surgery is needed when packages fail to advance or if there are signs of intestinal obstruction or rupture.

Management of foreign body-induced esophageal perforation

Surgery should be performed in patients with esophageal perforation, particularly when it is recognized late. The surgical approach depends on the location of perforation, the nature of the foreign body, underlying esophageal disease or other comorbidity, and the severity of local necro-inflammatory response assessed by CT scan and at surgery. Primary esophageal repair is preferable for perforations that are recognized early, but exclusion-diversion of the esophagus and thorough drainage may be needed. Rarely, nonoperative, conservative management may be adequate for small, contained perforations.

References

1. Webb WA, Taylor MB. Foreign bodies of the upper gastrointestinal tract. In Gastrointestinal Emergencies, 2nd edition, Taylor MB (ed), Lippincott Williams and Wilkins, pp 3–18, USA, 1997.
2. Eisen GM, Baron TH, Dominitz JA, et al. Guideline for the management of ingested foreign bodies. Gastrointest Endosc 2002; 55:802–6.
3. Webb WA. Management of foreign bodies of the upper gastrointestinal tract: Update. Gastrointest Endosc 1995; 41:39–50.
4. Bounds BC. Endoscopic retrieval devices. Techniques Gastrointest Endosc 2006; 8:16–21.
5. Li Z-S, Sun Z-X, Zou D-W, Xu G-M, Wu R-P, Liao Z. Endoscopic management of foreign bodies in the upper-GI tract: experience with 1088 cases in China. Gastrointest Endosc 2006; 64:485–92.
6. Desai TK, Stecevic V, Chang CH, et al. Association of eosinophilic inflammation with esophageal food impaction in adults. Gastrointest Endosc 2005; 61:795–801.

18 Esophageal Perforation

Peter D. Siersema

Introduction

Esophageal perforation is caused by a variety of disorders, of which iatrogenic perforation during endoscopic instrumentation or following surgery is the most common cause. In addition, perforation may occur spontaneously during vomiting (Boerhaave syndrome). Finally, esophageal leaks can be found in the context of a fistula as a consequence of radiation therapy or accompanied by a malignancy, most commonly of the esophagus.

Esophageal perforation is a serious injury with a high morbidity and mortality rate if left untreated [1]. Successful management depends on early diagnosis and prompt treatment. However, after a surgical procedure, a diagnosis of perforation is often difficult to establish, and, even more important, the diagnosis depends on the alertness of the physician.

The classic treatment option for esophageal perforation is a surgical approach. This is however not always possible in patients who present some time after a perforation, have a coexistent esophageal malignancy or develop an anastomotic dehiscence after esophageal surgery. Moreover, a substantial number of patients are old, fragile or are in a debilitated state, which may result in increased morbidity and a less favorable outcome following surgical management [2].

Repair of an esophageal perforation can also be accomplished by the use of endoscopic techniques and tools [3]. The aim is to close or seal an esophageal perforation from the luminal site. In addition, it is important to adequately drain the mediastinum, pleural cavities and/or peritoneal cavity, administer broad-spectrum antibiotics and routinely start nutritional support, preferably by the enteral route.

The aim of this chapter is to provide an overview of the endoscopic management of esophageal perforations. The management of esophageal fistulae, either benign or malignant, will not be discussed.

Clinical presentation

A high index of suspicion is critical to establish a diagnosis of esophageal perforation. A delay in the diagnosis is usually caused by the fact that the clinical picture is not typical for a perforation.

Clinical symptoms depend on the location of the perforation in the esophagus, and can be subdivided as follows [3]:

1. Cervical esophagus: neck pain, tachycardia, "early" dysphagia, symptoms of coughing following drinking or eating, dysphonia, bloody regurgitation and cervical crepitus.

2. Thoracic esophagus: chest pain, tachycardia, tachypnea, fever, pleural effusion, cardiac effusion, low blood pressure, sepsis and shock.

3. Esophagus around gastroesophageal junction: epigastric pain, back pain, inability to remain in a supine position, acute abdomen, sepsis and shock.

Diagnosis

A diagnosis of esophageal perforation is established if the clinical symptoms are suggestive and the radiological and/or endoscopic investigations show an esophageal perforation. A delay in the diagnosis is usually caused by the fact that the presenting symptoms, particularly in the case of a spontaneous perforation, are not conclusive enough to suggest the diagnosis.

Gastrointestinal Emergencies, 2nd edition. Edited by Tony Tham, John Collins and Roy Soetikno. © 2009 by Blackwell Publishing, ISBN: 978-1-4051-4634-0.

Etiology

In a series of 559 patients with esophageal perforation from the USA, iatrogenic injury to the esophagus was the most common cause of perforation with instrumentation accounting for 59% of patients [4] (Table 18.1). Other causes included Boerhaave syndrome (15%), foreign body ingestion (12%), trauma (9%), operative injury (2%), tumor (1%) and other causes (2%).

In a series of 122 patients with esophageal perforation who were referred for treatment to our unit in The Netherlands, operative injury was the most common cause of perforation (41%), which in two-thirds of cases was caused by anastomotic dehiscence after esophageal resection or wound dehiscence after resection of a diverticulum (Plate 18.1, Table 18.1). Other causes included endoscopic instrumentation (37%), with rigid esophagoscopy being responsible in 24% of these cases (Plate 18.2), bougie dilation in 22%, pneumatic dilation for achalasia in 19%, EUS in 19%, Zenker diverticulotomy in 8%, and EMR in 8%. Nonsurgical, nonendoscopic causes included Boerhaave syndrome (10%), trauma (5%), foreign body ingestion (4%) and other causes (3%).

As can be seen in Table 18.1, the difference in number of operative injuries accounted for the main difference between The Netherlands and USA series. This is probably explained by the fact that the Dutch center is one of the few national referall centers where esophageal cancer surgery is being performed.

Table 18.1 Causes of esophageal perforation in the USA [1] and in Rotterdam, Netherlands (unpublished series).

Cause of perforation	USA (%)	The Netherlands (%)
Instrumentation	59	37
Boerhaave's syndrome	15	10
Foreign-body ingestion	12	4
Trauma	9	5
Operative injury	2	41
Tumor	1	—
Other causes	2	3

Examination

Physical examination is often not conclusive. A diagnosis of esophageal perforation should however be suspected if a patient presents with cervical crepitus, pleural fluid, sepsis or shock in the presence of chest pain. In addition, if a patient has undergone an esophageal resection, resection of an esophageal diverticulum or has undergone upper endoscopy and develops fever one or more days after the procedure, an esophageal perforation should be suspected.

Investigations

If a patient presents with symptoms suggestive of an esophageal perforation, the first investigation is a chest radiograph, both posterioanterior and lateral. If this shows no signs of perforation, for example the presence of free air, pleural fluid or pneumonia, this can be followed by a gastrograffin swallow. We prefer gastrograffin and not barium as the former is water-soluble, whereas barium is not (Fig. 18.1).

In cases in which a high index of suspicion is present, for example in a patient with persisting fever

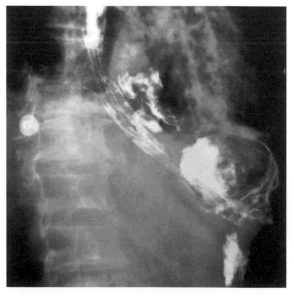

Figure 18.1 Barium swallow showing a perforation in the distal esophagus. We prefer Gastrografin as contrast medium and not barium in these cases, as the former is water-soluble, whereas barium is not.

following esophageal resection, a CT scan is the preferred investigation. This CT should include a scan of the neck, the chest, and, if indicated, the upper abdomen. This can be followed by upper endoscopy, as this will establish the exact location of a perforation, and also enable an endoscopic treatment to be performed during the same session.

Management

Figure 18.2 gives an outline summary of the management of esophageal perforation.

Surgery

The aim of surgery is the prevention of further contamination, elimination of the infectious tissue, restoration of the integrity of the esophagus, and establishing the intake of nutrients. Surgical treatment options include surgical repair, esophageal diversion and exclusion, or esophagectomy.

Primary surgical closure and mediastinal drainage, particularly if performed within 24 hours of the injury, has been shown to improve survival [5]. Repair of the perforation requires extensive mobilization of the esophagus to identify the perforation and to allow a tension-free repair. In addition, extensive drainage of the mediastinum with one or more chest tubes is required.

If primary repair is not possible, because of the extent of the paraesophageal inflammation, mediastinal drainage with diversion and exclusion (cervical esophagostomy for diversion, a gastrostomy for decompression and a jejunostomy for enteral feeding) or creation of a controlled esophagocutaneous fistula with T-tube drainage of the perforation can be performed [6]. This is a rather safe and uncomplicated approach as a first step but needs to be followed by reconstruction 6 months later. Esophagectomy is indicated for patients with perforation in a carcinoma, but also in cases where extensive necrosis is present or when the esophageal stricture is already difficult to manage (e.g. in cases with repeat dilation for caustic injury).

The mortality of a surgical procedure for esophageal perforation has been reported to vary between 10% and 20%. This mainly depends on the cause and location of the perforation, the interval between the perforation and initiation of therapy, the extent of contamination of the mediastinum, the type of surgery and the age and condition of the patient. A delay in diagnosis and therapy for more than 24 hours after the perforation can substantially increase mortality [7].

Endoscopy

An endoscopic approach to esophageal perforation has several advantages over surgery, as:
• closure of the perforation can be performed under direct observation;
• endoscopy can be performed under conscious sedation, which avoids the disadvantages of general anesthesia;
• trauma associated with a surgical approach by performing thoractomy, mediastinal exploration or extensive dissection can be avoided.

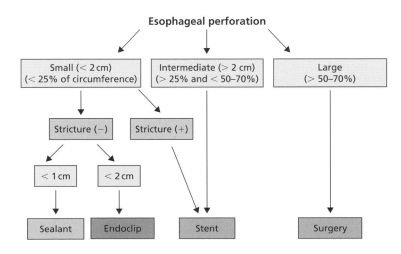

Figure 18.2 Management of patients with esophageal perforation.

In the last few years an increasing number of case reports and case series have reported on the endoscopic treatment of esophageal perforation. Most experience has been gained with the following endoscopic techniques and tools (Table 8.2):

1. Sealants (glue or graft) which will plug a defect.

2. Endoclips which will result in approximating the edges of a perforation.

3. Stents which are used to seal a perforation.

An endoscopic option should always be combined with drainage of the mediastinal cavity and/or pleural cavity. Drainage tubes can be placed percutaneously, or CT- or EUS-guided. Active lavage, irrigation and drainage of the abscess cavity are all important. In selected cases, endoscopic debridement of the abscess can be performed [8,9]. This should be supported by the administration of intravenous broad-spectrum antibiotics. We also administer intravenous proton pump inhibitors. Particularly in the initial stage, we advise fasting until a Gastrografin swallow has demonstrated that the perforation is adequately closed (sealant or clips) or sealed (stent). Finally, nutritional support should be initiated at an early stage. For this, we prefer enteral feeding by an endoscopically placed feeding tube in the distal duodenum, or, alternatively, total parental nutrition if enteral feeding is not possible.

Table 18.2 Endoscopic techniques or tools used for esophageal perforations.

Endoscopic sealants
a) Fibrin glue
- Tisseel (Baxter Westlake Village, CA)
- Hemaseel (Hemacure, Sarasota, FL)
b) Cyanoacrylates
- Histoacryl (B. Braun, Melsungen, Germany)
- Glubran (GEM, Viareggio, Italy)
- Dermabond (Ethocon, Somerville, NJ)
c) Tissue grafts
- Surgisis (Wilson-Cook, Winston-Salem, NC)

Endoclips
Endosclip or Quickclip (Olympus, Tokyo, Japan)
Triclip (Wilson-Cook, Winston-Salem, NC)
Resolution Clip (Boston Scientific, Natick, MA)

Stents
a) Metal
- Ultraflex stent (Boston Scientific)
- Wallstent (Boston Scientific)
- Flamingo Wallstent (Boston Scientific)
- Song stent (Medi-Tech, Seoul, Korea)
- Choo stent (M.I. Tech, Seoul, Korea)
- Niti-S stent (Taewong, Seoul, Korea)
b) Plastic
- Polyflex (Boston Scientific)

Endoscopic sealants

Sealants include fibrin glue, cyanoacrylates and tissue grafts [10,11]. These sealants are produced by different manufacturers (Table 18.2).

Most experience has been gained with fibrin glue, which has been reported to be successful in closure of esophageal perforations, but most often in all kinds of esophageal fistulae and anastomotic leaks. In one case report, the authors successfully used cyanoacrylate to close an esophageal fistula.

Before injecting fibrin glue into a fistulous opening, it is recommended to brush the fistulous tract or anastomotic leak. Subsequently, the catheter with fibrin glue is placed inside the orifice. Once fibrin is applied, it is important to avoid contact of the catheter with the fistulous tract. Repeat application, for example every 48 hours, for some weeks, is sometimes required to close a fistula or anastomotic leak.

Closing a fistula or leak is most successful if the diameter of the defect is not larger than 8–10 mm. Successful outcome of endoscopic closure is also dependent on the length and number of branches of the fistulous tract, the absence of active inflammation around the fistula or leak, and the absence of cancer or obstruction in the fistulous tract.

Endoscopic insertion of tissue grafts (Surgisis; Wilson-Cook, Winston-Salem, NC), an acellular matrix derived from porcine submucosa, is a relatively new method. It has successfully been reported in the closure of 12 of 17 refractory esophagogastric fistulae that had developed after bariatric surgery [11]. Although insertion of tissue grafts seems promising, it is often difficult to apply the tissue grafts into a fistula or leak by endoscopic means as no specific catheter system for this purpose is available yet.

Endoclips

Three types of endoclip devices are commercially available: Endoclip or Quickclip (Olympus, Tokyo, Japan), Triclip (Wilson-Cook), and Resolution clip (Boston Scientific, Natick, MA) (Table 18.2). So far, only published data are available on the use of the Quickclip in the treatment of esophageal perforations [3]. However, it seems likely that with the other available clips comparable results can be obtained.

All these clips have specific characteristics that make them useful in closing leaks or perforations, depending on the size and type, and the location in the esophagus. For this, no specific guidelines can be given. However, it is advisable to gain practical experience with at least one endoclip device in different situations as this will improve one's skills when clips are used to close a perforation.

Endoclip application has been shown to be successful in the closure of esophageal perforations from Boerhaave syndrome, foreign body ingestion, and following dilation of esophageal strictures, achalasia and anastomotic esophagojejunostomy strictures. In addition, endoclips have been shown to be highly successful in postoperative or post-EMR esophageal leakage.

In our experience, endoclips are particularly successful for the closure of acute perforations varying from a few millimeters to 1.5–2 cm, with the latter sizes always requiring multiple endoclips. However, closure of chronic esophageal fistulae in patients unfit to undergo surgery has been reported as well. In the case of a larger perforation, it is advisable to start clipping at the middle part of the perforation, and then work towards both lateral ends of the perforation. If the initial clip is placed at either end of the perforation, it is sometimes difficult at a later stage to approach the perforation at its middle part. In some instances, two or even three separate treatment sessions are required.

Closure of acute perforations is always within 3–7 days; however, a longer time (up to 2–4 weeks), may be required for more chronic perforations, or those that are associated with paraesophageal inflammation.

No complications have been reported with the use of endoclips. The placement of endoclips in the esophagus can be technically demanding as it may be difficult to approach the defect under direct view. In these situations, it is helpful to have a cap at the end of the endoscope.

Stents

Apart from several case reports, 13 studies, including our own experience, have reported on 159 patients who have been treated with various stent types, both metallic and plastic, to seal esophageal perforations resulting from postoperative complications (anastomotic or postresection leaks), endoscopic procedures, Boerhaave syndrome, and perforations associated with dilation of post radiation strictures and foreign body ingestion [8,12–22] (Table 18.3).

The stent types that were used included the uncovered Esophacoil stent, which is no longer commercially available, the partially covered Ultraflex stent (Boston Scientific), Wallstent (Boston Scientific) and Flamingo Wallstent (Boston Scientific), and the fully covered Song stent (Medi-Tech, Seoul, Korea), Choo stent (M.I. Tech, Seoul, Korea) and Niti-S stent (Taewong, Seoul, Korea). Most experience has however been gained with the fully covered plastic Polyflex stent (Boston Scientific). In our unit, we mainly use fully covered stents, particularly the Niti-S stent and the Polyflex stent (Fig. 18.3).

In most reported series, stents were almost always placed some time (1–83 days) after the first symptoms of the perforation (Table 18.3). This is of clinical importance as in these situations the paraesophageal tissues, i.e. the mediastinum, the pleural cavity, and the peritoneal cavity in selected cases, should be considered to be severely contaminated. Apart from placing a stent and placing drainage tubes in the mediastinum and/or pleural cavity and drains in abscesses in the peritoneum, some authors have added traditional surgical principles to their treatment algorithm [8,9].

Before stent placement, Schubert et al. [8] performed endoscopic cleansing of the fistula and the perianastomotic mediastinum at 2-day intervals. After a mean of 9 days, when the drains stopped producing purulent efflux and granulation tissue in the fistulous tract was observed, a stent was placed. In a study by Wehrmann et al. [9], paraesophageal abscesses that were present after esophageal perforation or postoperative leakage were treated with EUS-guided or mediastinal puncture. The abscess cavities were entered with an endoscope which allowed irrigation and drainage. Pleural effusions were treated with transthoracic drainage tubes. The esophageal defects were subsequently closed with endoclips ($n = 7$), fibrin glue ($n = 4$), stents ($n = 1$), or had spontaneously ($n = 3$) healed. It remains to be established whether endoscopic cleaning is indeed needed or whether adequate drainage of the mediastinum and/or pleural cavity in combination with immediate stent placement is sufficient. In our experience, which now includes 52

Table 18.3 Studies on the use of stents for the sealing of esophageal perforations.

First author (reference)	No. of patients	Etiology (n)	Interval to stent placement (days)	Size	Stent type (n)	Stent size [mm (n)]	Duration of stent placement (weeks)	Sealing (%)	Complications (n)	Stent removal (%)
Lee (12)	2	Boerhaave (1) Post-surgery (1)	n.a.	n.a.	Ultraflex (1) Esophacoil (1)	n.a.	8–12	100	None	50
Chung (13)	3	Boerhaave (3)	4–28	n.a.	Song (2) Ultraflex (1)	22 (1), 24 (1) 28 (1)	8–24	100	Migration (1)	100
Wadhwa (14)	5	Post-surgery (3) Boerhaave (1) Post-radiation (1)	n.a.	n.a.	Wallstent (1)	n.a.	6–32	60	Migration (1)	60
Siersema (15)	11	Boerhaave (5) Instrument. (3) Post-surgery (3)	1–28	15–30 mm	Flamingo (7) Ultraflex (4)	30 (7) 28 (4)	6–14	91	Migration (1) Fistula (1)	64
Doniec (16)	21	Post-surgery (18) Instrument. (2) Boerhaave (1)	3–81	25–100%	Ultraflex (21)	22 (7) 28 (14)	1–17	100 (closure: 80)	Migration (1) Stricture (5) Cover defect (7)	56
Evrard (17)	4	Post-surgery (4)	n.a.	n.a.	Polyflex (4)	n.a.	n.a.	100	Migration (3)	100

	N	Indication		Size	Stent				Complications	
Gelbmann (18)	9	Post-surgery (5), Instrument. (3), Boerhaave (1)	?-65	>50% (2); <50% (7)	Polyflex (9)	n.a.	mean: 19	78	Migration (3)	100
Hünerbein (19)	9	Post-surgery (9)	mean: 7.7	n.a.	Polyflex (9)	25 (9)	2; 2nd stent (7): 1–2	89	Migration (2)	100
Langer (20)	24	Post-surgery (24)	4–65		Polyflex (24)	20 (1) 23 (19) 25 (4)	n.a.	92	Perforation (2) Migration (9) Stricture (2) Food bolus (1) Reflux (1)	50
Radecke 21	15	Tumor (8), Post-surgery (5), Instrument. (2)	n.a.	n.a.	Polyflex (15)	n.a.	n.a.	73	n.a.	n.a.
Schubert (8)	12	Post-surgery (12)	3–12	20–70%	Polyflex (12)	25 (12)	2–8	92	Migration (2)	100
Peters (22)	3	Post-surgery (3)	7–83	n.a.	Choo stent (3)	24 (3)	7–10	100	Stricture (1)	100
Siersema (unpublished)	52	Post-surgery (18), Instrument. (21), Boerhaave (12), Foreign body ingestion (1)	1–35	<25%: 10 25–50%: 28 50–75%: 11 >75%: 3	Polyflex (21) Ultraflex (18) Flamingo (9) Niti-S (4)	23 (6) 25 (21) 26 (4) 28 (12) 30 (9)	2–21	88	Migration (4) Stricture (3) Fistula (1)	92

Boerhaave, Boerhaave syndrome; Instrument., Instrumentation. Size, size of perforation; n.a., not available

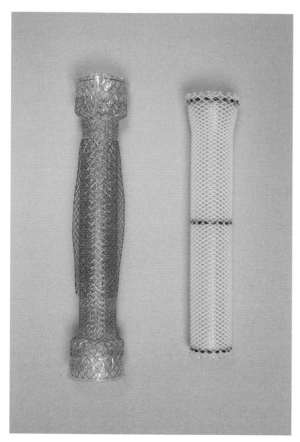

Figure 18.3 Fully covered stents for the sealing of esophageal perforations, with on the left a Niti-S stent made of nitinol and on the right a Polyflex stent made of silicone.

Nevertheless, in the two studies in which only large-diameter Polyflex stents were used [8,19], stent migration was observed in 4/21 (19%) placements. A practical solution could be to fix the stent with an endoclip in order to prevent the stent from migrating, as was suggested by Gelbmann et al. [19]. For this purpose, a small hole was cut through the silicone lining and the polyester mesh of the Polyflex stent before stent insertion. After positioning the stent, an endoclip was placed through the hole.

The length of time that a stent was left in the esophagus has shortened in the more recent studies (Table 18.3). In these studies [8,19] (and this is in line with our current experience) stents were removed after 2–4 weeks and only replaced if a perforation was still endoscopically present. In the reported studies using Polyflex stents for this indication, no difficulties were reported in stent retrieval. In fact, Gelbmann et al. [19] reported retrieval of Polyflex stents in 6 patients after a mean period of 19 weeks. In contrast, in a study using partially covered metal stents [15], two stents had to be removed in piecemeal fashion after a period of 11.5 and 14 weeks, respectively, because the uncovered stent parts were too firmly imbedded in the esophageal mucosa. A retained metallic strand in one of these patients resulted in a new fistula (Plate 18.3, which spontaneously closed after endoscopic removal of the strand (Fig. 18.4). It therefore seems preferable to use stents which are completely covered and easily removable. It remains to be established what type of stent material (metal, polyester, silicone, etc.) is most suitable for these benign indications. The pros and cons of the most commonly used stent types for sealing nonmalignant esophageal perforations are summarized in Table 18.4.

Summary

Based on this overview, it can be concluded that endoscopic therapy is an attractive modality for the treatment of esophageal perforation in the majority of patients with this complication. In our opinion, surgery should only be the first choice in patients who develop a perforation during instrumentation. Examples of this include patients with a perforation that:
• develops during the work-up of esophageal carcinoma, particularly if no evidence of metastatic disease is present;

patients with different types of esophageal perforation, adequate drainage alone and stent placement was successful in more than 85% of patients. The only way to definitely conclude that endoscopic cleansing is indeed indicated in these benign perforations is to perform a randomized study comparing stent placement alone vs. stent placement *plus* endoscopic cleansing of the paraesophageal tissues. This would however require a multicenter effort because of the relatively low number of cases per year, even in specialized centers.

In the majority of patients, large-diameter Polyflex stents were used to seal the anastomotic leak and minimize the risk of persisting contamination of the perianastomotic mediastinum (Table 18.3). In addition, it was expected that the use of large-diameter stents would minimize the risk of stent migration.

Table 18.4 Characteristics of the most commonly used stent types for the sealing of nonmalignant perforations of the esophagus.

	Ultraflex stent	Flamingo Wallstent	Polyflex stent	Niti-S stent
Maximum diameter(proximal/distal) (mm) stent	28/22	30/20	25/21	26/18
Diameter introduction catheter (mm)	5.3	6	14	7
Stent material	Nitinol	Metal	Plastic	Nitinol
Stent length (cm)	12	14	9, 12, 15	
Covered	Partially	Partially	Fully	Fully
Costs (%)*	100	125	100	60
Effectiveness in sealing†	+	+	+	+
Complications†	+/−	+/−	+/ −	+/−
Risk of migration†	+/−	+/−	+	−
Ease of removal†	−	−	+	+

*Expressed in percentages with the Ultraflex stent set on 100%
† Scale: −, negative/low; +/−, moderate; +, positive/high

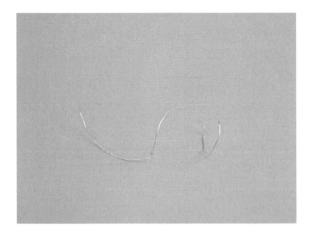

Figure 18.4 Same patient as in Figure 18.1, showing a Flamingo Wallstent in the distal esophagus covering the perforation (Plate 18.3). The stent was removed after 14 weeks, however a persisting fistula revealed a retained metallic strand which was endoscopically removed.

• develops after dilation of a refractory esophageal stricture, such as those following caustic ingestion;
• develops after pneumatic dilation of achalasia;
• persists under endoscopic therapy; or
• is larger than 50–70% of the circumference.

The remainder of esophageal perforation can be treated with an endoscopic technique or tool (Fig. 18.2). In summary, in patients with small leaks (<2 cm or less than 25% of the circumference), it is recommended to use an endoscopic sealant (<1 cm) or endoclips (<2 cm). However, if a stricture is also present it is preferable to use a (Polyflex) stent. When the perforation is larger than 2 cm or between 25% and 50–70% of the circumference, stent placement should be performed. If a perforation is larger than 50–70% of the circumference, for example in the case of an anastomotic dehiscence, a surgical procedure is often required.

Future developments

Is there anything new on the horizon? It would be a real step forward if we could endoscopically suture an esophageal perforation as our surgeon colleagues do. Recently, a case was reported on an esophagopleural fistula following complicated surgical repair of Boerhaave syndrome which was closed by a combination of fistula tract coagulation and endoscopic suturing using the Endocinch (CR Bard Interventional, Murray Hill, NJ) [23].

Covered biodegradable stents, with or without different drugs attached, are already being used by our cardiology and urology colleagues [24]. Moreover, an alternative could be the use of biodegradable formulations that can be used to cover fistulous tracts, cavities, etc.

References

1. Walker WS, Cameron EWS, Walbaum PR. Diagnosis and management of spontaneous transmural rupture of the oesophagus. Br J Surg 1985; 72:204–7.

2. Sawyer R, Philips C, Vakil N. Short- and long-term outcome of esophageal perforation. Gastrointest Endosc 1995; 41:130–4.

3. Raju GS, Thompson C, Zwischenberger JB. Emerging endoscopic options in the management of esophageal leaks. Gastrointest Endosc 2005; 62:278–86.

4. Brinster CJ, Singhal S, Lee L, Marshall MB, Kaiser LR, Kucharczuk JC. Evolving options in the management of esophageal perforation. Ann Thorac Surg 2004; 77:1475–83.

5. Zwischenberger JB, Savage C, Bidani A. Surgical aspects of esophageal disease. Perforation and caustic injury. Am J Respir Crit Care Med 2001; 164:1037–40.

6. Bufkin BL, Miller JI jr, Mansour KA. Esophageal perforation: emphasis on management. Ann Thorac Surg 1996; 61:1447–51.

7. Tilanus HW, Bossuyt P, Schattenkerk ME, Obertop H. Treatment of oesophageal perforation: a multivariate analysis. Br J Surg 1991; 78:582–5.

8. Schubert D, Scheidbach H, Kuhn R, Wex C, Weiss G, Eder F, et al. Endoscopic treatment of thoracic esophageal leaks by using silicone-covered, self-expanding polyester stents. Gastrointest Endosc 2005; 61:891–6.

9. Wehrmann T, Stergiou N, Vogel B, Riphaus A, Köckerling F, Frenz MB. Endoscopic debridement of paraesophageal, mediastinal abscesses: a prospective case series. Gastrointest Endosc 2005; 62:344–9.

10. Petersen B, Barkun A, Caroenter S, Chotiprasidhi P, Chuttani R, Silvermann W, et al. Tissue adhesives and fibrin glues. Gastrointest Endosc 2004; 60:327–33.

11. Maluf-Filho F, Moura E, Sakai P, Garrido JA, Ishioka S, Gama-Rodrigues J, et al. Endoscopic treatment of esophagogastric fistulae with an acellular matrix [abstract]. Gastrointest Endosc 2004; 59:AB151.

12. Lee JG, Hsu R, Leung JW. Are self-expanding metal mesh stents useful in the treatment of benign esophageal stenoses and fistulas? An experience in four cases. Am J Gastroenterol 2000; 95:1920–5.

13. Chung MG, Kang DH, Park DK, Park JJ, Park HC, Kim JH. Successful treatment of Boerhave's syndrome with endoscopic insertion of a self-expandable metallic stent: report of three cases and a review of the literature. Endoscopy 2001; 33:894–7.

14. Wadhwa RP, Kozarek RA, France RE, Brandabur JJ, Gluck M, Low DE, et al. Use of self-expandable metallic stents in benign GI diseases. Gastrointest Endosc 2003; 58:207–12.

15. Siersema PD, Homs MYV, Haringsma J, Tilanus HW, Kuipers EJ. Use of large-diameter metallic stents to seal traumatic nonmalignant perforations of the esophagus. Gastrointest Endosc 2003; 58:356–61.

16. Doniec JM, Schniewind B, Kahlke V, Kremer B, Grimm H. Therapy of anastomotic leaks by means of covered metallic stents after esophagogastrectomy. Endoscopy 2003; 35:652–8.

17. Evrard S, le Moine O, Lazaraki G, Dormann A, el Nakadi I, Devière J. Self-expanding plastic stents for benign esophageal lesions. Gastrointest Endosc 2004; 60:894–900.

18. Gelbmann CM, Ratiu, NL, Rath HC, Rogler G, Lock G, Schölmerich J, et al. Use of self-expandable plastic stents for the treatment of esophageal perforations and symptomatic anastomotic leaks. Endoscopy 2004; 36:695–9.

19. Hünerbein M, Stroszcynski C, Moesta KT, Schlag PM. Treatment of thoracic anastomotic leaks after esophagectomy with self-expanding plastic stents. Ann Surg 2004; 240:801–7.

20. Langer FB, Wenzl E, Prager G, Salat A, Miholic J, Mang T, et al. Management of postoperative esophageal leaks with the Polyflex self-expanding covered plastic stent. Ann Thorac Surg 2005; 79:398–404.

21. Radecke K, Gerken G, Treichel U. Impact of a self-expanding plastic esophageal stent on various esophageal stenoses, fistulas and leakages. Gastrointest Endosc 2005; 61:812–18.

22. Peters JH, Craanen ME, van der Peet DL, Cuesta MA, Mulder CJ. Self-expanding metal stents for the treatment of intrathoracic esophageal anastomotic leaks following esophagectomy. Am J Gastroenterol 2006; 101:1393–5.

23. Adler DG, McAfee M, Gostout CJ. Closure of an esophagopleural fistula by using fistula tract coagulation and an endoscopic suturing device. Gastrointest Endosc 2001; 54:652–3.

24. Tammela TL, Talja M. Biodegradable urethral stents. BJU Int 2003; 92:843–50.

Perforation of the Gastrointestinal Tract

John Moorehead, Ian McAllister

Peptic perforation

Introduction

The incidence of hospital admissions for peptic ulcer disease has been in decline since the 1970s, falling from 157 to 98 per 100 000 in Scotland [1]. In contrast, the admission rate for elderly women with perforated duodenal ulcers has almost doubled over the last 25 years [1,2]. The majority of deaths from peptic ulcer disease are as a result of perforation, specifically in elderly patients with gastric perforations.

Infection with *Helicobacter pylori* has been shown to be important in the development of peptic ulceration [3]. However, its role in the etiology of perforated peptic ulcer disease is less clear. A retrospective study by Gisbert et al. examined 16 consecutive patients with perforated peptic ulcer disease and compared the prevalence of *H. pylori* to 160 patients with uncomplicated peptic ulcers. They reported that only 62% of patients with perforated peptic ulceration were infected compared to 86% of patients with uncomplicated disease. However, when the patients also taking NSAIDs were excluded, the prevalence of infection was almost 90%, suggesting that *Helicobacter* may be an important risk factor for perforation in patients not prescribed NSAIDs [4].

The ingestion of nonsteroidal antiinflammatory drugs is associated with an increased risk of peptic ulcer perforation irrespective of *Helicobacter* infection [3,5]. It would appear that peptic ulcer disease and therefore perforation is rare in patients who are *Helicobacter* negative and non-NSAID users [3].

Gastrointestinal Emergencies, 2nd edition. Edited by Tony Tham, John Collins and Roy Soetikno. © 2009 by Blackwell Publishing, ISBN: 978-1-4051-4634-0.

In younger patients, smoking is a significant etiological factor, increasing the risk of peptic ulcer perforation by tenfold with a significant dose response correlation, but there is no additional risk for those who have managed to stop smoking [6].

Clinical presentation
History

Peptic ulcer perforation presents in over 90% of patients as severe, sudden upper abdominal pain. Over one-third of patients will have a prior history of peptic ulcer disease and many will have been prescribed various antacid medications. In excess of 40% of patients will be using NSAIDs or corticosteroids and a high proportion will be smokers [7]. A majority of patients will have other significant comorbidity, and up to 15% of patients are hospitalized for another complaint at the time of perforation [7].

Examination

The patients may exhibit signs of systemic inflammatory response syndrome with tachycardia, pyrexia and tachypnea. Upper abdominal peritonism is a reasonably consistent finding described in 60% of patients with loss of liver dullness on percussion suggestive of free air [7].

Care must be taken in the elderly patient who may present with vague symptoms such as mild abdominal pain, nausea, dyspepsia or anorexia. Clinical examination in the elderly may also be misleading with a significant proportion not exhibiting abdominal tenderness.

Investigations

Routine blood investigations often demonstrate a leukocytosis and elevated inflammatory markers in a case of peptic ulcer perforation.

An erect chest radiograph is an appropriate first-line investigation for the demonstration of free intra-peritoneal gas but in 50% of cases no free gas can be identified [8]. A combination of classical clinical findings and free air on an erect chest radiograph will often be sufficient to warrant proceeding straight to laparotomy. If diagnostic doubt persists, three other investigative modalities are open to the clinician in order to arrive at a diagnosis and a definitive treatment plan.

The addition of water-soluble contrast will confirm the presence of an intraperitoneal leak but is unable to differentiate between a patient without a perforation and one in whom the perforation has sealed [9].

Abdominal ultrasound may demonstrate evidence of intraperitoneal free fluid and reduced intestinal peristalsis but these findings are not specific for gastroduodenal perforation.

The advent of multidetector CT may assist the surgeon in differentiating between a sealed-off duodenal perforation and other causes of an acute abdomen. Some authors suggest that multidetector CT is the most reliable diagnostic method with which to assess gastrointestinal perforation as it allows detection of even small amounts of free air in the abdomen and has a high sensitivity in the detection of free fluid [10].

Management

Following patient resuscitation and optimization with nasogastric aspiration, pharmacological acid suppression and broad-spectrum antibiotics, the mainstay of treatment remains surgical intervention. In the next section we shall consider conventional surgical treatment, examine the role of minimally invasive surgery and discuss the nonoperative approach.

Conventional surgical treatment

Historically, perforated peptic ulcers were surgically managed by closing the perforation and surgically reducing acid secretion. In the 1940s the approach would have been to perform a truncal vagotomy and a drainage procedure to overcome delayed gastric emptying. By the 1960s the process was refined to a highly selective vagotomy which eliminated the requirement for a drainage procedure and hence reduced the postoperative morbidity. The long-term ulcer recurrence rates following these operations were in the region of 5–15%.

In 1999 an article by Chu et al. reported that recurrent ulcer disease in patients with a history of perforated duodenal ulcer and simple patch repair was related to *Helicobacter* infection [11]. A further investigation by Ng et al. concluded that eradication of *Helicobacter*, with acid suppression and antibiotics, following the simple surgical closure of a perforated peptic ulcer reduced the recurrence rate to less than 5% [12].

We therefore conclude that simple omental patch closure and peritoneal lavage alongside *Helicobacter* eradication reduces ulcer recurrence rates following perforation, thus consigning definitive ulcer surgery to the history books.

Minimally invasive surgery

Since 1990 laparoscopic techniques have been used to repair perforated peptic ulcers. However, there is still significant debate with regard to the merits of the minimally invasive approach. Laparoscopically, the perforation may be patched by suturing omentum as at open repair or equally well plugged with gelatine sponge and fibrin glue [13].

Siu et al. reported that laparoscopic patients had shorter operating times, reduced respiratory complications, shorter postoperative stay, earlier return to normal activity, required significantly less parenteral analgesia and had lower pain scores in the initial postoperative period. There was no difference in nasogastric aspirate and time to tolerating oral intake between the two approaches and there were more reoperations and intra-abdominal collections within the laparoscopic group in this study [14].

A meta-analysis of 13 studies comprising 658 patients reported similar findings, namely a reduction in postoperative pain and less analgesic requirements but again a significantly higher reoperation rate was noted with the laparoscopic approach [15].

A systematic review of the literature published in 2005 based on 1113 patients represented by 15 studies concluded that laparoscopic repair seemed better than open repair for low-risk patients, and that for high-risk patients with significant comorbidity the open approach may be more appropriate [15]. A recently published Cochrane review suggested that the laparoscopic approach probably reduced septic abdominal complications. However it was concluded that the laparoscopic results were not clinically different from those of open surgery [16].

On balance it would seem that minimally invasive surgery for perforated peptic ulcers confers some short-term benefits for the patient. However, this is traded against an increase in reoperation rates and no earlier return of gut function. Further studies are required to identify subgroups of patients, probably those of low risk, who may gain most from the minimally invasive approach.

Nonoperative approach

A randomized trial of nonoperative treatment for peptic ulcer perforation compared to standard surgical intervention has been published. A total of 83 patients were entered in the study; 40 patients were randomly assigned to conservative treatment consisting of intravenous fluid resuscitation, nasogastric suction, antibiotics and acid suppression. After 12 hours almost 30% did not improve and proceeded to emergency surgery. The overall morbidity and mortality between the two groups was similar but the hospital stay was 35% longer for those treated conservatively. There was a higher incidence of sepsis and intraabdominal abscess for the nonoperative approach and those patients over 70 years old were less likely to respond to conservative measures. Although conservative treatment is possible it may not optimal for patients with perforated peptic ulceration but should be reserved for those with a sealed perforation who are too frail for surgical intervention.

Special circumstances
Perforated gastric cancer

It has been estimated that less than 1% of gastric cancer cases will perforate and it has been reported that around 10–15% of all gastric perforations are caused by gastric carcinoma.

Patients will present with symptoms and signs similar to that of peptic ulcer perforation but may have additional symptoms such as anorexia, lethargy and weight loss. During emergency laparotomy it is often very difficult to identify the etiology of the perforation due to the surrounding edema and inflammation. It is therefore prudent to obtain tissue from the edges of the perforation for histopathological examination.

Management of perforated gastric malignancy involves two often incompatible aims: dealing with the peritonitis and performing an oncologically sound procedure. Roviello et al. identified factors which can help decide the most appropriate management option. Decisions should be made based on the general condition of the patient and the curability of the malignancy. If the patient's general condition is acceptable and the tumor is resectable then a radical total or subtotal gastrectomy should be performed. When the tumor is at an advanced stage and cure is unlikely but the patient is in a reasonable condition then a palliative gastrectomy is recommended. A simple patch repair as used for perforated peptic ulcers is reserved for patients who are too frail for surgical resection [17].

Most of these patients present with advanced disease and therefore the outlook is bleak. A number of patients do have an early-stage tumor, when a curative operation can be performed. Survival rates after gastric perforation are similar to the rates observed for elective patients [18].

Colonic perforation

Introduction

Perforation of the colon is associated with significant morbidity and high mortality. This is partly due to the systemic insult of fecal peritonitis and in part the group of patients involved, who are often elderly with significant comorbidity. Prompt, appropriate intervention is vital in improving survival and reducing long-term morbidity for this group.

Diverticular disease remains the single commonest cause for large bowel perforation, accounting for 40–60% of cases with a reported increase in the prevalence of perforated sigmoid diverticulitis from 2.4 per 100 000 in 1986 to 3.8 per 100 000 in 2000 [19]. Perforation of colonic carcinoma accounts for around 10–20% [20], and perforation due to ischemia approximately 10%. The remaining miscellaneous group comprise iatrogenic, trauma, foreign body and stercol perforation (see Table 19.1).

Table 19.1 Etiology of colonic perforation. From ref. 20.

Etiology	Number (%)
Diverticulitis	133 (63%)
Carcinoma	30 (14%)
Ischemia	20 (9.4%)
Iatrogenic	13 (6.1%)
Other	16 (7.5%)
Total	212

Perforation occurs in diverticular disease when a fecolith obstructs the neck of the diverticulum.

Perforation of the colon results in the escape of enteric organisms into the peritoneal cavity. The resulting peritonitis is always polymicrobial, containing a mixture of aerobic and anaerobic bacteria with a predominance of gram-negative organisms. Common pathogens include *E. coli, Enterobacter, Klebsiella* and anaerobic species including *Bacteroides, Clostridium* and anaerobic *Streptococcus.*

The release of bacteria into the normally sterile environment of the peritoneal cavity initiates the host defense to eliminate or indeed contain the infecting agent by compartmentalization. A reduction in fibrinolytic activity produces fibrinous exudates into which large numbers of bacteria are sequestered, limiting the spread of peritoneal contamination. The residual effect of this process is the formation of an abscess cavity which matures to protect the bacteria from the host's defense mechanisms. If a contained abscess cavity does not develop then generalized peritonitis will be the outcome, precipitating a more aggressive immune response. Activation of the systemic inflammatory cascade with the production of proinflammatory cytokines leads to systemic inflammatory response syndrome (SIRS) and, if unchecked, ultimately o multiple organ failure (MOF).

Diagnosis

The presentation of patients with colonic perforation varies from localized left lower quadrant pain to extreme circulatory collapse. Exactly where along this spectrum the patient presents is dependent on the degree of contamination, the site and etiogy of the perforation alongside the patient's comorbidity and duration of the symptoms.

History

A precise clinical history is important when considering the diagnosis of colonic perforation. Abdominal pain is evident in around 70% of patients diagnosed with colonic perforation with the time of onset, duration and localization of the pain all important [21]. A past history of left-sided abdominal pain over many years suggests possible diverticular disease, whereas a history of weight loss, altered bowel habit and rectal bleeding may indicate a colonic carcinoma.

Identifying immunocompromised patients, those with diabetes, peripheral vascular disease or colitis may facilitate the decision-making process with regard to management and prognosis.

Examination

Physical examination will reveal signs of systemic sepsis with tachycardia, hypotension, tachypnea and fever [21]. Abdominal palpation may elicit localized tenderness corresponding to the site of perforation. An immobile patient with a board-like abdomen, generalized tenderness on percussion and absent bowel sounds is suggestive of more widespread peritonitis.

Investigations

Routine laboratory tests often show evidence of leukocytosis and elevated inflammatory markers such as C-reactive protein. Evidence of renal dysfunction on the serum biochemistry would have a bearing on the operative management and indicate the possible need for renal support following any surgical intervention. In severe sepsis, hemostatic function may be deranged as evidenced by an abnormal clotting screen. A significant coagulopathy may therefore require correction before or during any surgical procedure.

Plain radiography demonstrates free air in only one-third of cases of colonic perforation and should not be relied upon for reassurance [22]. Contrast enemas are of limited value because the disease process is predominantly extraluminal. Computed tomography is safer and a more cost-effective alternative [23]. In suspected colonic perforation, multidetector computed tomography (MD-CT) with oral and intravenous contrast will identify free air in up to 100% of cases. Other MD-CT findings include the presence of an inflammatory phlegmon, pericolic inflammatory stranding, extraluminal fluid collection and bowel wall thickening around the perforation site [22]. A report by Lohrmann et al. demonstrated that CT identified the perforation site in 86% of patients with perforated sigmoid diverticulitis [24]. Multidectector CT has the added advantage that it may help differentiate between a neoplastic or diverticular perforation and possibly identify liver metastases. Reports suggest that the presence of enlarged pericolic lymph nodes, with a short (<10 cm) length of colonic wall thickening and a luminal mass, were findings more suggestive of carcinoma [25].

Table 19.2 Hinchey classification of peritoneal contamination in perforated diverticular disease. From ref. 26.

Stage I	Pericolic or mesenteric abscess
Stage II	Walled-off pelvic abscess
Stage III	Generalized purulent peritonitis
Stage IV	Generalized fecal peritonitis

Table 19.3 Mannheim peritonitis index. From ref. 27.

Risk factor	Score
Age >50	5
Female	5
Organ failure	7
Malignancy	4
Peritonitis >24 h preop	4
Origin of sepsis not colonic	4
Diffuse generalized peritonitis	6
Clear exudate	0
Purulent exudate	6
Fecal exudate	12

Classification

A classification proposed by Hinchey in 1978 offers a means to assess the inflammation and contamination following a diverticular perforation (Table 19.2) [26]. Although designed with diverticular disease in mind, the categories would also apply to nondiverticular perforations. Although the Hinchey classification describes the degree of contamination, it does not consider other factors which are important for prognostic evaluation.

The Mannheim peritonitis index (MPI) (Table 19.3) provides a reliable method of classification and risk assessment for patients with peritonitis of all causes and has been shown to be as efficient as APACHE II in predicting the risk of death [27]. The reliability of the MPI was assessed in a multicenter study of over 2003 patients in an effort to select high-risk patients for more aggressive intervention. The mortality rate for patients with an MPI score of <21 was 2.3%, 21–29 was 22.5% and MPI >29 was 59.1%; overall the index had an accuracy of 83% in predicting death [28].

Management
General measures

The initial management of a patient with a colonic perforation involves fluid resuscitation, intravenous antibiotics to cover aerobic and anaerobic organisms, a urinary catheter for monitoring output and, based on the clinical findings, a definitive treatment plan.

Conservative

If the patient is hemodynamically stable and the abdominal signs are localized, a medical approach may be indicated with a CT assessment as described above [29]. With this scenario antibiotics are continued and any small localized abscess (<5 cm) should resolve, whereas a larger abscess should be drained percutaneously under radiological guidance [30]. This approach should be coupled with regular clinical assessment to identify any deterioration in the patient's condition. Failure of medical management in association with percutaneous drainage warrants surgical intervention.

Surgical

A laparotomy is indicated without the need for a CT in the patient with signs of severe sepsis and generalized peritonitis. If the patient is relatively stable a CT may be useful to identify the exact site of perforation and the degree of intraabdominal contamination [24].

Having decided to operate, the next surgical dilemma is the selection of the most appropriate procedure. Essentially three options exist, namely a three-stage, two-stage or one-stage procedure; we shall consider the relative merits of each in turn.

Three-stage procedure

If, at laparotomy, the colonic perforation had precipitated purulent or fecal peritonitis, then traditionally this was managed in three stages. The first stage involved draining but not resecting the segment of perforated colon and diverting the fecal stream with a transverse loop colostomy. After a period of time the diseased segment of colon was excised and an anastomosis fashioned. Closure of the defunctioning colostomy with restoration of bowel continuity completed the final stage.

A review of the literature in 1984 by Krukowski identified a significant disadvantage in morbidity and a mortality rate approaching 25% when the diseased colon was retained [29]. Based on these findings a three-stage approach is best avoided.

Two-stage procedure

In the late 1970s, a number of units advocated the two-stage procedure which involved primary resection of the diseased segment, the formation of an end colostomy and oversewing of the rectal stump (Hartmann procedure) [31,32]. This was followed by reversal of the stoma, by anastomosis to the rectal stump when the intraabdominal sepsis had settled. The adoption of this two-stage approach more than halved the operative mortality [29].

The problem with the two-stage procedure is the colostomy reversal which can be a difficult and complex procedure. Often many patients tolerate and manage their colostomy well and up to 50% are satisfied not to pursue reversal [33]. Several authors have shown a high incidence of postreversal morbidity and therefore advocate the one-stage approach [34,35].

One-stage procedure

Primary resection and anastomosis has therefore found favor in an effort to reduce the morbidity associated with reversal of a Hartmann procedure. The procedure involves resection of the affected segment of colon followed by a primary colonic anastomosis. This approach has been mainly reserved for those patients without fecal peritonitis but a recent prospective non-randomized study demonstrated no difference in mortality between a one-stage and two-stage procedure; for patients with Hinchey stage III/IV diverticulitis [33].

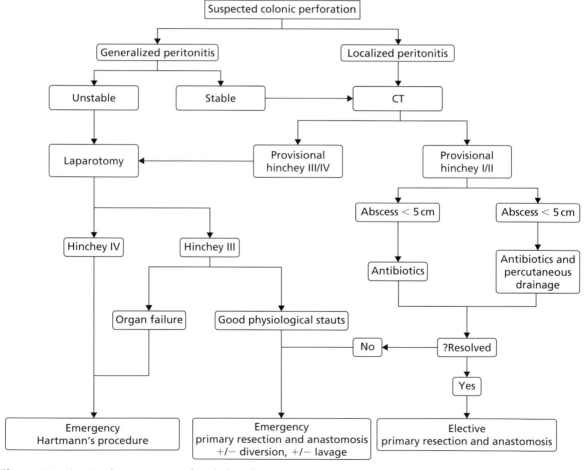

Figure 19.1 Algorithm for management of a colonic perforation.

Concerns remain about fashioning an anastomosis on an unprepared bowel in the presence of peritoneal contamination with edema in the colonic wall. Maneuvers such as on-table colonic lavage and formation of a defunctioning loop ileostomy have been utilized to reduce the likelihood and effects of an anastomotic leak. The evidence is weak, however, and some authors suggest that lavage and diversion may not be mandatory [36,37].

A systemic review by Constantinides et al. has recently been published. They performed a meta-analysis of 15 studies, only 2 of which were prospective and none was randomized. They demonstrated similar mortality rates for both one and two-stage procedures (14.1% vs 14.4%) for a colonic perforation with purulent or fecal peritonitis (Hinchey stage II). If the peritonitis was classified as Hinchey I/II then there was a significant improvement in mortality and morbidity for patients undergoing a one-stage procedure. However, the authors highlighted a significant selection bias in all of the papers examined as patients with significant peritoneal contamination and poor physiological status were often subjected to a Hartmann procedure.

It is therefore difficult to draw strong conclusions until a randomized controlled trial is performed comparing one- and two-stage procedures, in patient groups matched for age, sex, degree of contamination and physiological status.

Management algorithm

Based on the data available, a management algorithm has been constructed suggesting a management plan for the patient presenting with a suspected perforation of the colon (Fig. 19.1).

References

1. Jibril JA, Redpath A, Macintyre IM. Changing pattern of admission and operation for duodenal ulcer in Scotland. Br J Surg 1994; 81(1):87–9.
2. Higham J, Kang JY, Majeed A. Recent trends in admissions and mortality due to peptic ulcer in England: increasing frequency of haemorrhage among older subjects. Gut 2002; 50(4):460–4.
3. Huang JQ, Sridhar S, Hunt RH. Role of *Helicobacter pylori* infection and non-steroidal anti-inflammatory drugs in peptic-ulcer disease: a meta-analysis. Lancet 2002; 359(9300):14–22.
4. Gisbert JP, Legido J, Garcia-Sanz I, Pajares JM. *Helicobacter pylori* and perforated peptic ulcer: prevalence of the infection and role of non-steroidal anti-inflammatory drugs. Dig Liver Dis 2004; 36(2):116–20.
5. Armstrong CP, Blower AL. Non-steroidal anti-inflammatory drugs and life threatening complications of peptic ulceration. Gut 1987; 28(5):527–32.
6. Svanes C, Soreide JA, Skarstein A, Fevang BT, Bakke P, Vollset SE, et al. Smoking and ulcer perforation. Gut 1997; 41(2):177–80.
7. Gunshefski L, Flancbaum L, Brolin RE, Frankel A. Changing patterns in perforated peptic ulcer disease. Am Surg 1990; 56(4):270–4.
8. Miller RE, Nelson SW. The roentgenologic demonstration of tiny amounts of free intraperitoneal gas: experimental and clinical studies. Am J Roentgenol Radium Ther Nucl Med 1971; 112(3):574–85.
9. Wellwood JM, Wilson AN, Hopkinson BR. Gastrografin as an aid to the diagnosis of perforated peptic ulcer. Br J Surg 1971; 58(4):245–9.
10. Pinto A, Scaglione M, Giovine S, Romano S, Lassandro F, Grassi R, et al. Comparison between the site of multislice CT signs of gastrointestinal perforation and the site of perforation detected at surgery in forty perforated patients. Radiol Med (Torino) 2004; 108(3):208–17.
11. Chu KM, Kwok KF, Law SY, Tuen HH, Tung PH, Branicki FJ, et al. *Helicobacter pylori* status and endoscopy follow-up of patients having a history of perforated duodenal ulcer. Gastrointest Endosc 1999; 50(1):58–62.
12. Ng EK, Lam YH, Sung JJ, Yung MY, To KF, Chan AC, et al. Eradication of *Helicobacter pylori* prevents recurrence of ulcer after simple closure of duodenal ulcer perforation: randomized controlled trial. Ann Surg 2000; 231(2):153–8.
13. Lau WY, Leung KL, Kwong KH, Davey IC, Robertson C, Dawson JJ, et al. A randomized study comparing laparoscopic versus open repair of perforated peptic ulcer using suture or sutureless technique. Ann Surg 1996; 224(2):131–8.
14. Siu WT, Leong HT, Law BK, Chau CH, Li AC, Fung KH, et al. Laparoscopic repair for perforated peptic ulcer: a randomized controlled trial. Ann Surg 2002; 235(3):313–19.
15. Lunevicius R, Morkevicius M. Systematic review comparing laparoscopic and open repair for perforated peptic ulcer. Br J Surg 2005; 92(10):1195–207.
16. Sanabria AE, Morales CH, Villegas MI. Laparoscopic repair for perforated peptic ulcer disease. Cochrane Database Syst Rev 2005; (4):CD004778.
17. Roviello F, Rossi S, Marrelli D, De Manzoni G, Pedrazzani C, Morgagni P, et al. Perforated gastric

carcinoma: a report of 10 cases and review of the literature. World J Surg Oncol 2006; 4:19.

18. Cuschieri A, Weeden S, Fielding J, Bancewicz J, Craven J, Joypaul V, et al. Patient survival after d1 and d2 resections for gastric cancer: long-term results of the MRC randomized surgical trial. Surgical Co-operative Group. Br J Cancer 1999; 79(9–10):1522–30.

19. Makela J, Kiviniemi H, Laitinen S. Prevalence of perforated sigmoid diverticulitis is increasing. Dis Colon Rectum 2002; 45(7):955–61.

20. Biondo S, Pares D, Marti Rague J, De Oca J, Toral D, Borobia FG, et al. Emergency operations for nondiverticular perforation of the left colon. Am J Surg 2002; 183(3):256–60.

21. Gedebou TM, Wong RA, Rappaport WD, Jaffe P, Kahsai D, Hunter GC. Clinical presentation and management of iatrogenic colon perforations. Am J Surg 1996; 172(5):454–7; discussion 7–8.

22. Miki T, Ogata S, Uto M, Nakazono T, Urata M, Ishibe R, et al. Multidetector-row CT findings of colonic perforation: direct visualization of ruptured colonic wall. Abdom Imaging 2004; 29(6):658–62.

23. Janes SE, Meagher A, Frizelle FA. Management of diverticulitis. BMJ 2006; 332(7536):271–5.

24. Lohrmann C, Ghanem N, Pache G, Makowiec F, Kotter E, Langer M. CT in acute perforated sigmoid diverticulitis. Eur J Radiol 2005; 56(1):78–83.

25. Chintapalli KN, Chopra S, Ghiatas AA, Esola CC, Fields SF, Dodd GD, 3rd. Diverticulitis versus colon cancer: differentiation with helical CT findings. Radiology 1999; 210(2):429–35.

26. Hinchey EJ, Schaal PG, Richards GK. Treatment of perforated diverticular disease of the colon. Adv Surg 1978; 12:85–109.

27. Linder MM, Wacha H, Feldmann U, Wesch G, Streifensand RA, Gundlach E. [The Mannheim peritonitis index: an instrument for the intraoperative prognosis of peritonitis]. Chirurg 1987; 58(2):84–92.

28. Billing A, Frohlich D, Schildberg FW. Prediction of outcome using the Mannheim peritonitis index in 2003 patients. Peritonitis Study Group. Br J Surg 1994; 81(2):209–13.

29. Krukowski ZH, Matheson NA. Emergency surgery for diverticular disease complicated by generalized and faecal peritonitis: a review. Br J Surg 1984; 71(12):921–7.

30. Stabile BE, Puccio E, van Sonnenberg E, Neff CC. Preoperative percutaneous drainage of diverticular abscesses. Am J Surg 1990; 159(1):99–104; discussion.

31. Eng K, Ranson JH, Localio SA. Resection of the perforated segment: a significant advance in treatment of diverticulitis with free perforation or abscess. Am J Surg 1977; 133(1):67–72.

32. Rugtiv GM. Diverticulitis: selective surgical management. Am J Surg 1975; 130(2):219–25.

33. Keck JO, Collopy BT, Ryan PJ, Fink R, Mackay JR, Woods RJ. Reversal of Hartmann's procedure: effect of timing and technique on ease and safety. Dis Colon Rectum 1994; 37(3):243–8.

34. Bell C, Asolati M, Hamilton E, Fleming J, Nwariaku F, Sarosi G, et al. A comparison of complications associated with colostomy reversal versus ileostomy reversal. Am J Surg 2005; 190(5):717–20.

35. Aydin HN, Remzi FH, Tekkis PP, Fazio VW. Hartmann's reversal is associated with high postoperative adverse events. Dis Colon Rectum 2005; 48(11): 2117–26.

36. Patriti A, Contine A, Carbone E, Gulla N, Donini A. One-stage resection without colonic lavage in emergency surgery of the left colon. Colorectal Dis 2005; 7(4):332–8.

37. Ambrosetti P, Michel JM, Megevand JM, Morel P. [Left colectomy with immediate anastomosis in emergency surgery]. Ann Chir 1999; 53(10):1023–8.

20 Intestinal Obstruction

Andrew B.C. Crumley, Robert C. Stuart

Introduction

Intestinal obstruction is defined as the impedance or restriction to the normal passage of intestinal contents through the gastrointestinal tract. It is a common surgical emergency and is broadly classified into two categories – dynamic (mechanical) and adynamic (paralytic ileus). Dynamic obstruction occurs when intestinal peristalsis is actively working against a mechanical blockage. Adynamic obstruction is where there is a loss of normal peristalsis, without a mechanical blockage present.

Further subdivision and clinical presentation is based on:
- level of obstruction -high small bowel, low small bowel, large bowel;
- speed of onset – acute or chronic;
- etiology: mural, extrinsic, intraluminal;
- nature/pathophysiology – simple mechanical, strangulated, closed loop, volvulus, intussusception.

Clinical presentation varies depending on the site, speed of onset and etiology of the obstruction but broadly, the classical symptoms are: colicky abdominal pain, abdominal distension, constipation, and vomiting.

Etiology

Dynamic (mechanical) obstruction

Causes of dynamic or mechanical obstruction can be divided into three subgroups: extrinsic, mural (intrinsic), and intraluminal.

Gastrointestinal Emergencies, 2nd edition. Edited by Tony Tham, John Collins and Roy Soetikno. © 2009 by Blackwell Publishing, ISBN: 978-1-4051-4634-0.

Extrinsic

The most common cause of intestinal obstruction is extrinsic compression from adhesions. The incidence of adhesions causing obstruction is decreasing due to the use of powder-free gloves and improved operative tissue handling. Hernias also cause extrinsic obstruction by constricting the lumen of the intestine at the neck of the hernia sac. Inguinal hernias (due to the fact that they are the most common type of hernia) are responsible for most cases of obstruction due to a hernia. However, a greater percentage of femoral hernias present with obstruction, due to the tight neck at the entry to the femoral canal.

A volvulus is when a portion of the intestine twists around itself resulting in a closed-loop obstruction. A closed-loop obstruction refers to an obstruction where the intestine is obstructed at two points, i.e. there is no point of decompression. Volvulus can affect any part of the intestines, including a gastric volvulus, sigmoid volvulus, cecal volvulus or small bowel volvulus. The kink or twist that obstructs the lumen can also involve the blood supply resulting in ischemia, necrosis and perforation if untreated.

Mural or intrinsic

Lesions intrinsic to the bowel wall form strictures which obstruct the passage of intestinal contents. Malignant strictures are the most common cause of intrinsic lesions in adults but benign strictures from inflammatory bowel disease (most commonly Crohn's disease), diverticular disease and iatrogenic strictures following radiation or surgery are also found. In infants, congenital atresia or stenosis are the most common intrinsic cause of obstruction.

Intraluminal

Ingested foreign bodies can cause obstruction in particular in children and people with learning difficulties.

Fecal impaction can cause obstruction and in rare cases perforation from a stercoral ulcer. Gallstone ileus results when a large gallstone erodes through the gallbladder into the intestine via a fistula and then obstructs the lumen, typically at the ileocecal valve.

Adynamic obstruction (paralytic ileus)

Lack of transmission of normal peristalsis via the myenteric plexus causes an adynamic obstruction or paralytic ileus. Failure of contraction leads to stasis, and subsequent accumulation of gas and fluid. It is most commonly seen as a result of abdominal surgery and usually lasts no longer than 48–72 hours. Prolonged postoperative ileus should give rise to suspicion of another cause of ileus such as intra-abdominal sepsis, hemorrhage or metabolic upset. Other causes include pneumonia, retroperitoneal trauma or hemorrhage, drugs such as tricyclic antidepressants, mesenteric ischemia, and acute pancreatitis.

History

The level of the obstruction is important in determining the symptoms with which the patient will present. High small bowel obstruction tends to be of sudden onset while low small bowel obstruction has a more gradual onset. Large bowel obstruction usually has an insidious onset. The classical symptoms of mechanical obstruction are abdominal pain, vomiting, distension and constipation. In contrast, adynamic obstruction is usually painless.

The pain of obstruction is experienced as a colicky visceral pain. Patients tend to be restless with the pain and unable to find a position of relief. Pain which is relieved by lying still must raise the possibility of obstruction complicated with peritonitis. The area where the pain is felt is dependent on the embryological section of the intestine that is affected. Embryological mid-gut obstruction (second part of the duodenum to two-thirds along the transverse colon) presents with periumbilical discomfort, whereas hindgut obstruction (two-thirds transverse colon to anus) is felt as lower abdominal colic. Very high small bowel obstruction may be associated with a more continuous epigastric pain, relieved by vomiting.

The degree of abdominal distension described is also dependent on the level of obstruction. In all patients, there is overgrowth of both aerobic and anaerobic organisms, which results in increased gas production. Absorption of fluids and electrolytes by the intestine is inhibited, while production continues unabated. Intestine, proximal to the level of obstruction, therefore becomes dilated as a result of accumulation of fluid and gas. In distal obstruction therefore (colonic or distal small bowel), distension can be marked. In contrast, high small bowel, large bowel obstruction with a competent ileocecal valve, or any closed-loop obstruction, can present with minimal distension.

Absolute constipation is failure to pass either flatus or feces and is an early sign of large bowel obstruction. Patients with small bowel obstruction may still pass flatus or feces due to residual colonic matter and therefore the absence of constipation does not exclude intestinal obstruction. If the obstruction is partial the obstruction may be associated with diarrhea rather than constipation, for example fecal impaction, Richter hernia, gallstone ileus and colonic cancer.

Vomiting is an early feature of high small bowel obstruction and may result in relief from the associated pain. In general, the more distal the level of obstruction the later is the onset of vomiting as a feature. In some cases with distal colonic obstruction vomiting may even be absent. The longer the history of the obstruction the more feculent is the nature of the vomitus.

In taking the medical history of a patient with suspected intestinal obstruction, direct questioning concerning previous abdominal surgery and any lumps or hernias in the groin is essential. Care should also be exercised to inquire of respiratory symptoms, recent surgery, trauma and medications. It is important to inquire about any change in the nature of the pain as a shift from colicky pain to a more constant pain may indicate strangulation and ischemia with impending perforation.

Examination

In the early stages of intestinal obstruction the patient may look well and vital signs appear normal. Often by the time the patient presents for help, the intestinal obstruction however is advanced and he or she is severely ill. Persistent vomiting and diminished luminal absorption of fluid and electrolytes can lead to potentially fatal imbalances. Patients may exhibit signs of dehydration, with reduced skin turgor, dry mucous membranes, tachycardia and hypotension. If the temperature is raised, complications such as intestinal ischemia or perforation should be considered. Alternatively the temperature could be raised because the obstructing pathology involves inflammation, for example acute diverticulitis, pericolic abscess or inflammatory bowel disease.

Abdominal inspection focuses on the presence of scars from previous surgery, indicating a possible etiology from adhesions, and the presence of abdominal wall or groin hernias. Together they are the two commonest causes of obstruction. Abdominal distension is usual and the more distal the obstruction the more obvious it is. In some thin patients it may be possible to see visible peristalsis. Patients with gastric outlet obstruction may have an audible succussion splash.

Mild tenderness is commonly present. Marked tenderness indicates the progression to a complication such as ischemia or perforation. Palpation may reveal a mass such as in acute diverticulitis or an obstructing cancer. The need to carefully examine the hernial orifices cannot be overstated. Redness of the overlying skin or tenderness of the hernia may indicate strangulation.

On auscultation, the presence of high-pitched, tinkling, hyperactive bowel sounds indicate dynamic obstruction, whereas absent bowel sounds are indicative of adynamic obstruction.

Rectal examination is usually normal but may demonstrate an obstructing rectal cancer, fecal impaction or a ballooned, empty rectum in adynamic obstruction.

Investigations

In the early phase all laboratory investigations may be normal. A raised white blood cell count or C-reactive protein (CRP) may indicate an inflammatory cause for the obstruction or the development of complications such as ischemia or perforation. Dehydration is common in small bowel obstruction and pre-renal failure may be seen with a raised serum urea and creatinine. High small bowel obstruction with profuse vomiting may be associated with hypochloremic, hypokalemic alkalosis. A marked acidosis or raised serum amylase may indicate intestinal ischemia as a complication though these are not universally reliable.

Plain, supine abdominal radiography is the initial imaging modality of choice. This can be used to demonstrate the presence of obstruction and reveal the distinctive features of large and small bowel dilatation. Small bowel loops tend to be central in position and have striations that pass across the full width of the bowel. The large bowel, in contrast, tends to be peripherally located and its haustra (caused by the taenia coli) do not cover the whole width of the bowel. With a sigmoid volvulus, there is grossly dilated bowel which is seen to arise from the pelvis and extend into the upper abdomen. An erect chest radiograph, looking for subdiaphragmatic gas, is useful to help exclude perforation. An erect abdominal radiograph may demonstrate the presence of fluid levels, though these may also be caused by other nonobstructing conditions such as pancreatitis and abscess. In obstruction due to gallstone ileus, air in the biliary tree may be seen on abdominal radiography. Plain abdominal radiographs may not allow differentiation between mechanical and paralytic ileus.

If on clinical and radiological grounds the obstruction appears to be colonic, a water-soluble enema can be given to confirm and demonstrate the level of obstruction. Similarly if a subacute small bowel obstruction is suspected, a contrast follow-through can demonstrate, or exclude, the presence of a mechanical obstruction.

Increasingly CT scanning is being used early in cases of obstruction. The presence and level of obstructing lesions can be identified and in addition a scan can provide cancer staging information that may influence treatment. Rare causes of obstruction such as obturator hernias are also well defined on CT. The CT scan is particularly useful in defining other causes of the acute abdomen, the nature of inflammatory causes of obstruction, and assessing the likelihood of associated complications.

Management

The primary aim of initial management is aggressive resuscitation. Patients should be treated with oxygen, intravenous fluids, nasogastric tube insertion and a urinary catheter. Usually, successful resuscitation improves the patient's symptoms and signs and one should be careful not to be falsely reassured that surgery is not required. While surgery is often required early in the management of the mechanical obstruction there are some exceptions when it may be wiser to observe the patient expectantly. These include: multiple previous operations for obstruction, postoperative obstruction, abdominal carcinomatosis, previous abdominal or pelvic radiation treatment, and inflammatory bowel disease. The timing of any surgical intervention is dependent on the level of the obstruction, the assessment of whether the obstruction is simple or involves strangulated intestine, the degree or severity of electrolyte imbalance and the likelihood of the patient's condition and organ function being improved by delaying surgery.

High small bowel obstruction is rarely complicated by strangulation and the priority of management is correction of the fluid and electrolyte imbalances that are frequently severe due to the profuse vomiting. Often it is possible to defer surgery and investigate first using a combination of CT scanning, endoscopy and small bowel contrast radiology. Mid to lower small bowel obstruction is at a higher risk of strangulation or ischemia and surgery is more often required soon after the period of initial resuscitation. In the absence of any features of strangulation it is safe to defer surgery, investigate with CT scanning and occasionally a water-soluble oral contrast examination may prove therapeutic. Surgery for uncomplicated large bowel obstruction can usually be deferred until after investigations, to determine the underlying cause, can be performed. These investigations include a contrast enema, flexible sigmoidoscopy and CT scanning. Caution should be exercised when a closed-loop obstruction is suspected and right iliac fossa tenderness associated with colonic obstruction should prompt surgical intervention.

In a strangulated obstruction the viability of the bowel is threatened due to inadequate perfusion. Initially venous return is compromised, resulting in congestion and edema of the affected segment of bowel. As venous pressure is lower than arterial pressure, initially arterial supply is unaffected. However as the congestion and edema progresses, the pressure becomes greater than the arterial pressure, resulting in infarction. As the viability of the bowel mucosa is affected, there is a great loss of electrolytes and fluid, and spread of bacteria into the bloodstream with associated toxins, resulting in sepsis. Strangulation occurs most commonly secondary to hernias but is also found secondary to adhesive bands, internal hernias or volvulus. Differentiation between simple and strangulated hernias is clinically difficult. However, the absence of pyrexia, tachycardia, abdominal or hernia tenderness and leukocytosis make strangulation less likely.

Specific management is dependent on the etiology of the obstruction and the likelihood of strangulation. Adhesive obstruction is often treated successfully using the above conservative measures. A recent Cochrane review of small bowel adhesive obstruction states that passage of oral contrast to the cecum is a sensitive indicator that the obstruction will resolve spontaneously [1]. The limit of duration of observation is however controversial but should not be longer than 5 days [2,3].

Obstruction due to other mechanical causes should be treated surgically following appropriate preoperative resuscitation, and is tailored to the cause. For example, an obstruction due to an inguinal hernia requires reduction of the hernia, resection of nonviable intestine and hernia repair. Conventionally it is thought wise not to perform a mesh repair in the presence of infection but there is no evidence that this is necessarily the case [4]. Obstruction due to a femoral hernia should be repaired via the McKevedy approach, if ischemia is suspected, to allow a resection to be performed if required.

An exploratory laparotomy is required for cases due to conditions other than a hernia. Adequate exposure is by an incision appropriate for the suspected pathology. A previous incision is used if present and it is safest to enter the abdomen via an extension of the old wound where adhesions are least likely. The main considerations during the laparotomy are to determine the site and nature of the obstruction as well as the viability of the gut. Start at the cecum, if it is distended then colonic obstruction is the cause. If the cecum is collapsed then follow small bowel proximally to find cause. When colonic obstruction is suspected, begin the search for the obstruction distally and work upwards taking care not to miss a small annular cancer. Decompression of small bowel loops by milking contents back to stomach and aspiration via nasogastric tube is preferable to insertion of a Savage decompressor. Decompression of a massively distended colon can usually be accomplished using a large-bore needle connected to suction and inserted through one of the taenia coli. Particularly when the obstruction is due to adhesions, inflammatory bowel disease or diffuse cancer, it is important to examine the entire length of the small bowel as more than one level of obstruction may be present.

An obstructing colonic cancer without perforation can be treated with the appropriate resection, dependent on the site of the tumor. A primary anastomosis was traditionally performed for right-sided resections but many surgeons are reluctant to perform a primary anastomosis for emergency left colon resections. Evidence would suggest that the morbidity, mortality and leak rate for both left and right resections with anastomosis is however similar [5]. In addition, for obstructing left colon tumors, a segmental resection and anastomosis compared with subtotal colectomy has been shown to improve functional outcome and not to be associated with an increased rate of anastomotic leak or mortality [6].

In the presence of a perforated, obstructed tumor with contamination or when the viability of the bowel is questionable, convention states that a primary anastomosis should not be performed and the proximal bowel should be exteriorized. A review comparing a one-stage procedure (resection with primary anastomosis) with a two-stage procedure (Hartmann plus reversal) in patients with perforated diverticular disease, however, demonstrated no difference in morbidity or mortality [7].

In cases of obstruction due to irresectable disease a defunctioning stoma or bypass may be performed. For example, an obstructing cecal tumour can be palliatively bypassed with an ileo-transverse anastomosis. The palliative treatment of malignant colonic obstruction with expandable metal stents has also been shown to alleviate obstructive symptoms, without the need for surgery or a stoma [8,9]. Obstruction associated with diffuse intraabdominal malignancy can be treated with a combination of antiemetics, antisecretory drugs (octreotide or hyoscine) [10,11], analgesics and corticosteroids [12].

Adynamic or paralytic ileus is usually treated by conservative, nonoperative measures that rely on nasogastric decompression and resuscitation of fluid and electrolyte abnormalities. The aim should be to diagnose and treat the underlying medical or surgical cause of the problem. Surgery may be required if the cause is an acute abdominal problem such as peritonitis. Intraabdominal abscess as a cause of ileus is usually best managed by CT- or ultrasound-guided drainage.

References

1. Abbas S, Bissett IP, Parry BR. Oral water-soluble contrast for the management of adhesive small bowel obstruction. Cochrane Database Syst Rev 2005; CD004651.

2. Sosa J, Gardner B. Management of patients diagnosed as acute intestinal obstruction secondary to adhesions. Am Surg 1993; 59:125–8.

3. Seror D, Feigin E, Szold A, Allweis TM, Carmon M, Nissan S, Freund HR. How conservatively can postoperative small bowel obstruction be treated? Am J Surg 1993; 165:121–5.

4. Papaziogas B, Lazaridis C, Makris J, Koutelidakis J, Patsas A, Grigoriou M, Chatzimavroudis G, Psaralexis K, Atmatzidis K. Tension-free repair versus modified Bassini technique (Andrews technique) for strangulated inguinal hernia: a comparative study. Hernia 2005; 9:156–9.

5. Hsu TC. Comparison of one-stage resection and anastomosis of acute complete obstruction of left and right colon. Am J Surg 2005; 189:384–7.

6. The SCOTIA Study Group. Single-stage treatment for malignant left-sided colonic obstruction: a prospective randomized clinical trial comparing subtotal colectomy with segmental resection following intra-operative irrigation. The SCOTIA Study Group. Subtotal Colectomy versus On-table Irrigation and Anastomosis. Br J Surg 1995; 82:1622–7.

7. Salem L, Flum DR. Primary anastomosis or Hartmann's procedure for patients with diverticular peritonitis? A systematic review. Dis Colon Rectum 2004; 47:1953–64.

8. Lo SK. Metallic stenting for colorectal obstruction. Gastrointest Endosc Clin N Am 1999; 9:459–77.

9. Camunez F, Echenagusia A, Simo G, Turegano F, Vazquez J, Barreiro-Meiro I. Malignant colorectal obstruction treated by means of self-expanding metallic stents: effectiveness before surgery and in palliation. Radiology 2000; 216:492–7.

10. Ripamonti C, Mercadante S, Groff L, Zecca E, De Conno F, Casuccio A. Role of octreotide, scopolamine butylbromide, and hydration in symptom control of patients with inoperable bowel obstruction and nasogastric tubes: a prospective randomized trial. J Pain Symptom Management 2000; 19(1):23–34.

11. Mercadante S, Ripamonti C, Casuccio A, Zecca E, Groff L. Comparison of octreotide and hyoscine butylbromide in controlling gastrointestinal symptoms due to malignant inoperable bowel obstruction. Support Care Cancer 2000; 8(3):188–91.

12. Feuer DJ, Broadley KE. Corticosteroids for the resolution of malignant bowel obstruction in advanced gynaecological and gastrointestinal cancer (Cochrane Review). In: The Cochrane Library, Issue 1, 2003. Oxford: Update Software.

21 Acute Upper Nonvariceal Gastrointestinal Hemorrhage

Kelvin Palmer

The incidence of acute upper gastrointestinal hemorrhage ranges between 50 per 10000 and 190 per 10000 per year and is highest in areas of social deprivation. In Hong Kong, the incidence has decreased by 30% over the last 10 years. In contrast, the number of admissions for bleeding is stable or slightly increasing in elderly patients in the UK. The prevalence of *Helicobacter pylori*, use of nonsteroidal antiinflammatory drugs (NSAIDs) and prevalence of liver disease are important factors [1].

The mortality of patients admitted to hospital for acute gastrointestinal bleeding is about 10%. In the UK, crude mortality has not changed in more than half a century although the case mix has changed greatly over this time, and patients are now older and have greater medical disability than was the case 50 years ago [1].

Risk assessment

At the time of first assessment it is important to identify patients who have significant liver disease. Patients with liver disease are best managed at presentation by gastroenterologists (or hepatologists). Most will have a history of alcohol abuse or exposure to hepatotoxic viruses, have clinical evidence of liver disease and abnormal serum liver function tests. Management is discussed elsewhere (see Chapter 24, Variceal Hemorrhage).

Death following admission to hospital for gastrointestinal bleeding is almost invariably a consequence of decompensated comorbidity; it is seldom caused by exsanguination. Sudden blood loss and circulatory collapse may result in fatal cardiac or cerebrovascular events in patients with underlying vascular disease, and postoperative complications following emergency surgery are more likely in those with other conditions. Therefore, risk assessment is based on the:
- severity of the hemorrhage
- general health of the patient.

When patients present with acute upper gastrointestinal hemorrhage, it is crucial to define factors with prognostic value. Those at high risk of continuing bleeding or rebleeding need intensive monitoring and early endoscopic intervention, whereas low-risk patients should be "fast-tracked" towards early hospital discharge.

Rebleeding is associated with a tenfold increase in hospital mortality. In clinical trials, it is often used as an end point for defining success or failure of putative treatments. Mortality is particularly high in patients who bleed during a hospital stay for another serious disease (about 40% in published series, compared with 10–12% in patients admitted for gastrointestinal bleeding).

The Rockall score [2] (Table 3.3 and 3.4, Chapter 3) is a useful risk assessment tool. It was developed from a large audit of patients admitted to hospitals in England for acute upper gastrointestinal bleeding. Multivariant analysis identified age, shock, comorbidity and specific endoscopic findings as independent variables predicting rebleeding and death. The score has been validated by other groups; its major drawback in clinical practice is the need to undertake endoscopy before the score can be completed.

The Blatchford score [3] (Table 3.5 and 3.6, chapter 3) predicts outcome on the basis of clinical and laboratory factors, without the need for endoscopy and is therefore useful in the initial triage process.

Gastrointestinal Emergencies, 2nd edition. Edited by Tony Tham, John Collins and Roy Soetikno. © 2009 by Blackwell Publishing, ISBN: 978-1-4051-4634-0.

Endoscopy provides important prognostic information (Table 21.1). The presence of blood in the upper gastrointestinal tract, active spurting hemorrhage and a "nonbleeding visible vessel" are signs of a poor prognosis. Active ulcer bleeding implies an 80–90% risk of continuing hemorrhage or rebleeding. A visible vessel (representing adherent blood clot or a pseudoaneurysm over the arterial defect) is associated with a 50% risk of rebleeding during that hospital stay [4].

Therapeutic endoscopists attempt to wash the bleeding point vigorously to display these major endoscopic stigmata of recent hemorrhage, using washing catheters and snares to remove blood clot. These maneuvers risk provoking further bleeding, but this can usually be managed by one of the techniques described below. Sometimes, the clot cannot be removed, and the presence of nonadherent blood clot carries an intermediate risk of further bleeding.

Table 21.1 Endoscopic stigmata and the risk of rebleeding.

Endoscopic finding	Risk of rebleeding (%)
Clean base	3
Flat spots	7
Oozing only	10
Adherent clot	33
Nonbleeding visible vessel	50
Active bleeding	90

Management: general principles

An algorithm for the management of acute gastrointestinal hemorrhage is shown in Fig. 21.1.

Resuscitation

The principles of "airway, breathing and circulation" apply. Patients presenting with major bleeding are often elderly and have significant cardiorespiratory,

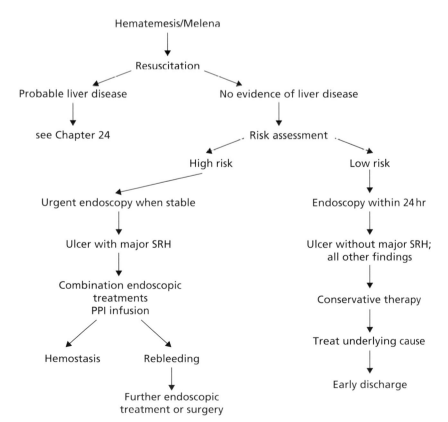

Figure 21.1 Algorithm for acute gastrointestinal bleeding. SRH stigmata of recent hemorrhage; PPI proton pump inhibitors.

117

renal and cerebrovascular comorbidity. It is vital that these conditions are recognized and supported.

Intravenous fluid replacement to maintain blood pressure and urine output is the first step in management, coupled with appropriate management of cardiac and respiratory disease. Central venous pressure (CVP) monitoring is useful in the elderly and in many patients with cardiac disease, to optimize decisions concerning volume of fluid replacement. Intravenous fluids should be given through a large cannula inserted in an antecubital vein. Crystalloids (principally normal saline) are used to normalize blood pressure and urine output; colloids (e.g. Gelofusine) are often used in the presence of major hypotension. Saline should be used with care in patients with liver disease since these patients retain salt and water and may develop pulmonary edema in addition to ascites.

Blood transfusion is administered to patients who are shocked and bleeding actively. Blood is also transfused when the hemoglobin concentration is less than 10 g/dL. The evidence for this transfusion threshold is relatively poor, but it is known that a hemoglobin concentration of less than 7 g/dL has significant adverse cardiac effects in the intensive care setting, and it is reasonable to preempt this by using a level of 10 g/dL in bleeding patients.

Patients with liver disease present specific problems. Hepatic encephalopathy, renal failure and ascites may all develop or worsen as a consequence of bleeding and warrant specific management. All liver disease patients who develop bleeding should receive antibiotics to prevent life-threatening sepsis.

Monitoring

Monitoring includes measurement of pulse, blood pressure, urine output (through an indwelling catheter) and CVP. Actively bleeding patients with evidence of shock (defined as pulse >100 bpm and/or systolic blood pressure <100 mmHg) are best managed in a high-dependency environment.

Endoscopy

Endoscopy is the primary diagnostic investigation and is undertaken after optimum resuscitation has been achieved. In most cases, it is best performed within 24 hours of admission, on the first available elective list. Out-of-hours emergency endoscopy is occasionally required in actively bleeding, shocked patients. Endoscopy has three purposes.

1. It provides an accurate diagnosis. Certain diagnoses greatly influence management; for example, esophageal varices and active bleeding from peptic ulcers require specific endoscopic and pharmacological interventions.

2. Prognostic information helps direct the patient to the high-dependency unit, the general ward or, in some very low-risk cases, immediate hospital discharge.

3. Most importantly, endoscopy facilitates application of specific therapies to high-risk bleeding lesions.

Endoscopic therapy

At least 80% of patients admitted to hospital for hematemesis and melena have an excellent prognosis; bleeding stops spontaneously and supportive therapy is all that is required. Endoscopic therapy is indicated in the following situations:

- bleeding esophageal varices;
- peptic ulcer with major stigmata of recent hemorrhage (active spurting bleeding, a nonbleeding visible vessel and nonadherent clot);
- vascular malformations, including actively bleeding arteriovenous malformations, gastric antral vascular ectasia and Dieulafoy lesion;
- rarely, active bleeding from a Mallory–Weiss tear.

Specific treatments

The frequency in which the various causes of acute upper gastrointestinal hemorrhage are encountered are listed in Table 21.2.

Table 21.2 Causes of hematemesis and melena.

Cause	Proportion of patients (%)
Peptic ulcer (duodenal, gastric and stomal)	30–35
Varices	5–10
Esophagitis	10–15
Mallory–Weiss tear	5
Erosions (gastric and duodenal)	10–15
Tumors (benign and malignant)	2–4
Vascular malformations	1–3
Small bowel and colonic	5
None found	2–20

Peptic ulcer is the most frequent cause of major, life-threatening acute gastrointestinal bleeding. Significant hemorrhage results from erosion of an underlying artery, and the magnitude of bleeding is directly related to the size of the arterial defect and the diameter of the artery. Consequently, bleeding may be particularly severe from large, posterior duodenal ulcers eroding the gastroduodenal artery and high, lesser curve gastric ulcers involving branches of the left gastric artery. Most patients present with little or no history of dyspepsia. A history of aspirin or NSAID use is common. The management of peptic ulcer bleeding is discussed below (page 121).

Esophagogastric varices are a less common cause, but because of the severity of bleeding and of underlying liver disease in the majority of patients, their impact upon service utilization is disproportionately great. The portal pressure is greater than 12 mmHg, usually as a consequence of cirrhosis, occasionally from portal vein occlusion. At the time of diagnosis of cirrhosis, varices are present in 60% of decompensated and 30% of compensated patients and their presence and size is associated with the severity of liver disease and continued alcohol abuse. The management of varices is discussed in Chapter 24.

Mallory–Weiss tears occur at the esophagogastric junction and are a consequence of prolonged retching. Alcohol abuse is the usual cause, but other causes of nausea and vomiting (e.g. chemotherapy, digoxin toxicity, renal failure, advanced malignancy) may be responsible. Bleeding usually stops spontaneously and active endoscopic or surgical intervention is required only in the presence of continuing active bleeding. Endoscopic application of clips is the treatment of choice; underrunning of the tear at open surgery is very rarely necessary.

Esophagitis is common in elderly patients presenting with "coffee-ground" hematemesis. Bleeding is seldom life-threatening; in most cases, conservative supportive therapy combined with proton pump inhibitor drugs is all that is necessary. However, it is important to be aware that, in this group of patients, coffee-ground vomiting may have another cause (drug toxicity, underlying renal or cardiac failure, pancreatitis or colon cancer), even when esophagitis is proven at endoscopy. Although the natural history of the bleeding event may be benign, the prognosis is often dictated by comorbidities.

Gastritis, duodenitis and gastroduodenal erosions are associated with NSAIDs and *H. pylori* infection. In most patients, supportive therapy and cessation of NSAID use or *H. pylori* eradication therapy achieve a favorable outcome.

Vascular anomalies may present with hematemesis and melena.

• Small arteriovenous malformations are often found at routine endoscopy during investigation for dyspepsia, and in this situation should be ignored. In other cases, large or multiple arteriovenous malformations can cause significant bleeding. This usually leads to insidious development of iron deficiency anemia, but occasionally major acute hemorrhage occurs. Most arteriovenous malformations have no obvious cause and present in elderly patients; in younger patients, they are sometimes caused by hereditary hemorrhagic telangiectasia. Other patients have valvular heart disease or an artificial heart valve, and bleeding may be exacerbated by anticoagulant drugs. Thermocoagulation by the heater probe or bipolar coagulation is the preferred treatment of choice.

• Gastric antral vascular ectasia is an uncommon vascular anomaly characterized by linear, readily bleeding red streaks radiating from the pylorus into the gastric antrum. It is occasionally associated with liver disease. Most patients present with iron deficiency anemia rather than acute bleeding, and some require frequent blood transfusion. The most convenient treatment modality is argon plasma coagulation. This usually requires multiple sessions.

• Portal hypertensive gastropathy results from venous congestion of the gastric mucosa; in most patients, this is caused by portal hypertension from cirrhosis. Endoscopic therapy has no significant therapeutic role and treatment is based upon reduction of portal pressure using propanolol, transjugular intrahepatic portosystemic shunt (TIPS) or (rarely) portacaval shunt surgery.

• Dieulafoy lesion is an unusual cause of acute bleeding in which a superficial submucosal artery is eroded. The diagnosis can be made only when endoscopy is undertaken during active bleeding; though the arterial damage is probably caused by a small ulcer, no mucosal lesion can be identified after bleeding has ceased. The most common site of a Dieulafoy lesion is the gastric fundus; it may also develop in the duodenum or other parts of the stomach. The optimum endoscopic therapy is unclear, but application of clips or thermocoagulation have been used with success.

Esophagogastric tumors are a relatively uncommon cause of acute upper gastrointestinal hemorrhage. The most important benign type is gastrointestinal stromal cell tumor (previously termed 'leiomyoma'), which arises from the muscle layers of the gastric or duodenal wall. Erosion through the mucosa gives a characteristic umbilicated endoscopic appearance. These tumors erode underlying arteries and may cause major bleeding. Rarely, large tumors become malignant. Surgical resection is indicated.

Carcinomas and lymphomas of the stomach tend to present with other upper gastrointestinal symptoms and iron deficiency anemia rather than with hematemesis and melena. Thermocoagulation using argon plama coagulation may reduce blood loss in patients who have unresectable disease.

Aortoduodenal fistula should be considered in all patients presenting with major upper gastrointestinal bleeding after aortic graft insertion. Bleeding occurs from the second part of the duodenum, is massive and may recur over hours or days. All such patients should be referred to a vascular unit immediately after initial resuscitation. Endoscopic findings are nonspecific and usually comprise either massive acute bleeding or a blood clot. The main purpose of endoscopy is to exclude other causes prior to surgical referral; there are no specific endoscopic features and the optimum diagnostic modality is CT scanning which usually reveals an inflammatory mass associated with the graft, as it abuts upon the third part of the duodenum.

Small bowel or right-sided colonic disease sometimes presents with melena and rarely with hematemesis. Colonoscopy, barium radiology and enteroscopy are used to identify the underlying tumor or vascular anomaly when upper gastrointestinal endoscopy fails to identify a bleeding source. In young patients, a bleeding Meckel diverticulum should be considered. The management will depend on the specific underlying cause of bleeding.

Management of peptic ulcer hemorrhage

The evidence supporting endoscopy therapy is based on clinical trials for peptic ulcer hemorrhage. Three categories of direct endoscopic treatment have been evaluated; each attempts to seal the arterial defect created by the ulcer.

Injection

Direct injection of fluids into the bleeding ulcer using disposable needles is technically straightforward. Its efficacy is proven by many clinical trials, though the mechanism of benefit remains speculative; tamponade by compressing the artery within the fibrous confines of the chronic ulcer, vasoconstriction induced by epinephrine, endarteritis caused by sclerosants or alcohol, and a direct effect on blood clot formation from fibrin glue or thrombin may all be relevant.

The most widely used injection fluid is 1:10000 epinephrine. This stops active bleeding in more than 90% of patients, but 15–20% rebleed [5]. Epinephrine injection is extremely safe and has no significant complications. Addition of sclerosants (polidocanol, sodium tetradecyl sulfate, ethanolamine) or alcohol does not reduce the risk of rebleeding and carries a risk of life-threatening necrosis of the injected area; for these reasons, they should not be used. Fibrin glue (a mixture of thrombin and fibrinogen injected through separate channels of a sophisticated needle) and human thrombin are probably the most effective injection materials, have a low complication rate but are not freely available.

Heat energy

In this method, devices are applied directly to the bleeding point at endoscopy, to cause coagulation and thrombosis. The heater probe is pushed firmly onto the bleeding lesion to apply tamponade, and defined pulses of heat energy are then given to coagulate the vessel. Clinical trials have shown the device to be as effective and as safe as injection therapy. Bipolar coagulation, in which electrical energy is conducted between multiple probes on the tip of an endoscopically positioned catheter, is as effective as the heater probe. The argon plasma coagulator also appears to be effective in arresting bleeding in limited clinical trials. Thermal treatments can cause perforations but this risk is very low.

Mechanical devices

"Endoclips" can be applied to visible vessels. They can be difficult to deploy on awkwardly positioned ulcers, but may be the best option for treatment of major bleeding ulcers. Arterial defects of more than 1 mm diameter do not usually respond to injection therapy, but an adequately positioned clip can stop bleeding from relatively large arteries. The major hazard is exacerbation of bleeding, should application prove unsuccessful.

Combinations of endoscopic therapy

Although the exact modes of action of these endoscopic therapies are largely speculative, it is clear that each achieves hemostasis by a different mechanism. A metaanalysis of published trials shows that combination of injection and thermal treatments is superior to single modality treatment [6].

Rebleeding after endoscopic therapy

Endoscopic therapy can achieve primary hemostasis in most patients with a bleeding ulcer. However, rebleeding occurs in 15–20% of cases, usually within the first 24 hours. It is most common when the initial bleeding episode was severe; thus, shocked patients presenting with active, spurting hemorrhage from large, posterior duodenal ulcers are the group most likely to rebleed.

Management following rebleeding is often difficult and is largely based on clinical judgment and local expertise. Discussion between endoscopist and gastrointestinal surgeon is vital. In most patients, it is appropriate to repeat the endoscopy and re-treat the bleeding lesion. A trial from Hong Kong showed that the mortality and blood transfusion requirements of patients who rebled after initially successful endoscopic therapy were similar whether they were treated with urgent surgery or repeat endoscopic therapy [7].

Once adequate hemostasis is achieved by endoscopic retreatment, an expectant policy is reasonable. The place of second-look endoscopy, performed once primary endoscopic hemostasis has been achieved, remains controversial. It is entirely appropriate to repeat endoscopy if there is doubt regarding the adequacy of endoscopic treatment, or if blood clot prevented therapy and in these circumstances the repeat procedure should be done within 24 hours of the initial endoscopy since approximately 80% of rebleeding episodes occur within this time frame. Some experts routinely repeat endoscopy in all patients who receive endoscopic therapy for major stigmata, and a metaanalysis of published trials shows this to have marginal benefits [6].

Drug therapy

A range of drugs have been evaluated with the aim of reducing further bleeding once endoscopic hemostasis has been achieved. Of these, only acid suppressive therapy has a strong evidence base. The rationale is based upon the observation that the stability of blood clot is low in an acid environment. It is crucial that gastric pH does not fall below 6, and the only practical means of achieving this is constant infusion of a proton pump inhibitor. This can be achieved most readily by intravenous infusion of a proton pump inhibitor drug (e.g. omeprazole or pantoprazole, 80 mg bolus followed by an 8 mg/hour infusion for 72 hours). Metaanalyses have demonstrated that this significantly reduces the risk of rebleeding and need for emergency surgery, although it has not been shown to significantly reduce mortality [8]. Other regimens have also been shown to reduce the rate of ulcer rebleeding; these include high-dose oral omeprazole and high-dose intravenous famotidine, and both approaches need more study.

Somatostatin and tranexamic acid are also sometimes used to reduce ulcer rebleeding although the evidence base for their use is less secure.

Drug therapies are only valuable in patients at high risk of further bleeding (i.e. those with major stigmata of recent hemorrhage); ulcers without major stigmata have an excellent prognosis without specific intervention. While the council of perfection is therefore only to use these drugs after endoscopy (and endoscopic therapy), it has become standard practice to start proton pump inhibitor infusions in all bleeding patients at the time of initial resuscitation, particularly if there are likely to be significant delays in undertaking endoscopy. A Cochrane review suggests that the oral route of administration of proton pump inhibitors may be just as effective as the intravenous route as long as a high dose is used.

Surgical intervention

For patients with ulcer bleeding, emergency surgery is undertaken when endoscopic therapy combined with pharmacological intervention fails to secure permanent hemostasis, as follows:

• Active bleeding cannot be controlled by endoscopic therapy because torrential hemorrhage obscures the bleeding point, or active bleeding continues despite successful application of endoscopic therapy.

• Rebleeding follows initially successful endoscopic treatment (it is reasonable to repeat endoscopic therapy on one occasion after rebleeding, providing local expertise is available and only after discussion between endoscopist and surgeon).

The type of operation depends on the site of the ulcer. Bleeding duodenal ulcers are treated by underrunning the ulcer, sometimes with pyloroplasty. Gastric ulcers are treated with partial gastrectomy or simple ulcer excision. Vagotomy is no longer undertaken because proton pump inhibitor drugs abolish acid secretion.

Secondary prophylaxis

After hemostasis has been achieved, it is important to prevent late recurrent hemorrhage. For ulcer patients eradication of *H. pylori* almost abolishes the risk of late rebleeding. In patients who need, for good reason, to continue NSAID therapy, the following should be considered.

• Use the least toxic NSAID that controls the arthritic symptoms.

• Co-prescribe a proton pump inhibitor with the NSAID.

• Consider use of a COX-2-specific antiinflammatory drug rather than a conventional NSAID. These are associated with significantly fewer recurrent ulcer-related adverse events (both hemorrhage and perforation) although concerns concerning increased vascular events have largely precluded their use.

• The management of patients with *H. pylori* who need to continue taking an NSAID remains controversial. Gastritis (an inevitable consequence of *H. pylori* infection) induces mucosal prostaglandin production, and this may protect the gastroduodenal mucosa from the harmful effects of NSAIDs. However, current studies suggest that the magnitude of prostaglandin production is unlikely to outweigh the deleterious effects of *H. pylori*, and that eradication therapy is indicated in patients with a bleeding ulcer who are *H. pylori* positive and require NSAID therapy.

References

1. Church NC, Palmer KR. Non-variceal gastrointestinal haemorrhage. In: Evidence-based Gastroenterology and Hepatology, 2nd edition. McDonald JWD, Burroughs AK, Feagan BG (eds). Oxford, Blackwell Publications, 2004; 139–59.
2. Rockall TA, Logan RFA, Devlin HB, Northfield TC. Risk assessment following acute upper gastrointestinal haemorrhage. Gut 1996; 38:316–21.
3. Blatchford O, Murray WR, Blatchford M. A risk score to predict need for treatment for upper gastrointestinal haemorrhage. Lancet 2000; 356:1319.
4. Bornman PC, Theodorou N, Shuttleworth RD et al. Importance of hypovolaemic shock and endoscopic signs in predicting recurrent haemorrhage from peptic ulceration: a prospective evaluation. Brit Med J 1985; 291:245–7.
5. Chung SCS, Leung JWC, Steele RJC. Endoscopic injection of adrenaline for actively bleeding ulcers: a randomised trial. Brit Med J 1988; 296:1631–3.
6. Calvet X, Vergara M, Brullet E et al. Addition of a second endoscopic treatment following epinephrine injection improves outcome in high-risk bleeding ulcers. Gastroenterology 2004; 126:441–50.
7. Lau JY, Sung JJ, Lam YH et al. Endoscopic retreatment compared with surgery in patients with recurrent bleeding after initial endoscopic control of bleeding ulcers. N Eng J Med 1999;340: 751–4.
8. Leontiadis GI, Sharma VK, Howden CW. Proton Pump Inhibitor treatment for acute peptic ulcer bleeding The Cochrane data base of systematic reviews: Review 2006 Issue 1.

22 Acute Pancreatitis

David R. Lichtenstein

Introduction

Acute pancreatitis is best defined as an acute inflammatory process of the pancreas that may also involve peripancreatic tissues and remote organ systems. The overall incidence is 1 in 4000 for the general population. Most patients with acute pancreatitis have a mild course and recover with restoration of normal pancreatic function and gland architecture. However, in 10–20%, the various pathways that contribute to increased intrapancreatic and extrapancreatic inflammation result in what is generally termed systemic inflammatory response syndrome (SIRS). In some instances, SIRS predisposes to multiple organ dysfunction and/or pancreatic necrosis. Early steps in the management of patients with acute pancreatitis can decrease severity, morbidity and mortality. Prevention of the septic and nonseptic complications in patients with severe acute pancreatitis depends largely on monitoring, vigorous hydration, and early recognition of pancreatic necrosis and choledocholithiasis.

Clinical presentation and complications (see Table 22.1)

Abdominal pain is virtually always present and may be severe and refractory to analgesics. Pain is located generally in the epigastrium, often radiates to the back and is usually worse when supine. The onset may be swift with pain reaching maximum intensity within 30 min, is frequently unbearable, and characteristically

persists for more than 24 h without relief. The pain is often associated with nausea and vomiting. Physical examination usually reveals severe upper abdominal tenderness at times associated with guarding. Ileus occurs when there is extension of the inflammatory process into the small intestinal and colonic mesentery or a chemical peritonitis occurs.

With acute pancreatitis, a variety of toxic substances including pancreatic enzymes, vasoactive materials (e.g. kinins), and other toxic substances (e.g. elastase, phospholipase A2) are liberated by the pancreas and extravasate along fascial planes in the retroperitoneal space, lesser sac and peritoneal cavity [1]. These materials cause chemical irritation and contribute to third space losses of protein-rich fluid, hypovolemia and hypotension. These toxic substances may also reach the systemic circulation by lymphatic and venous pathways and contribute to subcutaneous fat necrosis and end-organ damage, including shock, renal failure and respiratory insufficiency (atelectasis, effusions and acute respiratory distress syndrome). Grey Turner's sign (ecchymosis of the flank) or Cullen's sign (ecchymosis in the periumbilical region) may be seen in association with hemorrhagic pancreatitis.

Metabolic problems are common in severe disease and include hypocalcemia, hyperglycemia and acidosis. Hypocalcemia is most commonly caused by concomitant hypoalbuminemia [2]. Other mechanisms may include complexing of calcium to released free fatty acids, protease-induced degradation of circulating parathyroid hormone (PTH), and failure of PTH to release calcium from bone. Local spread of inflammation leads to effects on contiguous organs that include gastritis and duodenitis, splenic vein thrombosis, colonic necrosis, and external compression of the common bile duct leading to biliary obstruction. Trypsin can activate plasminogen to plasmin and induce clot lysis. Conversely,

Gastrointestinal Emergencies, 2nd edition. Edited by Tony Tham, John Collins and Roy Soetikno. © 2009 by Blackwell Publishing, ISBN: 978-1-4051-4634-0.

Table 22.1 Clinical presentation and complications of acute pancreatitis.

Mild ↓ Severe	**Pancreatic autodigestion**	■ Edema, hemorrhage, necrosis, atrophy ■ Reduced exocrine function ■ Reduced endocrine function
	Local spread	■ Fat necrosis ■ Peripancreatic fluid ✓ ascites, pseudocyst, abscess ■ Retroperitoneal hemorrhage ■ Enteric erosion or obstruction
	Systemic	■ Hypovolemia, hypoalbuminemia ■ Coagulopathies ■ Pulmonary dysfunction (ARDS) ■ CNS ■ Renal

trypsin can activate prothrombin and thrombin and produce thrombosis, leading to disseminated intravascular coagulation.

Extrapancreatic fluid collections [3] occur when fluid extravasates from the pancreas or surrounding leaky tissues. They are located in or near the pancreas, and lack a wall of granulation or fibrous tissue. Acute fluid collections occur more commonly with severe pancreatitis. Most of these lesions regress spontaneously and almost all remain sterile.

Pancreatic pseudocysts [3] (Fig. 22.1) are defined as encapsulated nonepithelial lined collections of pancreatic juice, either pure or containing debris, single or multiple, small or large, and can be located in or adjacent to the pancreas. Fluid collections must be present for a minimum of 4 weeks from the onset of pancreatitis to be termed a pseudocyst. While most pseudocysts remain asymptomatic, presenting symptoms may include abdominal pain, early satiety, nausea, and vomiting due to compression of the stomach or gastric outlet. Rapidly enlarging pseudocysts may rupture, hemorrhage, obstruct the extrahepatic biliary tree, erode into surrounding structures, extend into the mediastinum, and become infected. Most pseudocysts less than 6 cm in diameter will resolve over time and a third of lesions less than 10 cm in diameter remain asymptomatic or resolve. Indications for pseudocyst drainage include suspicion of infection or progressive enlargement with associated symptoms described above. Asymptomatic pseudocysts should be followed. Pseudocysts can be

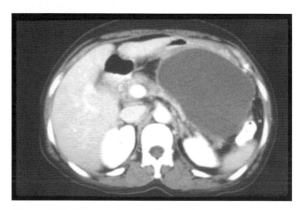

Figure 22.1 CT scan of pancreatic pseudocyst.

drained surgically, percutaneously or endoscopically. The choice of treatment for symptomatic pseudocysts is frequently determined by the locally available expertise and by clinician preference since no method has been shown to be superior to the others.

Pancreatic abscesses [3] are circumscribed intraabdominal collections of pus, usually in proximity to the pancreas. They contain little or no pancreatic necrosis. A pancreatic abscess usually does not occur until 4 to 6 weeks after the onset of acute pancreatitis.

Pancreatic fistulae [4] occur as a result of duct disruption and are treated with parenteral nutrition, endoscopic stenting and somatostatin analogue. Surgical intervention may be needed if this conservative approach is unsuccessful.

Table 22.2 Diagnosis of acute pancreatitis.

Signs and symptoms	Labs	Differential diagnosis
• Abdominal pain	• ↑ WBC	• Cholecystitis
• Abdominal tenderness	• ↑ Serum amylase	• Peptic ulcer disease
• Nausea and vomiting	• ↑ Serum lipase	• Diverticulitis
• Fever		• Intestinal ischemia
• Tachycardia		• Intestinal obstruction
		• Salpingitis
		• Ectopic pregnanacy

Diagnosis: clinical and imaging

The diagnosis of acute pancreatitis (Table 22.2) is based on a combination of clinical, biochemical, and radiological factors. There is general acceptance that a diagnosis of acute pancreatitis [3] requires two of the following three features: (1) abdominal pain characteristic of acute pancreatitis, (2) serum amylase and/ or lipase ≥ 3 times the upper limit of normal, and (3) characteristic findings of acute pancreatitis on CT scan.

Increases in serum pancreatic enzymes may occur in a variety of other conditions including bowel perforation, obstruction, mesenteric ischemia, tuboovarian disease and renal failure [2]. In general, serum lipase is thought to be more sensitive and specific than serum amylase in the diagnosis of acute pancreatitis. Serum lipase may be preferable because it remains normal in some nonpancreatic conditions associated with an elevation of serum amylase including macroamylasemia, parotitis and tuboovarian disease. Serum lipase remains elevated longer than serum amylase and therefore may be helpful if a patient delays seeking medical attention [2]. Repeated measurements of pancreatic enzymes have little value in assessing clinical progress of the illness or ultimate prognosis. Moreover, the magnitude of serum amylase or lipase elevation does not correlate with the severity of pancreatitis.

Transabdominal ultrasound and computed tomography are the two imaging modalities most frequently used in patients with acute pancreatitis. These techniques tend to be complementary. Ultrasound is very good at detecting gallbladder stones (accuracy of 90%); however, the reported sensitivity of ultrasound for the detection of common bile duct stones is limited and ranges from 20% to 75%, although specificity is quite high if they are identified. Dilation of the common bile duct alone is neither sensitive nor specific for the detection of common bile duct stones. Visualization of the pancreas with ultrasound in the face of ongoing acute pancreatitis tends to be poor due to overlying intestinal gas. Occasionally, the pancreas is adequately visualized by abdominal ultrasound to reveal features that are consistent with the diagnosis of acute pancreatitis including diffuse glandular enlargement, hypoechoic texture of the pancreas reflective of edema, and ascites.

Contrast-enhanced CT (CECT) scan [1–3,5] is best used to exclude conditions that masquerade as acute pancreatitis and to confirm a diagnosis of pancreatitis (pancreatic enlargement, peripancreatic inflammatory change and extrapancreatic fluid collections). Additionally, CECT scans may prove useful in evaluating complications (acute fluid collections, abscess, pseudocyst and necrosis) and assessing severity of disease (see below). Note that a normal CT scan is present in 15–30% of those with mild disease. There is controversy as to whether the use of intravenous contrast agents may result in adverse outcomes in patients with acute pancreatitis during the initial 24 to 48 hours. Decreased pancreatic capillary flow rates after intravenous contrast administration have been observed in two animal studies. Since prospective and randomized human studies are not available, it is reasonable to reserve CECT scans for patients with severe acute pancreatitis, patients with smoldering acute pancreatitis that is slow to improve, patients with suspected local complications, and patients with an unclear etiology of the attack of pancreatitis.

MRI scanning is similar to CT with respect to imaging the inflamed pancreas and may be preferred in individuals at risk for contrast-induced injury (e.g. contrast allergy or renal insufficiency). However, recent studies also indicate the potential for gadolinium-induced nephrotoxicity with MRI examinations [6]. MRI is also sensitive for the detection of necrosis [7] and small neoplasms when these are under consideration. MRCP is a noninvasive means of imaging the pancreaticobiliary tree and has a sensitivity of greater than 90% for common bile duct stones.

Assessment of severity and outcome

Clinical and laboratory data

Despite the importance of recognizing severe disease early in the course, many patients initially identified as having mild disease progress to severe disease indolently over the initial 48 to 72 hours. The overall mortality rate for acute pancreatitis is 5–10%. Early deaths within the first two weeks are frequently due to multisystem organ failure caused by the release of inflammatory mediators and cytokines. Late deaths are more likely to result from local or systemic infection. The risks of infection and death correlate with severity of disease and the presence and extent of pancreatic necrosis. Therefore, patients should be stratified into 'mild' or 'severe' levels of illness based on clinical assessment, scoring systems, serum markers, and CECT (contrast enhanced computerized tomography) scanning [1–3]. Patients with mild acute pancreatitis constitute 80% of all attacks and less than 5% of mortality. Mild acute pancreatitis usually runs an uneventful self-limited course. Scoring systems such as Ranson's criteria or the Acute Physiologic and Chronic Health Evaluation (APACHE II) system are used by some clinicians but they have limitations, particularly since the scores cannot be finalized until 48 hours into the hospitalization. With increasing scores, the likelihood of a complicated, prolonged and often fatal course increases. Ranson's 11 prognostic indicators include five that are available on admission which in general reflect the severity of the acute inflammatory process (age >55 years, WBC >16000/mm³, glucose >200 mg/dL, LDH >350 IU/L, AST >250 U/L) whereas the six that are measured at the end of the first 48 hours reflect the systemic effects of circulating

Table 22.3 Simplified Glasgow prognostic scoring criteria.

During initial 48 hours	
Age	>55 years
WBC	>15,000 mm³
LDH	>600 IU/L
Glucose	>180 mg/dL (10 mmol/L)
Albumin	<32 g/L
Calcium	<8 mg/dL (2.0 mmol/L)
PaO₂	<60 mmHg (8 kPa)
Urea	>45 mg/dL (16 mmol/L)
>3 signs indicates severe attack	

Table 22.4 Indicators of organ failure.

Hypotension	Systolic BP <90 mmHg
Hypoxia	PaO₂ ≤60 mmHg
Renal failure	Creatinine >2 mg/dL
GI bleeding	>500 mL/24 hours

enzymes including respiratory failure, renal failure and fluid sequestration (Hct decreased >10, BUN >5 mg/dL, PO₂ <60 mmHg, base deficit >4 mEq/L, serum calcium <8 mg/dL, and estimated fluid sequestration >6L). In many series, mortality is approximately 10–20% when there are three to five signs, and >50% when there are six or more Ranson's signs. A simplified version of the Ranson criteria is the Glasgow prognostic scoring criteria (Table 22.3).

Other cytokine markers (e.g. CRP, TAP, elastase, etc.) as well as the initial hematocrit as a surrogate marker of hemoconcentration will assist in predicting the prognosis.

Any presence of organ dysfunction predicts severe disease (Table 22.4).

Pancreatic imaging: interstitial vs. necrotizing disease

CECT is useful for assessing severity of pancreatitis. A CT severity index (Table 22.5) grades severity of pancreatitis by the number of peripancreatic fluid collections and amount of necrosis on dynamic scanning. The distinction between interstitial and necrotizing acute pancreatitis has important prognostic implications (Fig. 22.2). Approximately 20–30% of patients

Table 22.5 CT severity index for acute pancreatitis.

Unenhanced CT Finding	Grade	Score	Enhanced CT Necrosis	Score
Normal	A	0	0	0
Pancreatic enlargement	B	1		
Peripancreatic stranding	C	2	<33%	2
Single peripancreatic collection	D	3	33-50%	4
Multiple peripancreatic collections	E	4	>50%	6

CT severity index equals unenhanced CT score plus necrosis score: maximum=10, greater than or equal to 6=severe disease
Adapted from Balthazar EJ. Radiology 2002;223:603

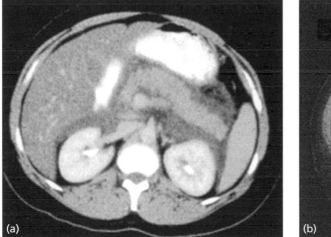 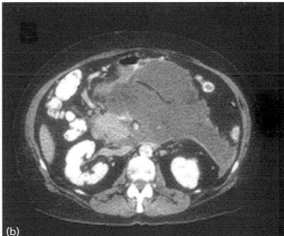

Figure 22.2 Contrasted CT scans demonstrating interstitial pancreatitis (a) and necrotizing pancreatitis (b).

with acute pancreatitis have necrotizing pancreatitis; the remainder has interstitial pancreatitis, which is defined by an intact microcirculation and uniform enhancement of the gland on CECT. Necrotizing pancreatitis is characterized by disruption of the pancreatic microcirculation such that large areas do not enhance on CECT following bolus intravenous administration of contrast material. The clinical significance of pancreatic necrosis is that it predicts a worse severity of pancreatitis, and increased risk of infection in the necrotic pancreatic tissue termed infected necrosis. In one series, those with necrosis had a morbidity of 82% and a mortality of 23%, whereas those without necrosis (interstitial) had a morbidity of 6% and a mortality of 0% [14]. Pancreatic infection develops in 30–50% of patients with acute necrotizing pancreatitis but rarely in those with interstitial disease (<1%). Translocation of bacteria from the colon is likely the most important cause of infected necrosis. The necrosis should be considered sterile during the early days following admission. Aspiration of suspected infected pancreatic necrosis to guide surgical intervention typically becomes of importance after the first week to 10 days. The overall mortality in severe acute necrotizing pancreatitis triples if there is infected necrosis (10% vs. 30%) [14].

Etiology of acute pancreatitis

The pathogenesis of acute pancreatitis remains incompletely understood. Based on experimental models, the initiating event in acute pancreatitis is intraacinar activation of trypsin from trypsinogen, resulting in acute intracellular injury, pancreatic autodigestion, and the potential for profound systemic complications once activated enzymes are leaked into the bloodstream. Initiating events may include obstruction of the pancreatic duct (e.g. gallstones, pancreatic tumor), overdistention of the pancreatic duct (e.g. from ERCP), reflux of biliary or duodenal juices into the pancreatic duct, changes in permeability of the pancreatic duct, ischemia of the organ, and toxin-induced cholinergic hyperstimulation.

During the initial hospitalization for acute pancreatitis, reasonable attempts to determine etiology is appropriate, and in particular those causes that may affect acute management. The cause for acute pancreatitis is readily identified in 70–90% of patients after an initial evaluation consisting of history, physical examination, focused laboratory testing, and routine radiological evaluation. Relevant historical clues include any previous diagnosis of biliary tract disease or gallstones, cholecystectomy, other biliary or pancreatic surgery, acute or chronic pancreatitis or their complications, use of ethanol, medications and the timing of their initiation, recent abdominal trauma, weight loss or other symptoms suggesting a malignancy, or a family history of pancreatitis. Blood tests within the first 24 h should include liver chemistries, calcium and triglycerides. There are an extensive number of potential etiologies for acute pancreatitis as indicated below (Table 22.6). Approximately 80% of those with acute pancreatitis are due to alcohol or gallstones.

Alcohol

Acute alcoholic pancreatitis is the most common cause of pancreatitis. Only a minority of individuals who abuse alcohol will develop pancreatitis. The discrete mechanism by which alcohol may induce pancreatitis remains unclear. Many patients with otherwise

Table 22.6 Causes of acute pancreatitis.

Obstructive Causes
Gallstones
Tumors—ampullary or pancreatic tumors
Parasites—*Ascaris* or *Clonorchis*
Developmental anomalies—pancreas divisum, choledochocele, annular pancreas
Periampullary duodenal diverticula
Hypertensive sphincter of Oddi
Afferent duodenal loop obstruction

Toxins
Ethyl alcohol
Methyl alcohol
Scorpion venom—excessive cholinergic stimulation causes salivation, sweating, dyspnea, and cardiac arrhythmias; seen mostly in the West Indies
Organophosphorus insecticides

Drugs
Definite association (documented with rechallenges): azathioprine/6-MP, valproic acid, estrogens, tetracycline, metronidazole, nitrofurantoin, pentamidine, furosemide, sulfonamides, methyldopa, cytarabine, cimetidine, ranitidine, sulindac, dideoxycytidine
Probable association: thiazides, ethacrynic acid, phenformin, procainamide, chlorthalidone, L-asparaginase

Metabolic Causes
Hypertriglyceridemia, hypercalcemia, end-stage renal disease

Trauma
Accidental—blunt trauma to the abdomen (car accident, bicycle)
Iatrogenic—postoperative, ERCP, endoscopic sphincterotomy, sphincter of Oddi manometry

Infectious
Parasitic—ascariasis, clonorchiasis
Viral—mumps, rubella, hepatitis A, hepatitis B, non-A, non-B hepatitis, coxsackievirus B, echo, adenovirus, cytomegalovirus, varicella, Epstein-Barr, human immunodeficiency virus
Bacterial—mycoplasma, *Campylobacter jejuni*, tuberculosis, *Legionella*, leptospirosis

Vascular
Ischemia—hypoperfusion (such as after cardiac surgery) or atherosclerotic emboli
Vasculitis—systemic lupus erythematosus, polyarteritis nodosa, malignant hypertension

Idiopathic
10–30% of pancreatitis; up to 60% of these patients have occult gallstone disease (biliary microlithiasis or gallbladder sludge); other less common causes include sphincter of Oddi dysfunction and mutations in the cystic fibrosis transmembrane regulator

Miscellaneous
Penetrating peptic ulcer
Crohn's disease of the duodenum
Pregnancy associated
Pediatric association—Reye's syndrome, cystic fibrosis

idiopathic acute relapsing pancreatitis will deny or minimize their alcohol use and this can only be established with careful questioning.

Gallstone pancreatitis

Among patients with gallstones, the incidence of acute pancreatitis is 0.17% per year. The presence of gallstones, however, increases the relative risk of pancreatitis up to 25- to 35-fold. It is theorized that gallstone passage causes transient obstruction of the pancreatic duct, precipitating acute pancreatitis. Acute gallstone pancreatitis should be suspected when associated with transient elevation in liver-associated enzymes and in particular ALT >150 IU [8]. Most stones pass spontaneously from the ampulla and do not require intervention.

Microlithiasis

Microlithiasis may be identified in up to 30–65% of patients with idiopathic acute relapsing pancreatitis [9]. Bile collected from the biliary tree during ERCP or aspirated from the duodenum after administration of cholecystokinin should be examined for cholesterol monohydrate crystals or calcium bilirubinate granules under a polarizing light microscope. Several important issues limit the use of bile analysis. Many patients (29–34%) with gallstones (who all should be expected to have microlithiasis or crystals) have a negative bile analysis. Moreover, the technique is not standardized, and in particular the quantity of crystals needed to define a positive result differs among institutions. However, most believe that the presence of even a small number of crystals is abnormal. Prospective controlled trials in patients with acute relapsing pancreatitis have demonstrated that when microlithiasis is identified, treatment with cholecystectomy, biliary sphincterotomy or dissolution therapy can prevent recurrence of pancreatitis.

Hereditary pancreatitis

A number of studies have identified genetic mutations in patients with idiopathic pancreatitis, including mutations in the genes encoding cationic trypsinogen (PRSS1), pancreatic secretory trypsin inhibitor (serine protease inhibitor Kazal type 1 or SPINK-1) and cystic fibrosis transmembrane conductance regulator (CFTR) [10]. In general, the role of genetic testing in idiopathic acute pancreatitis is controversial. Diagnosis of these genetic disorders currently contributes little to direct patient management since no specific therapy is available. Similarly, inadvertent disclosure of the results of genetic testing might have significant negative effects on the patient and the ability to obtain health insurance. On the other hand, one could argue that the identification of an underlying genetic cause may obviate the need for further testing, might allow more informed family planning, and might allow better surveillance for complications including pancreatic cancer. The decision to pursue genetic testing is one that should only be made with the advice and involvement of an experienced counselor.

Pancreas divisum

Pancreas divisum is present in 5–10% of the general population. Pancreas divisum is diagnosed by pancreatography via ERCP (Fig. 22.3) or MRCP. Therapeutic maneuvers to increase drainage through the accessory papilla by endoscopic papillotomy or surgical sphincteroplasty may reduce the incidence of recurrent pancreatitis.

Hyperlipidemia

The breakdown products of triglycerides include toxic free fatty acids which are theorized to injure the endothelial lining of the small pancreatic blood vessels. Triglyceride levels greater than 1000 mg/dL are usually required to induce acute pancreatitis. In addition to primary hyperlipidemia, hypertriglyceridemia may result from therapy with estrogens and other pharmacological agents. Once patients recover from the acute

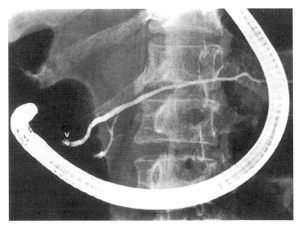

Figure 22.3 Pancreas divisum is diagnosed by pancreatography by ERCP via the minor papilla.

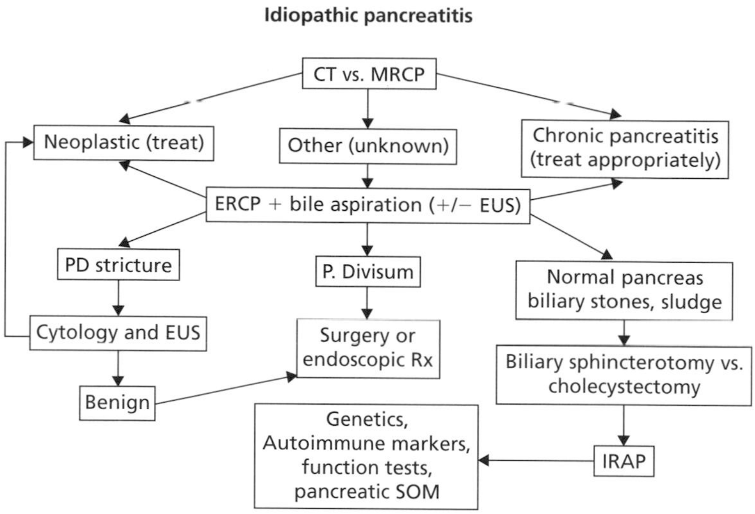

Idiopathic pancreatitis

Figure 22.4 Algorithm for evaluation of idiopathic pancreatitis.
SOM = sphincter of Oddi manometry, IRAP = idiopathic recurrent acute pancreatitis.

episode, treatment with lipid lowering agents and diet can effectively reduce the rate of recurrence.

Post-ERCP pancreatitis

Iatrogenic pancreatitis attributed to manipulation of the major papilla during ERCP is becoming an increasingly common cause of pancreatitis. In some series this is the third most common cause following gallstones and alcohol use. Post-ERCP pancreatitis is more apt to occur following Sphincter of Oddi manometry, biliary sphincterotomy, pancreatic duct manipulation, and in patients with a history of unexplained acute relapsing pancreatitis. Post-ERCP pancreatitis occurs in 3–25% of patients. Studies evaluating the use of corticosteroids and noniodinated contrast agents have failed to demonstrate a reduction in risk. Studies using intravenous Gabexate prior to ERCP demonstrate a decreased risk of post-ERCP pancreatitis. However, the cost and relative unavailability of this drug have contributed to its failure to achieve a significant clinical penetration.

Autoimmune pancreatitis

Autoimmune pancreatitis [11] is a benign disease characterized by irregular narrowing of the pancreatic duct, swelling of parenchyma, lymphoplasmacytic infiltration and fibrosis, and a favorable response to corticosteroid treatment. In this condition, the whole pancreas is diffusely affected; however, a few cases with focal mass lesions mimicking pancreatic adenocarcinoma are reported. Patients with autoimmune pancreatitis have high serum antinuclear antibody levels and serum IgG4 concentrations, providing a useful means of distinguishing this disorder from other diseases of the pancreas or biliary tract.

Idiopathic pancreatitis

Patients in whom an initial evaluation does not reveal an underlying etiology are classified as having 'idiopathic' acute pancreatitis. It is in these patients where one can consider a more extensive evaluation. In most analyses, the most common explanations which are identified with a more extensive evaluation include microlithiasis, sphincter of Oddi dysfunction (SOD), pancreas divisum and other congenital abnormalities, pancreatic and ampullary neoplasm, and genetic causes (Fig. 22.4) [12].

Up to 10–20% of adults with pancreatitis are termed idiopathic, although this classification is expected to become less common as factors of genetic predisposition and environmental susceptibility are elucidated. The serum amylase and lipase levels are used to help establish the diagnosis of acute pancreatitis but also may provide some insight into the underlying etiology. Pancreatitis resulting from gallstones, microlithiasis or drugs is typically associated with the highest levels of amylase and lipase and the degree of elevation of amylase tends to be greater than lipase. Elevations of liver chemistries are seen most commonly in patients with acute pancreatitis due to a biliary source, i.e.

gallstones, pancreatic or ampullary neoplasm, micro-lithiasis, choledochal cyst, choledochocele and SOD. An elevation of the ALT of greater than or equal to 150 IU/L (approximately a 3-fold elevation) is associated with a 95% probability of biliary pancreatitis [8]. Similarly, a bilirubin level greater than 2.0 mg/dL is predictive of biliary pancreatitis [13].

Treatment of acute pancreatitis

The treatment of acute pancreatitis (Fig. 22.5) depends on the severity of the disease, as well as the presence of any complications.

Supportive care

The goals of medical therapy include supportive care, limitation of systemic complications, and prevention of pancreatic infection once necrosis takes place. Patients with mild disease are treated supportively with intravenous hydration, parenteral analgesics, and bowel rest. Nasogastric tube suction is indicated for symptomatic relief in patients with nausea, vomiting and ileus. Severe acute pancreatitis with its inherent increased morbidity and mortality requires monitoring in an intensive care unit, aggressive fluid and electrolyte monitoring and replacement. There are no specific treatments proven to be effective in limiting systemic complications. Agents that put the pancreas to rest (e.g. somatostatin,

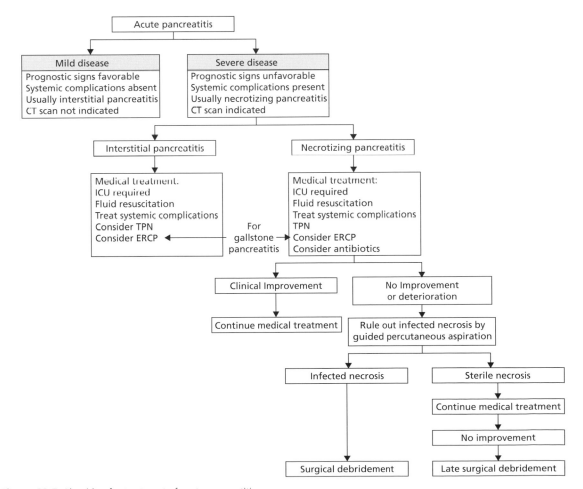

Figure 22.5 Algorithm for treatment of acute pancreatitis.

calcitonin, glucagon, nasogastric suction, H$_2$ blockers) and enzyme inhibitors (e.g. aprotinin, gabexate mesylate) have not been shown to lower morbidity and mortality [1–3].

Nutritional care

As most patients with acute pancreatitis have mild disease and resume oral feeding within several days, it is difficult to recommend nutritional support in all patients with acute pancreatitis. Ensuring adequate nutrition is important in patients with severe or complicated pancreatitis, but the optimal means of doing so remains controversial. To meet metabolic demands and rest the pancreas, nutrition can be provided by total parenteral nutrition (TPN) through central venous access or preferably as enteral feeding through a nasoenteric feeding tube placed into the jejunum. In general, it is reasonable to conclude from small, prospective, nonblinded studies that enteral feeding is safer and less expensive than TPN [15,16]. A metaanalysis of six randomized trials involving a total of 263 patients demonstrated improved outcomes with enteral nutrition, including decreased rates of infection, surgical intervention, a reduced length of hospital stay, and reduced costs (20% of the costs associated with total parenteral nutrition) [17]. However, no reduction in organ failure or mortality was demonstrated. Enteral feeding is usually well tolerated in patients with ileus. However, total parenteral nutrition may be necessary for patients with nasogastric tube discomfort, those who cannot obtain sufficient calories through enteral nutrition or in whom enteral access cannot be maintained.

ERCP in gallstone pancreatitis

Urgent ERCP with identification and clearance of bile duct stones is recommended for patients with evidence of ongoing biliary obstruction, as suggested by clinical and laboratory data. ERCP may also be considered for patients with severe, acute pancreatitis within 24 to 48 hours of the onset of the attack, although this remains controversial due to conflicting data from endoscopic studies [18]. MRCP and EUS can be used when there is a lower suspicion for common bile duct stones.

The risk of gallstone pancreatitis recurrence is as high as 50–75% in patients with an intact gallbladder

within the subsequent 6 months; therefore cholecystectomy is generally recommended. Biliary sphincterotomy leaving the gallbladder in situ is considered an effective alternative for those not considered to be candidates for cholecystectomy.

Prevention of infected necrosis

The proper role of antibiotics in acute pancreatitis remains controversial. No antibiotics are indicated in mild cases. However, infectious complications are an important concern in severe cases, especially those with pancreatic necrosis. A potential role for prophylactic antibiotics in severe pancreatitis was initially given support by a randomized trial demonstrating that the administration of imipenem reduced infectious complications, including central line sepsis, pulmonary infection, urinary tract infection, and infected pancreatic necrosis [19]. Subsequent trials yielded mixed, but generally confirmatory, results. However, a recent randomized trial [20] and metaanalysis [21] failed to demonstrate differences in outcome among patients treated with antibiotics as compared with placebo. As a result, most experts no longer recommend prophylactic antibiotics in acute necrotizing pancreatitis, with the added concern that prolonged use of potent antibiotic agents may lead to the emergence of resistant organisms and fungal infections in the necrotic pancreas. Under circumstances with necrotizing pancreatitis associated with fever, leukocytosis and/or organ failure, antibiotics should be administered while appropriate cultures (including culture of CT-guided percutaneous aspiration of the pancreas) are obtained. Antibiotics can be discontinued if no source of infection is found. Some centers use antifungal therapy in addition to antibacterial therapy, but this practice has not been validated by randomized trials.

Surgical management

Sterile pancreatic necrosis is generally treated medically during the first several weeks even in the presence of multisystem organ failure. Eventually, after the acute pancreatic inflammatory process has subsided and coalesced into an encapsulated structure, frequently called organized necrosis, debridement may be required for intractable abdominal pain, vomiting caused by extrinsic compression of stomach or duodenum, or systemic toxicity. Debridement can be performed by surgical, endoscopic or radiological techniques [1–3,17].

Surgical intervention is indicated in patients with infected pancreatic necrosis [17]. In most cases, the diagnosis is confirmed by fine-needle aspiration before surgical intervention, but because false negative results can occur (reported sensitivity, 88%), surgery also warrants consideration when there is a high index of suspicion of infected necrosis even if infection is not documented. Surgery within the first few days after the onset of severe acute pancreatitis is associated with rates of death up to 65%. Furthermore, there is no clear demarcation between viable and nonviable tissue early in the course of acute pancreatitis. Observational data support delaying surgical debridement of necrotic tissue for at least 2 weeks if possible while the patient's medical condition is optimized and viable pancreatic tissue becomes evident. This approach appears to improve survival and maximize organ preservation. Patients who are medically unfit for open surgical debridement can be treated with less invasive surgical techniques, radiological techniques, and, at times, endoscopic techniques in medical centers with these capabilities.

References

1. Pandol SJ, Saluja AK, Imrie CW, Banks PA. Reviews in basic and clinical gastroenterology. acute pancreatitis: bench to bedside. Gastroenterology 2007; 132:1127–51.

2. Forsmark CE, Baillie J. AGA Institute Technical Review on Acute Pancreatitis. Gastroenterology 2007; 132:2022–44.

3. Banks PA, Freeman ML and the Practice Parameters Committee of the American College of Gastroenterology. Am J Gastroenterol 2006; 101:2379–400.

4. Telford JJ, Farrell JJ, Saltzman JR, et al. Pancreatic stent placement for duct disruption. Gastrointest Endosc 2002; 56:18–24.

5. Balthazar EJ. Acute pancreatitis: assessment of severity with clinical and CT evaluation. Radiology 2002; 223:603–13.

6. Laissy JP, Idee JM, Fernandez P, et al. Magnetic resonance imaging in acute and chronic kidney disease: present status. Nephron Clin Pract 2006; 103:50–7.

7. Arvvanitakis M, Delhave M, De Maertelaere VD, et al. Computed tomography and magnetic resonance imaging in the assessment of acute pancreatitis. Gastroenterology 2004; 126:715–23.

8. Tenner S, Dubner H, Steinberg W. Predicting gallstone pancreatitis with laboratory parameters: a meta-analysis. Am J Gastroenterol 1994; 89:1863–9.

9. Saraswat VA, Sharma BC, Agarwal DK, et al. Biliary microlithiasis in patients with idiopathic acute pancreatitis and unexplained biliary pain: response to therapy. J Gastroenterol Hepatol 2004; 19:1206–11.

10. Witt H, Apte MV, Keim AV, Wilson JS. Chronic pancreatitis: challenges and advances in pathogenesis, genetics, diagnosis, and therapy. Gastroenterology 2007; 132:1557–73.

11. Kim KP, Kim MH, Song MH, et al. Autoimmune pancreatitis. Am J Gastroenterol 2004; 99:1605–16.

12. Dragnov P, Forsmark CE. Idiopathic pancreatitis. Gastroenterology 2005; 128:756–63.

13. Cohen ME, Slezak L, Wells CK, et al. Prediction of bile duct stones and complications in gallstone pancreatitis using early laboratory trends. Am J Gastroenterol 2001; 96:3305–11.

14. Vege SS, Baron TH. Management of pancreatic necrosis in severe acute pancreatitis. Clin Gastroenterol Hepatol 2005; 3:192–6.

15. Olah A, Pardavi G, Belagyi T, et al. Early nasojejunal feeding in acute pancreatitis is associated with a lower complication rate. Nutrition 2002; 18:259–62.

16. Petrov MS, Kukosh MV, Emelyanov NV. A randomized controlled trial of enteral versus parenteral feeding in patients with predicted severe acute pancreatitis shows a significant reduction in mortality and in infected pancreatic complications with total enteral nutrition. Dig Surg 2006;23:336–45.

17. Marik PE, Zaloga GP. Meta-analysis of parenteral nutrition versus enteral nutrition in patients with acute pancreatitis. BMJ 2004; 328:1407.

18. Mark DH, Lefevre F, Flamm CR, et al. Evidence-based assessment of ERCP in the treatment of pancreatitis. Gastrointest Endosc 2002; 56(6 suppl):S249–54.

19. Pederzoli P, Bassi C, Vesentini S, et al. A randomized multicenter trial of antibiotic prophylaxis of septic complications in acute necrotizing pancreatitis with imipenem. Surg Obstet Gynecol 1993; 176:480–3.

20. Isenmann R, Nzi MR, Kron M, et al. Prophylactic antibiotic treatment in patients with predicted severe acute pancreatitis: a placebo-controlled, double-blind trial. Gastroenterology 2004;126:997–1004.

21. Bai Y, Gao J, Zou D, Li Z. Prophylactic antibiotics cannot reduce infected pancreatic necrosis and mortality in acute necrotizing pancreatitis: evidence from a meta-analysis of randomized controlled trials. Am J Gastroenterol 2008; 103:104–10.

23 Biliary Emergencies

Bhavani Moparty, David L. Carr-Locke

Biliary emergencies include biliary colic, acute chole-cystitis, choledocholithiasis, cholangitis, gallstone pancreatitis (covered in Chapter 22), and bile leaks.

Biliary 'colic'

Clinical presentation

Biliary colic is a common misnamed manifestation of gallstone disease. Patients present with intermittent biliary pain that resolves after a few hours. It is usually constant and not typically colicky.

Diagnosis

It is important to differentiate biliary colic from other etiologies of pain such as cholecystitis, peptic ulcer disease, gastroesophageal reflux disease, pancreatitis, musculoskeletal pain, irritable bowel syndrome and cardiovascular disease.

Etiology

Biliary colic occurs due to intermittent obstruction of the cystic duct by stones.

History

The patient complains of right upper quadrant or epigastric pain. The pain gradually increases in intensity and then plateaus and resolves within a few hours. A longer duration of pain may be suggestive of another etiology.

Examination

There may be mild to moderate right upper quadrant tenderness or normal examination.

Gastrointestinal Emergencies, 2nd edition. Edited by Tony Tham, John Collins and Roy Soetikno. © 2009 by Blackwell Publishing, ISBN: 978-1-4051-4634-0.

Investigations

Laboratory findings are usually normal. An ultrasound of the abdomen should be performed to assess for gallstones and other gallbladder/biliary etiologies.

Management

In the patient with documented gallstones, an elective cholecystectomy should be recommended.

Acute cholecystitis

Clinical presentation

Patients present with constant right upper quadrant or epigastric pain which may radiate to the back or right shoulder. This pain may be associated with nausea, vomiting, fevers and leukocytosis. There is often a history of biliary colic. The pain of acute cholecystitis differs from biliary colic in that generally the pain is of longer duration and of more severe intensity. Acalculous cholecystitis accounts for about 10% of cases and is typically noted to occur in critically ill patients. Complications from cholecystitis are due to secondary infection leading to empyema, gangrene, perforation, emphysematous cholecystitis and gallstone ileus. The overall mortality is about 3% [1].

Diagnosis

The diagnosis is established with imaging studies revealing evidence of acute cholecystitis. See Table 23.1 for differential diagnosis.

Etiology

The pathogenesis is not completely understood. Bile stasis occurs due to cystic duct obstruction from gallstones, parasites, hemobilia, or tumor. As many as 90% of cases are due to gallstones. Acalculous cholecystitis can result

Table 23.1 Differential diagnosis of acute cholecystitis.

Differential diagnosis
Biliary colic
Acute appendicitis
Acute pancreatitis
Hepatitis
Peptic ulcer disease
Renal disease
Right-sided pneumonia
Fitz-Hugh Curtis syndrome (ascending pelvic infection and inflammation of the liver capsule or diaphragm)
Coronary artery disease
Intraabdominal abscess

from decreased gallbladder motility which can occur in severely ill patients typically who have been fasting, bedridden, receiving total parenteral nutrition, or mechanically ventilated.

History
Patients typically report a history of steady, severe pain which may have been precipitated after a fatty meal. Most patients also have a history of gallstones or biliary colic.

Examination
The physical examination may be significant for an ill appearing patient, who is febrile and has peritoneal signs (rebound tenderness, guarding). A Murphy's sign (pain on palpation of the right upper quadrant while the patient is inspiring deeply) can be present. If so, the diagnostic accuracy for cholecystitis is 80%. A patient who develops complications from cholecystitis such as empyema, gangrene, perforation, emphysematous cholecystitis and gallstone ileus appears more toxic in appearance with worsening of symptoms.

Investigations
Laboratory studies
Complete blood count should be checked to evaluate for leukocytosis. *Liver function tests* may be mildly elevated. If biliriubin, transaminases or alkaline phosphatase are significantly elevated, there may be a coexisting bile duct stone or Mirizzi syndrome (bile duct compression from impacted cystic duct stone). *Blood cultures* should be obtained.

Imaging
Abdominal radiography can be performed to assess for other etiologies of abdominal pain such as obstruction or perforation. It may occasionally show calcified stones. It can demonstrate free air, air in the biliary tree or gallbladder lumen indicating complications such as perforation, gallstone ileus or emphysematous cholecystitis respectively.

Ultrasound of the right upper quadrant may reveal gallstones, gallbladder wall thickening (4–5 mm), pericholecystic fluid, and a "sonographic Murphy's sign." In a review of 30 studies, the sensitivity and specificity for diagnosis of acute cholecystitis on ultrasound was 88% and 80%, respectively [2].

Cholescintigraphy (HIDA scan) can be performed if ultrasound is not diagnostic. A positive test occurs when the gallbladder is not visualized after the isotope is given, suggesting cystic duct obstruction. This finding may also occur in those with severe liver disease, prior biliary sphincterotomy or prolonged fasting.

Magnetic resonance cholangiography (MRC) and *CT scan* are not routinely used for diagnosing cholecystitis, but may be of use in assessing for related complications.

Management
- Admit to the hospital
- Intravenous hydration
- Nil per mouth
- Analgesics
- Antibiotics
  - Mild cases – 7 days treatment with a second-generation cephalosporin
  - Severe cases – broad-spectrum antibiotics such as ampicillin with gentamicin and metronidazole.

Surgery
Definitive therapy is based on severity of symptoms. If the patient is unstable and there is evidence of complications such as abscess, gangrene or perforation, an emergent cholecystectomy should be considered.

Low-risk patients
In a metaanalysis of 12 controlled studies, it was suggested that early cholecystectomy (immediate cholecystectomy within 7 days of symptoms) is preferred [3]. This approach was associated with decreased hospital stay, complications and death rate. Laparoscopic cholecystectomy is preferred unless there is underlying

liver disease, coagulopathy, generalized peritonitis or gallbladder cancer.

High surgical risk, critically ill patients

Conservative measures to stabilize should initially be undertaken. Percutaneous cholecystostomy can be considered and once symptoms resolve then elective cholecystectomy can proceed. If cholecystectomy is not feasible due to the high risk of the procedure, then the surgeon can opt for stent placement into the gallbladder via endoscopic retrograde cholangiopancreatography (ERCP).

Mirizzi syndrome

This syndrome occurs when there is common hepatic duct compression from an impacted cystic duct stone. The original classification describes two types of Mirizzi syndrome, but other classifications also exist.
- Type I: an impacted stone in the cystic duct causes compression of the common hepatic duct.
- Type II: there is erosion of the stone through the lumen, resulting in a fistula.

Patients present with obstructive jaundice, fever and right upper quadrant pain. There is usually an elevation in bilirubin and alkaline phosphatase. Ultrasound can show a stone impacted in the gallbladder neck, along with proximal biliary dilation with a normal caliber duct below the stone. ERCP is generally diagnostic and helps delineate the anatomy. Type I Mirizzi syndrome is managed with a cholecystectomy. Endoscopic treatment can be used as a temporizing measure prior to surgery or as definitive treatment in high surgical risk patients. Type II Mirizzi syndrome is managed with a cholecystocholedochoduodenostomy.

Choledocholithiasis

Clinical presentation

Choledocholithiasis occurs in 10–20% of those who have gallstones and more frequently in those with symptomatic gallstones [4]. Patients can present with abdominal pain, cholangitis, or biliary pancreatitis or be noted to have an incidental finding on imaging. The emergency scenario exists when pain and/or jaundice persists despite conservative management.

Diagnosis

The diagnosis is readily made in those with obstructive jaundice, cholangitis or pancreatitis. In those with nonspecific liver test abnormalities or those that are asymptomatic, it may more difficult to diagnose.

Etiology

Primary bile duct stones develop de novo in the ducts. They are generally more common in Asians and are believed to arise as result of bile stasis or parasitic infection. Secondary bile duct stones are thought to have migrated from the gallbladder.

History

Patients may be asymptomatic or present with right upper quadrant pain and jaundice.

Examination

Examination may reveal jaundice and abdominal tenderness.

Investigations

Ultrasound of the abdomen is the first imaging test used and may reveal duct dilation or stone. The sensitivity of ultrasound for detection of dilated bile ducts ranges from 55% to 90%, and ranges from 20–75% for the detection of bile duct stones [5].

Endoscopic ultrasound (EUS) is an endoscopic procedure that can be used for imaging the biliary tree and has accuracy around 98% for the detection of common bile duct stones [6].

Magnetic resonance cholangiopancreatography (MRCP) is a noninvasive technique for imaging the biliary tree. The accuracy is not as good compared to EUS for stones less than 6 mm [7]. The sensitivity for the detection of stones was 80% for EUS compared to 40% for MRCP, with similar specificity at about 95%.

Helical CT cholangiography has also been used to detect common bile duct stones. The sensitivity, specificity and accuracy for stone detection on helical CT were 85%, 88% and 86%, respectively, compared to 91%, 100% and 94% on EUS. ERCP was used as the gold standard [8].

Intraoperative cholangiography (IOC) can be performed at the time of laparoscopic cholecystectomy to assess for stones. If present, bile duct exploration or ERCP can performed for stone extraction.

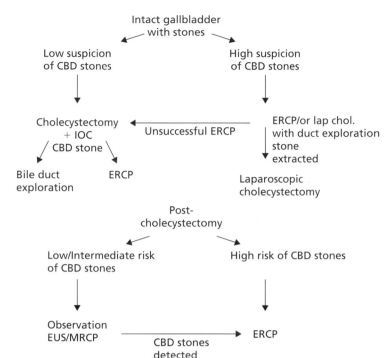

Figure 23.1 Algorithm for the management of bile duct stones. From ref. 10.
CBD = common bile duct, IOC = intraoperative cholangiogram.

ERCP is generally the gold standard for demonstrating the presence of stones. The National Institute of Health (NIH) consensus statement on ERCP for diagnosis and therapy concluded that MRCP, EUS and ERCP have comparable sensitivity in the diagnosis of common bile duct stones [9]. Currently ERCP is used more for therapy (i.e. stone extraction), rather than diagnosis, since there are other less invasive modalities to use for diagnostic purposes.

Management

Figure 23.1 provides an algorithm for the management of bile duct stones [10].

Cholangitis

Clinical presentation

Cholangitis occurs due to infection of an obstructed bile duct, secondary to stones, stricture or an occluded biliary stent. The syndrome manifesting as the Charcot triad of fever, jaundice and right upper quadrant pain occurs in 50–75% of patients [11]. If there is associated hypotension and confusion, this is referred to as the Reynold pentad and carries a grave prognosis

without emergent intervention. The mortality rate for cholangitis ranges from 7% to 40%.

Diagnosis

The clinical presentation, along with an elevated white cell count, and cholestatic liver pattern is suggestive of cholangitis. Ultrasound should be performed initially to evaluate the common bile duct for dilation and stones. ERCP can be diagnostic and therapeutic. Differential diagnosis includes cholecystitis, pancreatitis, hepatic abscess and right lower lobe pneumonia. These can be differentiated on physical examination and imaging. Other biliary etiologies can include bile leaks, stricture, cholecystitis, Mirizzi syndrome or infected choledochal cyst.

Etiology

Table 23.2 lists the causes of cholangitis. Bacteria implicated include *Escherichia coli, Enterococci, Klebsiella, Pseudomonas, Proteus* species, *Bacteroides fragilis* and *Clostridium perfringens.*

History

Prior history of gallstones and/or biliary colic.

Table 23.2 Etiology of acute cholangitis.

Iatrogenic (biliary instrumentation)
Choledocholithiasis
Benign biliary stricture
Malignant biliary obstruction
Sump syndrome
Mirizzi syndrome
Sclerosing cholangitis
Ampullary obstruction
AIDS cholangiopathy
Oriental cholangiohepatitis

Examination

Examination can reveal fever, right upper quadrant tenderness and jaundice.

Investigations

Laboratory studies

Complete blood count usually shows leukocytosis. *Liver enzymes* are elevated in a cholestatic pattern (elevated bilirubin, and alkaline phosphatase). Transaminases can also be elevated, suggestive of hepatocyte necrosis. *Amylase* and *lipase* may be elevated if there is associated pancreatitis. *Blood cultures* may be positive. *Coagulopathy* may result from associated sepsis.

Imaging

An abdominal ultrasound should be the initial test; if normal consider CT, MRCP or EUS. If there is a high index of suspicion proceed to ERCP. Percutaneous transhepatic cholangiography (PTC) can be considered if ERCP is not possible or difficult due to surgically altered anatomy.

Management

Figure 23.2 provides an algorithm for the management of acute cholangitis.
- Admit to hospital.
- Support with intravenous fluids, nil by mouth, correct coagulopathy.
- Blood cultures.
- Broad-spectrum antibiotics to cover gram-negative organisms and enterococci (fluoroquinolone, ampicillin and gentamicin, carbopenems).

If there is no improvement of symptoms within 12 hours after starting antibiotics, as manifested by persistent fever, or persistent abdominal pain, this would require urgent biliary decompression.

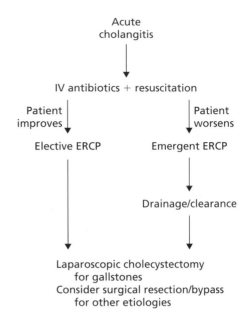

Figure 23.2 Algorithm for treatment of acute cholangitis.

ERCP can achieve biliary decompression by sphincterotomy and stone extraction or stent placement. Generally, bile/pus is aspirated to decompress the ducts prior to injecting contrast to minimize bacteremia. The bile can be sent for gram stain and culture. A cholangiogram is performed to localize the site of obstruction. If the patient is critically ill, a stent can be placed and further intervention delayed until the patient is stabilized. Otherwise, a sphincterotomy is done and stone extraction is performed by balloon or basket or, if larger stones, by mechanical or electohydraulic lithotripsy. If all stones are not removed in the initial procedure, a stent is placed to provide drainage until further extraction of residual stones. ERCP has been shown to have lower morbidity and mortality than surgical bile duct exploration [12–14]. ERCP is successful for stone extraction in 90–95%.

If ERCP is unsuccessful, percutaneous drainage, nasobiliary catheter or surgical approaches can also be considered. Surgery should be reserved for those who fail endoscopic therapy since there is a higher mortality [15].

Definitive management varies based on the etiology of the cholangitis. Choledocholithiasis is managed as above. Benign biliary strictures may require biliary dilation and plastic stent placement. Malignant biliary obstruction would require treatment of the malignancy along with metal stent placement. Sump syndrome can be treated by endoscopic sphincterotomy. Mirizzi's syndrome is managed as described above. Primary sclerosing cholangitis can be managed by stenting of the dominant stricture, and using ursodeoxycholic acid, but definitive treatment would involve liver transplant. Ampullary obstruction secondary to stenosis can be managed with a sphincterotomy or may require ampullectomy or surgery if malignant obstruction is present. AIDS cholangiopathy commonly causes papillary stenosis which can be relieved with sphincterotomy. Oriental cholangiohepatitis may be managed initially with antibiotics and endoscopic clearance of stones, but may require hepatic lobectomy.

Bile leak

The incidence of reported iatrogenic biliary tract injuries during laparoscopic cholecystectomy ranges from 0 to 1% compared to 0.1–0.2% during open cholecystectomy. Classification of bile duct injuries is shown in Table 23.3.

Clinical features

The time period for clinical presentation and recognition of bile duct injuries is highly variable and dependent on the nature of the injury.

A *bile leak* usually presents early. The mean period to postoperative detection is 8 days. The patient may complain of severe, diffuse abdominal pain, nausea, bloating and fatigue. There may be a low-grade pyrexia and mild leukocytosis.

Biliary strictures usually present later, as long as 3 months after cholecystectomy. They may present with jaundice, cholangitis, elevated liver enzymes or abdominal pain.

Management

• Morbidity and mortality are minimized when successful management of bile duct injuries is accomplished early.
• Abdominal ultrasound or CT assesses whether or not there is extrahepatic biliary obstruction and the presence or absence of bile collections.
• If a bile collection is found in the right upper quadrant, it should be drained percutaneously.

Table 23.3 Classification of bile duct injuries.

	Type of injury
Type A	Bile leaks from the cystic duct and ducts of Luschka (from right hepatic lobe in the gallbladder fossa to right hepatic or common bile duct)
Type B	Occlusion of aberrant right hepatic duct
Type C	Leakage of right hepatic duct
Type D	Lateral trauma to the main bile duct causing leakage
Type E	Involves common and main hepatic ducts and correspond to Bismuth classification types 1 to V

• If a leak or obstruction is present, an ERCP should be undertaken to define the site and extent of the biliary injury with endoscopic therapy if indicated. An exception may be the situation where bile drainage through the drain decreases suggesting healing of the leak and no further intervention may be required.
• The most common is leakage from the cystic duct stump (type A) followed by junction of the cystic duct with the bile duct (type D) and duct of Luschka (type A).
• Leaks can be treated by endoscopic stent placement or sphincterotomy. If there are associated common bile duct stones, they should be removed following a sphincterotomy. Complete bile duct occlusion from a clip or ligature precludes endoscopic therapy. Type E is most severe and requires expert management by a hepatobiliary team. A Roux-en-Y hepaticojejunostomy is the procedure of choice for complete ductal transection or for high-grade stricture.

References

1. Reiss, R, Deutsch, AA. State of the art in the diagnosis and management of acute cholecystitis. Dig Dis 1993; 11:55.
2. Shea, JA, Berlin, JA, Escarce, JJ, et al. Revised estimates of diagnostic test sensitivity and specificity in suspected biliary tract disease. Arch Intern Med 1994; 154:2573.
3. Papi, C, D'Ambrosio, L, Capurso, L. Timing of cholecystectomy for acute calculous cholecystitis: a meta-analysis. Am J Gastroenterol 2004; 99:147.

4. Ko CW, Lee S. Epidemiology and natural history of common bile duct stones and prediction of disease. Gastrointest Endosc 2002, 56(Suppl 6):S165–S169.

5. Pasanen A Partanen K, Pikkarainen PH et al. A comparison of ultrasound, computed tomography and endoscopic retrograde cholangiopancreatography in the differential diagnosis of benign and malignant jaundice and cholestasis. Eur J Surg 1993, 159:23–9.

6. Napoleon B, Dumortier J, Keriven-Souquet O, et al. Do normal findings at biliary endoscopic ultrasonography obviate the need for endoscopic retrograde cholangiography in patients with suspicion of common bile duct stone? A prospective follow-up study of 238 patients. Endoscopy 2003, 35:411–15.

7. Scheiman JM, Carlos RC, Barnett JL, et al. Can endoscopic ultrasound or magnetic resonance cholangiopancreatography replace ERCP in patients with suspected biliary disease? A prospective trial and cost analysis. Am J Gastroenterol 2001, 96:2900–4.

8. Polkowski M,Palucki J Regula J, Tilszer A, Butruk E. Helical computed tomographic cholangiography versus endosonography for suspected bile duct stones: a prospective blinded study in non-jaundiced patients. Gut 1999; 45(5):744–9.

9. NIH state-of-the-science statement on endoscopic retrograde cholangiopancreatography (ERCP) for diagnosis and therapy. NIH Consens State Sci Statements 2002; 19:1–26.

10. Eisen GM, Dominitz JA, Faigel DO, et al. An annotated algorithm for the evaluation of choledocholithiasis. Gastrointest Endosc 2001, 53:864–6.

11. Saik RP, Greenberg AG, Farris JM. Spectrum of cholangitis. Am J Surg 1975; 130:143.

12. Cotton PB. Endoscopic retrograde cholangiopancreatography and laparoscopic cholecystectomy. Am J Surg 1993; 165:474.

13. Leese T, Neoptolemos JP, Baker AR, Carr-Locke DL. Management of acute cholangitis and the impact of endoscopic sphincterotomy. Br J Surg 1986; 73(12):988–92.

14. Hui CK, Lai KC, Wong WM, et al. A randomised controlled trial of endoscopic sphincterotomy in acute cholangitis without common bile duct stones. Gut 2002; 51(2):245–7.

15. Lai ECS, Tam PC, Paterson IA et al. Emergency surgery for severe acute cholangitis: the high risk patient. Ann Surg 1990; 211: 55–9.

24 Variceal Hemorrhage

Yan Zhong, Stefan Seewald, Nib Soehendra

Acute esophagogastric variceal hemorrhage is a life-threatening emergency that is still associated with a high mortality. This is especially true when advanced cirrhosis of the liver is the underlying disease, in particular if the cirrhosis of the liver is caused by alcoholism that most likely has also damaged other organs such as the kidney and heart. The management in the acute stage is therefore a complex issue requiring close multidisciplinary cooperation.

Clinical presentation

Patients suffering from an acute variceal hemorrhage usually present with hematemesis followed by melena. Depending on the severity of blood loss, hemodynamic instability, and the stage of the underlying liver disease, bleeding may be associated with encephalopathy, ascites, jaundice, hepatorenal syndrome and infection.

Physical inspection may reveal skin lesions such as palmar erythema, and spiders, particularly in the areas of face, neck, shoulders and arms suggesting the presence of advanced liver disease related to alcoholism.

Diagnosis

Endoscopy is well established as the primary approach to acute upper gastrointestinal bleeding because it provides diagnosis and therapy at the same time (see Chapter 3). To improve therapeutic results, precise diagnosis of the bleeding source is of major importance. Patients with already known portal hypertension may bleed from other sources than varices [1,2]. The use of balloon tamponade in a patient suffering from Mallory–Weiss bleeding that is not uncommon in alcoholic patients would be disastrous. The success

of endoscopic examination strongly depends on the experience of the endoscopist and the completeness of the armamentarium.

Thorough upper gastrointestinal endoscopy is mandatory to exclude presence of multiple bleeding sources. In the case of bleeding from the esophagus (varices, Mallory–Weiss tears), immediate hemostasis should be first performed prior to completion of the endoscopic investigation. A stomach full of blood obscures the view and carries a risk of aspiration. Complete evacuation of blood clots from the stomach and duodenum is required to obtain a precise diagnosis, and in addition may reduce the risk of development of encephalopathy. The use of a therapeutic endoscope with a working channel of 6.0mm (GIF-XTQ 160, Olympus Optical Corp., Tokyo, Japan) is recommended to enable quick suction. An additional powerful suction pump is required to evacuate oropharyngeal secretion preventing aspiration. A water pump is used for flushing through the additional water jet channel of the endoscope (Fig. 24.1). Such a targeted cleansing of the stomach is more efficient than any other method such as lavage or erythromycin administration.

Regarding timing of endoscopy in patients with upper gastrointestinal hemorrhage, cost-effective indication criteria for urgent endoscopy must be considered (see Chapters 3 and 21). Symptoms of acute bleeding such as hematemesis, melena and hemodynamic instability are valid indications for emergency upper gastrointestinal endoscopy that can be carried out immediately after stabilizing the hemodynamic condition of the patient. The importance of airway management cannot be overstressed. Endotracheal intubation may be necessary to prevent aspiration and also to facilitate emergency endoscopy in those with massive bleeding.

The initial severity of bleeding with significant blood loss and early rebleeding are independent risk factors that are prognostically related to mortality. Rebleeding

Gastrointestinal Emergencies, 2nd edition. Edited by Tony Tham, John Collins and Roy Soetikno. © 2009 by Blackwell Publishing, ISBN: 978-1-4051-4634-0.

is the most decisive of all the determinants. The effectiveness of any endoscopic method has therefore to be assessed by two parameters, i.e. initial hemostasis and rebleeding rate. Ultimately, definitive initial bleeding control is the most important goal, in order to improve outcome.

Therapy

Management of acute hemorrhage from esophagogastric varices is still a challenging issue. All hemostatic treatment modalities are considered palliative, as they are unable to alter the underlying disease. Only liver transplantation may provide cure for advanced liver disease.

The outcome of acute hemorrhage depends not only on the initial hemostasis, but also on the emergency general management of the patient: hemodynamic and respiratory resuscitation, and prevention and treatment of complications, such as aspiration, infection, coagulopathy, encephalopathy and renal failure.

Pharmacotherapy

The role of pharmacotherapy is debatable. However, vasoactive drugs are recommended as an initial treatment if an immediate endoscopy is not available. Terlipressin (glypressin), a long-acting analogue of vasopressin, is the most commonly used drug to decrease the portal venous pressure; 1–2 mg is given intravenously every 4–6 hours. A metaanalysis suggests that terlipressin can reduce mortality. Somatostatin and its synthetic analogue octreotide have a similar portal pressure decreasing effect with fewer side effects compared to vasopressin. It is administered by intravenous infusion (somatostatin 250 μg/hour, octreotide 50–100 μg/hour) following a bolus of 250 μg somatostatin or 50 μg octreotide. Vasoactive drugs may transiently control variceal bleeding in around 50% of cases. Definitive endoscopic treatment (bleeding control and secondary prophylaxis) should therefore follow as soon as possible. Patients with massive variceal bleeding, however, are unlikely to benefit from pharmacotherapy alone.

Balloon tamponade

Tamponade of the esophagus using the double-balloon Sengstaken–Blakemore balloon or tamponade of the gastric fundus and cardia using the single-balloon Linton–Nachlas balloon in case of acute variceal hemorrhage represents an ultimate treatment when endoscopy fails to control bleeding. It is very infrequently used today because of its high complication rate (see Chapter 10), in contrast to the effectiveness of endoscopic hemostatic methods. Like pharmacotherapy, balloon tamponade is also used when immediate endoscopy is not available.

The use of balloon tamponade requires some precautions, in order to prevent complications (Fig. 24.2):
1. Ensure the placement of the gastric balloon in the stomach radiologically prior to inflating the gastric

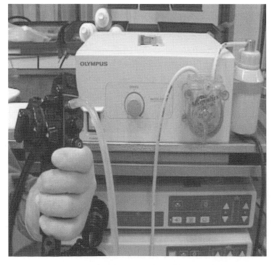
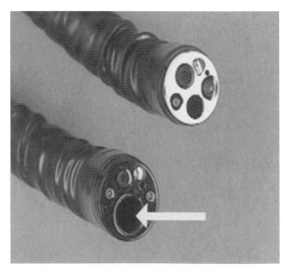

Figure 24.1 Endoscopic armamentarium for gastrointestinal hemorrhage. Therapeutic upper GI endoscope with 3.7 and 6.0 mm working channel (right). A water pump attached to the water jet channel (left).

balloon of the Sengstaken–Blakemore tube with at least 150 mL air or water (400 mL for the Linton–Nachlas balloon).

2. Put the tube under gentle external traction before inflating the esophageal balloon with maximum 80 mL

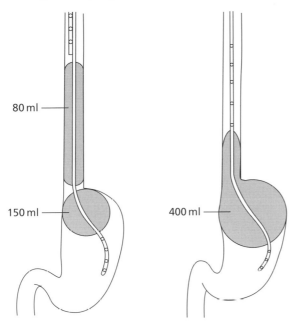

Figure 24.2 Placement of Sengstaken–Blakemore balloon tube for esophageal variceal bleeding (left), Linton–Nachlas balloon tube for variceal bleeding from the cardia and fundus (right).

air or water. The Linton–Nachlas balloon is first inflated with 150 mL air or water, and then filled up to 400 mL under gentle traction. External traction is maintained during the entire application.

Placement of a Sengstaken–Blakemore balloon tube in case of endoscopically uncontrolled esophageal variceal bleeding may be cumbersome or even impossible. Additionally, patients treated with balloon tamponade are at high risk of aspiration, and therefore usually require tracheal intubation. In such cases, the use of a newly designed removable covered self-expandable metal stent (SX-Ella-Danis stent, Ella-CS s.r.o. Czech Republic) has been recommended, as it is easier to insert and does not obstruct the esophagus. The stent has a length of 135 mm and a diameter of 25 mm. A balloon attached at the distal end of the delivery catheter allows for precise stent placement without fluoroscopic monitoring. The stent is introduced over an endoscopically placed guidewire. Once the tip is deeply advanced into the stomach, the balloon is inflated, and the delivery catheter is slowly withdrawn until the inflated balloon comes across the cardia. The stent can then be deployed under gentle traction in the usual manner. In the preliminary report of Hubmann et al. [3], the stent was left for 5–7 days. As for balloon tamponade, it is advisable to remove the stent as early as possible because of the potential risk of damaging

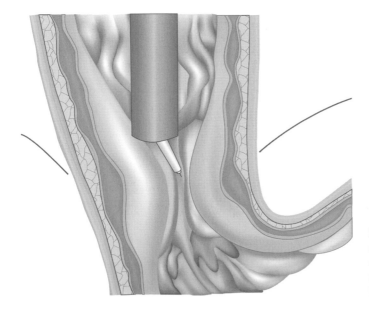

Figure 24.3 Para- or perivariceal injections of sclerosant for controlling mild hemorrhage from an esophageal varix. Injections are performed as close as possible to the variceal wall, in order to compress the bleeding site and to induce thrombosis of the varix.

the esophageal wall. Endoscopic treatment should immediately follow to eradicate the varices. For this purpose, band ligation is preferred over sclerotherapy because of its lower rates of complications, rebleeding and mortality [4].

Sclerotherapy

Injection sclerotherapy using ethanolamine oleate 3%, polidocanol 1%, sodium morrhuate 5% etc. is effective in controlling mild variceal bleeding of the esophagus. Injection is performed para- or perivariceally with a

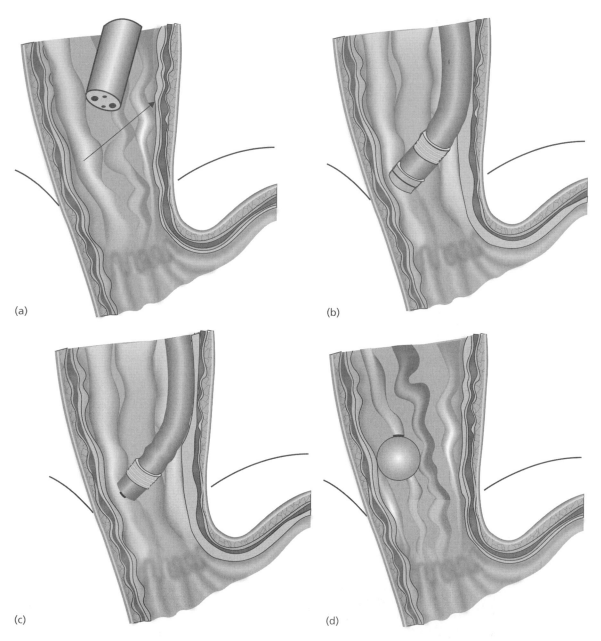

(a)

(b)

(c)

(d)

Figure 24.4 Band ligation of an acutely bleeding esophageal varix. (a) Following the identification of the bleeding site, the endoscope is withdrawn in order to attach the band ligation device. (b) The bleeding site is targeted and sucked into the attached cylinder. (c) The band is released. (d) The bleeding is stopped, and the bleeding site is seen on the ligated varix.

22–25 G needle depending on the viscosity of the sclerosant used (Fig. 24.3). The length of the needle should not exceed 5 mm to prevent transmural injections. Use of large amount of sclerosant must be avoided because of the risk of wall necrosis that may lead to further complications (see Chapter 10). Sclerotherapy is therefore not particularly suitable for severe bleeding from large esophageal varices because of the high volume of sclerosant needed. The hemostatic effect of endoscopic sclerotherapy in esophageal varices is based on initial mechanical compression of the bleeding site and thereafter thrombosis of the varix by chemical endothelial irritation. In patients with advanced cirrhosis of the liver and coagulopathy, sclerotherapy is therefore unlikely to achieve definitive hemostasis. In a randomized trial comparing sclerotherapy with cyanoacrylate obliteration, sclerotherapy showed an immediate hemostasis rate of only 56% with a an early rebleeding rate of 56%, and most of early rebleeding occurred within the first 2 weeks, caused by sclerotherapy-induced ulcers [5].

Sclerotherapy is also not indicated for huge fundic varices because of the high risk of torrential early rebleeding from sclerotherapy-induced ulcers, as it is unable to obliterate all the tributaries in one session. Most patients with bleeding gastric varices treated with sclerotherapy will die from uncontrolled rebleeding within the first 30 days [6].

Band ligation

Endoscopic variceal ligation has proved to be effective in acute esophageal variceal bleeding. Its major drawback is that one has to withdraw the endoscope after identifying the bleeding source, in order to attach the device to the tip of the endoscope (Fig. 24.4).

In the case of severe variceal bleeding visibility and suction are limited due to the cap. If the bleeding spot cannot be well identified, placement of several rubber bands using the multiband ligator at the most distal portion of the esophagus is recommended to reduce the blood flow, thus controlling the bleeding (Fig. 24.5).

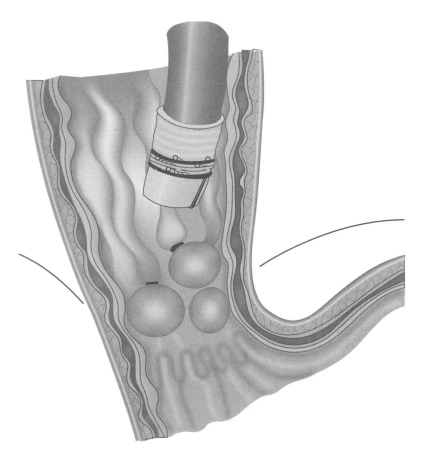

Figure 24.5 Control of an endoscopically unidentifiable esophageal variceal bleeding using a multiband ligator. Bleeding is controlled by placing several bands at the most distal esophagus.

Following the control of bleeding, endoscopy should be repeated as soon as possible, in order to achieve complete eradication of the varices hence minimizing the rate of early rebleeding. Second endoscopic treatment can usually be performed after 4 days. Ligation can be cautiously applied to the still patent varices despite the presence of fresh ligation-induced necroses. Further ligations should be consistently repeated every 3–4 weeks

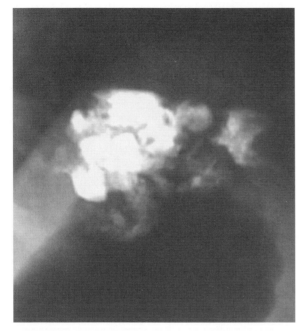

Figure 24.6 Endoscopic picture of huge fundic varices (see Plate 24.1). Venography obtained after complete obliteration therapy using a total of 6 mL Histoacryl-Lipiodol mixture (b).

until complete eradication of the varices is achieved. Compared to sclerotherapy, band ligation has shown a higher recurrence rate of variceal formation after initial eradication. Sclerotherapy using small amount of sclerosant may be required to eradicate remaining varices untreatable by band ligation. Metachronous combination of band ligation and low-volume sclerotherapy has been proved to significantly reduce variceal recurrence and recurrent bleeding rates [7,8].

Endoscopic variceal ligation should not be used for huge bleeding fundic varices for the same reason as for the sclerotherapy. Acute bleeding from smaller fundix varices may be controlled by band ligation. However, band ligation is unable to obliterate all the tributaries of huge fundic varices, hence carrying a high risk of massive rebleeding due to the ligation-induced ulcers after 2–3 days [9]. Figure 24.6 (see also Plate 24.1) shows the venography of extensive conglomeration of collateral vessels of fundic varices behind the gastric wall emphasizing the phenomenon "the tip of the iceberg."

Cyanoacrylate obliteration

Endoscopic variceal obliteration using N-butyl-2-cyanoacrylate (Histoacryl®, Braun-Melsungen, Germany, Glubran®, GEM, Italy) is undoubtedly more effective than other treatment modalities for massive esophageal and fundic variceal hemorrhage [10–13]. It represents the only endoscopic option to effectively control bleeding from sclerotherapy or EVL-induced ulcers (Plate 24.2a, b). Cyanoacrylate obliteration is also widely accepted as the current best treatment

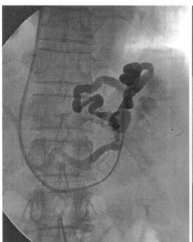
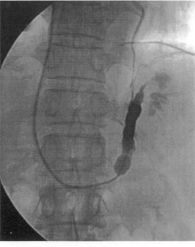

Figure 24.7 Radiographs illustrating the principle of balloon retrograde transjugular obliteration of fundic varices (courtesy of Dr Murakami, Japan).

Table 24.1 Technique of endoscopic variceal obliteration using N-butyl-2 cyanoacrylate.

Mix Histoacryl® with Lipiodol® in 0.5:0.8 ratio

Inject directly into the varix

Lubricate the injector with Lipiodol

Measure the dead space of the injector

Use distilled water of the same volume to flush out cyanoacrylate

Continue flushing the injector after injection to maintain the injector patency

Apply not more than 0.5 mL of glue per injection in esophagus and 1.0 ml in fundus to avoid embolization

Obliterate all visible fundic varices in one session to prevent rebleeding

modality for controlling acute hemorrhage from huge fundic varices (Plate 24.3a, b).

Balloon-occluded retrograde transvenous obliteration (B-RTO) is widely used for eradication of fundic varices in Japan [14]. Figure 24.7 shows the technique of transjugular approach of B-RTO.

Following the European approval of N-butyl-2-cyanoacrylate for endoscopic application, the tissue glue has attracted more interest in many countries of the world because it is easier and highly effective in controlling both esophageal and fundic variceal hemorrhage.

The tissue glue N-butyl-2-cyanoacrylate is an aqueous solution which polymerizes and hardens within 20 seconds in a physiological milieu and almost instantaneously upon contact with blood. To prevent

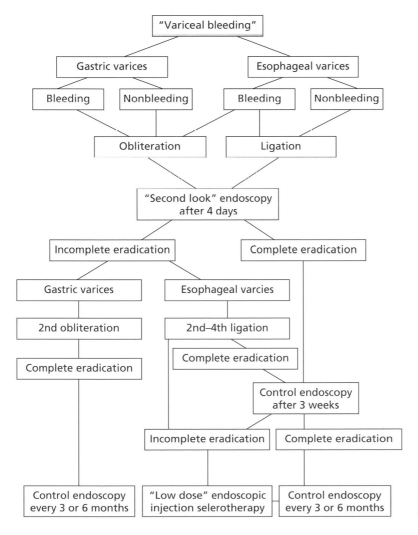

Figure 24.8 Algorithm of endoscopic management of acute esophagogastric variceal hemorrhage.

cyanoacrylate from solidifying too quickly, it is necessary to dilute it with the oily contrast agent Lipiodol® (Guerbert Villepinte, France) in a ratio of 0.5 : 0.8. Lipiodol is not only compatible with the tissue adhesive but also allows fluoroscopic monitoring of the glue injection. N-butyl-2-cyanoacrylate is injected strictly into the lumen of the varix.

The most serious potential risk of intravariceal injection of N-butyl-2-cyanoacrylate is embolism. There have been several case reports on embolization of the glue from the varices into the lung, spleen, brain and pelvic region [15]. These serious complications are rare. Usually, N-butyl-2-cyanoacrylate polymerizes and solidifies in the vessel instantaneously, so that an embolism is very unlikely. In the case of patent foramen ovale or other right-to-left shunting in the mediastinum, this rare, serious complication may occur. To prevent such complications, the amount of N-butyl-2-cyanoacrylate per injection should be limited to a maximum of 0.5 mL for esophageal varices and 1 mL for large fundic varices. If greater amounts are needed due to the large size of the varices, injection should be performed in succession. The details of the cyanoacrylate injection technique are described in Table 24.1.

Our algorithm of endoscopic management of esophagogastric variceal bleeding is shown in Fig. 24.8.

In acute variceal hemorrhage, transjugular intrahepatic portosystemic shunt (TIPS) has a role if endoscopic treatment fails [16]. Surgical shunt has been widely abandoned because of its very high perioperative morbidity and mortality.

References

1. Dagradi AE, Mehler R, Tan DT, et al. Sources of upper gastrointestinal bleeding in patients with liver cirrhosis and large esophagogastric varices. Am J Gastroenterol 1970; 54:458–63.

2. Gilbert DA, Silverstein FE, Tedesco FJ, et al. The national ASGE survey on upper gastrointestinal bleeding. III. Endoscopy in upper gastrointestinal bleeding. Gastrointest Endosc 1981; 27:94–102.

3. Hubmann R, Bodlaj G, Czompo M, et al. The use of self-expanding metal stents to treat acute esophageal variceal bleeding. Endoscopy 2006; 38:896–901.

4. Laine L, Cook D. Endoscopic ligation compared with sclerotherapy for treatment of esophageal variceal bleeding: a meta-analysis. Ann Intern Med 1995; 123:280–7.

5. Maluf-Filho F, Sakai P, Ishioka S, et al. Endoscopic sclerosis versus cyanoacrylate endoscopic injection for the first episode of variceal bleeding: a prospective, controlled, and randomized study in Child–Pugh class C patients. Endoscopy 2001; 33:421–7.

6. Trudeau W, Prindiville T. Endoscopic injection sclerosis in bleeding gastric varices. Gastrointest Endosc 1986; 32:264–8.

7. Lo GH, Lai KH, Cheng JS, et al. The additive effect of sclerotherapy to patients receiving repeated endoscopic variceal ligation: a prospective, randomized trial. Hepatology 1998; 28:391–5.

8. Masumoto H, Toyonaga A, Oho K, et al. Ligation plus low-volume sclerotherapy for high-risk esophageal varices: comparisons with ligation therapy or sclerotherapy alone. J Gastroenterol 1998; 33:1–5.

9. Seewald S, Seitz U, Yang AM, et al. Variceal bleeding and portal hypertension: still a therapeutic challenge? Endoscopy 2001; 33:126–39.

10. Feretis C, Dimopoulos C, Benakis P, et al. N-butyl-2-cyanoacrylate (Histoacryl) plus sclerotherapy versus sclerotherapy alone in the treatment of bleeding esophageal varices: a randomized prospective study. Endoscopy 1995; 27:355–7.

11. Thakeb F, Salama Z, Salama H, et al. The value of combined use of N-butyl-2-cyanoacrylate and ethanolamine oleate in the management of bleeding esophagogastric varices. Endoscopy 1995; 27:358–64.

12. Lo GH, Lai KH, Cheng JS, et al. A prospective, randomized trial of butyl cyanoacrylate injection versus band ligation in the management of bleeding gastric varices. Hepatology 2001; 33:1060–4.

13. Sarin SK, Jain AK, Jain M, et al. A randomized controlled trial of cyanoacrylate versus alcohol injection in patients with isolated fundic varices. Am J Gastroenterol 2002; 97:1010–15.

14. Chikamori F, Kuniyoshi N, Shibuya S, et al. Urgent transjugular retrograde obliteration for prophylaxis of rebleeding from gastric varices in patients with a spontaneous portosplenorenal shunt. Dig Surg 2000; 17:23–8.

15. Wahl P, Lammer F, Conen D, et al. Septic complications after injection of N-butyl-2-cyanoacrylate: report of two cases and review. Gastrointest Endosc 2004; 59:911–16.

16. Barange K, Peron JM, Imani K, et al. Transjugular intrahepatic portosystemic shunt in the treatment of refractory bleeding from ruptured gastric varices. Hepatology 1999; 30:1139–43.

25 Acute Liver Failure

Aijaz Ahmed, Emmet B. Keeffe

Introduction

Acute liver disease may cause rapidly evolving hepatic decompensation characterized by coagulopathy and hepatic encephalopathy, a syndrome known as acute liver failure [1–3]. Patients with acute liver failure typically present with nonspecific symptoms that are promptly followed by jaundice and altered mental status. The changes in mental status can progress from mild confusion to coma over a short period of time. The abnormalities in laboratory tests include markedly elevated serum aminotransferase levels, hyperbilirubinemia and hypoprothrombinemia. Hypoglycemia, renal failure and metabolic acidosis are poor prognostic indicators in the setting of acute liver failure. In patients who develop multiorgan failure, the mortality rate ranges from 50% to 90%.

An illness resulting in sudden hepatocyte dysfunction is the basic mechanism that leads to acute liver failure. The most common causes of acute liver failure include drug-induced liver injury (acetaminophen/paracetamol, isoniazid, etc.) and acute viral hepatitis. Up to 50% of cases of acute liver failure are due to acetaminophen hepatotoxicity. Rarely, acute liver failure is the initial manifestation of an underlying chronic liver disease (Wilson disease, autoimmune hepatitis or reactivation of chronic hepatitis B). Treatment of acute liver failure should be individualized. In general, aggressive supportive care may buy time and allow for hepatic regeneration and recovery to take place. However, clinical features and diagnostic tests indicative of poor prognosis necessitate timely liver transplantation.

Definitions

Acute liver failure

Acute liver failure is characterized by marked coagulopathy and defined as a prothrombin time or factor V level of less than 50% of normal in the setting of acute liver disease (Table 25.1).

Fulminant hepatic failure

Trey and Davidson [4] defined fulminant hepatic failure in 1970 as the acute onset of liver disease with coagulopathy, development of hepatic encephalopathy within 8 weeks of the onset of illness, and no prior evidence of liver disease. There is disagreement regarding the time interval between the onset of symptoms and hepatic encephalopathy. Some experts have proposed a time interval between the onset of jaundice, rather than symptoms, and the development of hepatic encephalopathy to define acute liver failure [5]. Bernuau and colleagues [5] at the Hôpital Beaujon define fulminant hepatic failure as the development of hepatic encephalopathy within 2 weeks of the onset of jaundice (Table 25.1).

Subfulminant hepatic failure

Subfulminant hepatic failure constitutes acute liver failure characterized by the development of encephalopathy 2 weeks to 3 months after the appearance of jaundice.

Late-onset hepatic failure

Late-onset hepatic failure is characterized by an interval of 8 weeks to 6 months between the onset of illness and development of hepatic encephalopathy.

Gastrointestinal Emergencies, 2nd edition. Edited by Tony Tham, John Collins and Roy Soetikno. © 2009 by Blackwell Publishing, ISBN: 978-1-4051-4634-0.

Table 25.1 Definitions of acute liver failure.

Acute liver failure	Acute liver disease, with prothrombin time or factor V less than 50% of normal
Fulminant hepatic failure	Acute liver failure with hepatic encephalopathy, developing less than 2 weeks[1] (or 8 weeks)[2] after onset of jaundice[1] (or illness)[2]
Subfulminant hepatic failure[3]	Acute liver failure with hepatic encephalopathy, developing from 2 weeks[1] (or 8 weeks)[2] to 3 months[1] (or 6 months)[2] after onset of jaundice[1] (or illness)[2]

[1]Criteria from ref. 5.
[2]Criteria from ref. 4 and ref. 17.
[3]Also called late-onset hepatic failure.
Reproduced from ref. 1.

Hyperacute, acute and subacute hepatic failure

O'Grady and colleagues [6] from King's College Hospital classified acute hepatic dysfunction into three subgroups based on time interval between the onset of jaundice and hepatic encephalopathy. In hyperacute liver failure, the time interval was less than 7 days; in acute liver failure, the time interval was 8 and 28 days, and in subacute liver failure, time interval was between 5 and 12 weeks [6]. The classifications by Bernuau et al. [5] and O'Grady et al. [6] label patients with previously stable, chronic liver disease who develop sudden hepatic decompensation as acute liver failure. Patients with the shortest time interval between the onset of jaundice and development of hepatic encephalopathy have the best prognosis. Therefore, patients with fulminant (hyperacute or acute) may benefit from prompt diagnosis and appropriate management, including evaluation for liver transplantation if necessary.

Epidemiology

The actual incidence of acute liver failure remains unknown. It is estimated that approximately 2000 individuals develop acute liver failure annually in the United States, with 200 to 300 undergoing liver transplantation [7]. It is suspected that referral bias influences the reported etiology and outcome of acute liver failure.

Etiology

The causes of acute liver failure are diverse and the distribution varies according to the geographic region.

The most common causes of acute liver failure include drug-induced liver injury and viral hepatitis. These two causes account for 80% to 85% of all cases for which a cause can be determined (Table 25.2). The etiology of acute liver failure has been variable over the years. Current data from the Acute Liver Failure Study Group (ALFSG) demonstrates that drug-induced liver injury is the most common cause of acute liver failure. According to the ALFSG registry, acetaminophen accounted for 32% of cases of acute liver failure in 1998 and 47% in 2005 [8]. Earlier studies showed that viral hepatitis accounted for the majority of cases between 1960 and 1980. A report from the University of Pittsburgh spanning from 1983 to 1995 showed a 19% incidence of acetaminophen hepatotoxicity and 18% incidence of hepatitis B as the cause of acute liver failure [9]. A report from ALFSG in a prospective analysis from 17 centers between 1998 and 2001 showed drug-induced hepatotoxicity (acetaminophen toxicity 39% and idiosyncratic drug reaction 13%) as the leading cause, with hepatitis A and B accounting for 11% of cases with acute liver failure [10–12].

Other unusual etiologies of acute liver failure include toxins, metabolic diseases, vascular events, tumors and allograft rejection. In the developed geographic regions, such as US and Europe, drug-induced hepatotoxicity, particularly acetaminophen-related, is the most common etiology. On the other hand, acute viral hepatitis is the most common etiology in developing countries. A large series from King's College Hospital in London reported that 56% of 763 patients developed acetaminophen-related fulminant hepatic failure. A study from the US reported 38% of acute liver failure was caused by acetaminophen. It is

Table 25.2 Known causes of acute liver failure.

Viral hepatitis
  Hepatitis A, B, C, D and E viruses
Hepatitis due to other viruses
  Herpesviruses 1, 2, and 6
  Adenovirus
  Epstein–Barr virus
  Cytomegalovirus
Drug-induced liver injury
  Acetaminophen overdose
  Idiosyncratic drug reaction
Toxins
  Amanita phalloides
  Organic solvents
  Phosphorus
Metabolic disorders
  Acute fatty liver of pregnancy
  Reye syndrome
Vascular events
  Acute circulatory failure
  Budd–Chiari syndrome
  Veno-occlusive disease
  Heat stroke
Miscellaneous disorders
  Wilson disease
  Autoimmune hepatitis
  Massive infiltration with tumor
  Liver transplantation with primary graft nonfunction

Reproduced from ref. 1.

estimated that the increase in acute liver failure in US is associated with the use of excessive therapeutic doses of acetaminophen by heavy drinkers of alcohol.

Drugs

Drug-induced liver injury is the leading cause of acute liver failure in the developed countries. It accounts for more than 50% of all cases of acute liver failure in the US and the UK. Drug-induced acute liver failure may complicate as many as 20% cases of drug-induced hepatitis. It is estimated that more than 50 000 emergency room visits and nearly 500 deaths in the US occur annually as a result of acetaminophen-related hepatotoxicity. Drug-induced liver injury is more prevalent in women and individuals older than 40 years of age. Drug-related hepatotoxicity has been divided into two groups, namely dose-dependent (predictable) and idiosyncratic (unpredictable). Dose-dependent hepatotoxicity is predictable and presents with a typical pattern. In contrast, idiosyncratic hepatotoxicity affects less than 1% of users of an individual drug and lacks a characteristic pattern. Idiosyncratic drug reactions account for 10–15% of cases of acute liver failure, but are associated with high mortality rate.

Acetaminophen-induced hepatotoxicity occurs in a dose-dependent, predictable fashion. Acetaminophen is generally safe within the recommended dosage of 3–4 g/d, and its sulfate or glucuronide metabolites are not hepatotoxic. A minor fraction of an acetaminophen dose is metabolized by P-450 enzymes to a reactive metabolite that is conjugated by glutathione to a nontoxic compound. Acetaminophen hepatotoxicity consistently results in hyperacute liver failure. Serum aminotransferase levels are markedly elevated in patients with acetaminophen hepatotoxicity, with values typically exceeding 3000–4000 IU/L. Acute liver failure is triggered by acetaminophen overdose when more than 10 g is ingested or with use of high therapeutic doses by alcoholics who have induced cytochrome P-450 enzymes. In addition, alcoholics may have reduced glutathione stores due to poor nutrition, leaving more toxic intermediates available to cause cell injury. These toxic intermediate metabolites accumulate and bind to cytoplasmic proteins within hepatocytes leading to cell death. Acetaminophen overdose can be associated with up to 50% mortality, whereas excessive ingestion of acetaminophen by alcoholics is associated with an approximate 20% mortality rate.

Examples of drugs that may be associated with idiosyncratic hepatotoxicity resulting in acute liver failure include halothane, isoniazid, disulfiram, valproate, phenytoin, sulfonamides, methyldopa, propylthiouracil, nonsteroidal antiinflammatory drugs, bromfenac and troglitazone. In most cases, presumed idiosyncratic abnormalities in hepatic drug metabolism are the main underlying mechanisms of this type of injury. In patients with idiosyncratic drug-induced hepatotoxicity, eosinophilia and/or the presence of a rash are indicative of hypersensitivity reaction, although these findings are uncommon.

Viral hepatitis

All five hepatotropic viruses have been associated with acute liver failure. However, acute hepatitis C is more likely to result in chronic liver disease rather than cause fulminant hepatitis. In the past, patients with fulminant hepatic failure and unknown cause of acute liver failure were labeled as non-A, non-B hepatitis. It was suspected that hepatitis C virus, or some other viral agent, was the likely etiology. Subsequently, hepatitis C virus RNA and/or antibody to hepatitis C virus were found to be undetectable in the majority of patients labeled as cryptogenic fulminant hepatic failure. It is important to know that less than 1% of patients with acute viral hepatitis will develop fulminant liver failure. Patients who develop fulminant hepatic failure secondary to acute hepatitis A and acute hepatitis B present with a hyperacute course. Typically, jaundice is rapidly followed within 1 week by hepatic encephalopathy. Acute hepatitis A causes fulminant hepatic failure in 0.1% to 0.5% of cases and is common in intravenous drug users. Patients with fulminant hepatitis A usually fare well with a survival rate of 60%. Fulminant hepatitis A is more severe in older patients and individuals with preexisting chronic liver disease. Acute hepatitis B is the most common viral cause of fulminant hepatic failure. Rapid clearance of hepatitis B virus has been reported in 30% to 50% of patients with acute hepatitis B-related fulminant hepatic failure as a result of major immunological attack on infected hepatocytes. These patients may have undetectable levels of HBsAg within a few days of onset of illness and have been wrongly labeled as cryptogenic liver disease. Hepatitis D virus is a rare cause of acute liver failure, is more prevalent in injection drug users, and typically presents in the setting of fulminant hepatitis B. Acute coinfection with hepatitis B and hepatitis D virus or superinfection with hepatitis D virus in a patient with chronic hepatitis B may precipitate fulminant hepatic failure, and coinfected patients are at higher risk for fulminant hepatic failure than patients with acute hepatitis B monoinfection [13]. Fulminant hepatic failure is infrequently associated with hepatitis E infection, but hepatitis E virus-related epidemics have been associated with fulminant hepatic failure in pregnant women. The mortality rate is approximately 40% in pregnant patients with hepatitis E-induced fulminant hepatic failure. Hepatitis caused by other viruses, including herpes viruses 1, 2 and 6, adenovirus, Epstein–Barr virus and cytomegalovirus rarely results in acute liver failure (Table 25.2).

Toxins

Several toxins have been implicated in patients with acute hepatic failure. Organic solvents, such as fluorinated hydrocarbons trichloroethylene and tetrachloroethane, can induce hepatotoxicity and acute liver failure.

Metabolic conditions

Metabolic conditions associated with acute liver failure include acute fatty liver of pregnancy and Reye syndrome. Both of these conditions present with liver biopsy findings of microvesicular fatty infiltration as compared to massive hepatic necrosis that is uniformly noted in other causes of fulminant hepatic failure. Typically, acute fatty liver of pregnancy presents in the third trimester with rapid onset of jaundice, hypoglycemia, coagulopathy and hepatic encephalopathy. Serum aminotransferase levels are usually below 1000IU/L. Emergent delivery of the fetus is recommended. Acute liver failure can also be associated with Wilson disease and autoimmune hepatitis.

Miscellaneous

Vascular complications can also lead to the development of acute liver failure (Table 25.2). Myocardial infarction or cardiomyopathy with acute circulatory failure can precipitate acute liver failure. Rarely, hepatic venous outflow obstruction following acute Budd–Chiari syndrome or venoocclusive disease can result in acute liver failure. Heat exhaustion-related reversible liver failure can develop in high-risk population, such as miners and long-distance runners. Metastatic tumor causing massive hepatic infiltration characterized by intrasinusoidal invasion can precipitate acute liver failure. Primary allograft nonfunction within a few days following liver transplantation can present as acute liver failure necessitating retransplantation.

The above-mentioned causes of acute liver failure may be characterized by a fulminant or subfulminant course of hepatic failure (Table 25.3). Fulminant hepatic failure (hyperacute or acute) is the usual presentation of liver failure in patients with acute hepatitis (types A, B, D and E), *Amanita phalloides* poisoning, acetaminophen overdose, and acute fatty liver of pregnancy. In contrast, patients with cryptogenic acute liver failure, drug-induced liver injury, hepatic venous outflow obstruction, Wilson disease and autoimmune hepatitis typically present with subfulminant hepatic

Table 25.3 Course of acute liver failure according to cause.

Predominantly fulminant (hyperacute > acute[1]) hepatic
   failure:
   Hepatitis A, B, D and E
   Amanita phalloides
   Acetaminophen overdose
   Acute fatty liver of pregnancy
Predominantly subfulminant (or subacute[1]) hepatic failure:
   Indeterminate or sporadic
   Drug-induced liver injury
   Budd–Chiari syndrome
   Veno-occlusive disease
   Wilson disease
   Autoimmune hepatitis

[1]Acute liver failure terminology (hyperacute vs acute vs
subacute) of O'Grady et al. (ref. 6).
Reproduced from ref. 1.

failure. The survival rate in patients affected by fulminant hepatic failure (40% to 60%) is significantly
better than that in patients with subfulminant hepatic
failure (10% to 30%).

Clinical manifestations

The classic presentation of acute liver failure constitutes a triad of jaundice, hepatic encephalopathy and
coagulopathy [1–3]. The progression of acute liver
failure is characterized by metabolic irregularities,
renal dysfunction (50% of patients), cardiopulmonary
failure and sepsis. Patients are susceptible to bacterial
infections (80% of patients) or fungal infections (30%
of patients).

Symptoms and signs

The initial symptoms of acute liver failure are constitutional and include complaints such as malaise or nausea. These symptoms are rapidly followed by jaundice.
Mental status changes develop days to weeks after
the onset of jaundice. The severity of hepatic encephalopathy is divided into four grades. The diagnosis of
grade 1 hepatic encephalopathy requires a high index
of suspicion and is characterized by mild confusion,
poor concentration ability and subtle neurological

impairment. Grade 2 hepatic encephalopathy is characterized by asterixis and dysarthria. Other clinical
findings in grade 2 include drowsiness, personality
changes and inappropriate behavior. During grade
3, most patients are disoriented and somnolent, but
arousable. In grade 4, patients develop hepatic coma
and are unarousable. Patients who develop grade 4
hepatic encephalopathy have a less than 20% survival
rate. Physical examination is characterized by jaundice, easy bruising, changes in mental status and
decreased or absent hepatic dullness on hepatic percussion. The findings on physical examination vary
with the time of presentation.

Laboratory findings

Laboratory findings noted in patients with acute liver
failure vary with severity of underlying liver disease
and include marked elevation in serum aminotransferase levels, hyperbilirubinemia, hypoprothrombinemia, hypoglycemia and respiratory alkalosis preceding
metabolic acidosis. Coagulopathy in acute liver failure
is characterized by a prolonged prothrombin time and
a factor V level of less than 50% of normal. Other
electrolyte abnormalities that are common and may
require correction include hyponatremia, hypophos-
phatemia, hypocalcemia and/or hypomagnesemia.

Management of complications

Acute liver failure may be incorrectly diagnosed
as sepsis or a drug overdose during its initial stages.
Prompt diagnosis and timely intervention can change
the outcome of acute liver failure. Patients with acute
liver failure are at increased risk for life-threatening
complications. The identification of the cause of acute
liver failure can help streamline the management
(acetylcysteine for acetaminophen overdose), predict
the need for liver transplantation and estimate the
prognosis of the underlying condition.

General measures

Patients with acute liver failure should be admitted to
the intensive care unit and transferred to a hospital
with a liver transplant program [14]. Patients should
undergo an expedited liver transplant evaluation and
listed for transplantation on the United Network for
Organ Sharing (UNOS) transplant waiting list or its

Table 25.4 Contraindications to liver transplantation for acute liver failure.[1]

Seropositivity for human immunodeficiency virus
Active alcohol or drug abuse
Advanced cardiopulmonary disease
Uncontrolled sepsis
Widespread thrombosis of portal and mesenteric veins
Irreversible brain damage
Sustained elevation of intracerebral pressure to >50 mmHg
Cerebral perfusion pressure <40 mmHg for >2 hours
Improving hepatic function

[1]Modified from ref. 18.
Reproduced from ref. 1.

European equivalents if there are no contraindications (Table 25.4). Patients may need placement of Swan–Ganz and intraarterial catheters, a urinary catheter and a nasogastric tube. Invasive measurement of intracerebral pressure and prompt treatment of cerebral edema may be required to prevent permanent neurological damage. Mechanical ventilation is recommended in patients with grade 3 or grade 4 hepatic encephalopathy.

Hepatic encephalopathy and cerebral edema

Liver transplantation is contraindicated in at least 30% of patients with acute liver failure as a result of neurological complications (Table 25.4). The underlying pathogenetic mechanisms for hepatic encephalopathy and cerebral edema are different. Hepatic encephalopathy is triggered by the accumulation of toxic substances in the central nervous system. The toxic agents implicated include ammonia and endogenous benzodiazepine agonists. Patients with grade 1 and grade 2 hepatic encephalopathy have a favorable outcome. Grade 3 and grade 4 hepatic encephalopathy are associated with poor prognosis. Cerebral edema is usually fatal following uncal herniation. The underlying mechanism for cerebral edema in the setting of acute liver failure remains unclear. Grade 4 hepatic encephalopathy is complicated by cerebral edema in approximately three-quarters of patients. Cerebral edema is the most common cause of death in patients with grade 4 hepatic encephalopathy. The

blood–brain barrier is disrupted by cerebral edema. Cerebral ischemia develops if cerebral perfusion pressure (mean arterial pressure minus intracerebral pressure) drops below 40 mmHg.

Hepatic encephalopathy associated with fulminant hepatic failure should be managed in an intensive care unit. It is recommended that the patient head be elevated at 20–30°. Lactulose is not as effective in patients with fulminant hepatic failure. Lactulose should be instituted by nasogastric tube or by rectal enema. Lactulose dose should be titrated with a goal for two to four loose bowel movements per day. The role of antibiotics in hepatic encephalopathy secondary to fulminant hepatic failure is not well defined. Hepatic encephalopathy can deteriorate following gastrointestinal bleeding, hypokalemia or sepsis. These aggravating conditions should be promptly diagnosed and immediately treated.

The clinical features of cerebral edema include hypertension, bradycardia, abnormal pupillary reflexes, decerebrate rigidity and posturing, and brainstem respiratory patterns and apnea. The clinical manifestations occur late and indicate poor prognosis. It is recommended that intracerebral pressure be monitored closely and maintained below 20 mmHg. CT scan of the head may be needed to exclude other intracerebral complications such as hemorrhage or other structural lesions to assess candidacy for liver transplantation. CT scan and/or magnetic resonance imaging of the head are unreliable in predicting the intracerebral pressures.

Intracranial pressure should be monitored with subdural or epidural transducers. Epidural transducers have lower sensitivity than subdural monitors but are safer to place. The benefits of intracerebral pressure transducers outweigh the risk of hemorrhage. The transducer measurements should be closely monitored to maintain intracerebral pressure below 20 mmHg and cerebral perfusion pressure above 50 mmHg. Patients with a persistently elevated intracerebral pressure greater than 40 mmHg despite aggressive therapy are poor candidates for orthotopic liver transplantation.

Mannitol is the drug of choice to treat cerebral edema. Mannitol is used intravenously at a dose of 0.5–1 g/kg over 5 minutes and the same dose can be reinstituted to maintain the intracerebral pressure. Mannitol use is contraindicated if serum osmolality rises above 320 mosm/L. Mannitol should be used in conjunction with hemodialysis or continuous arteriovenous hemofiltration in patients with renal failure. In patients who are refractory to mannitol, pentobarbital can be used with boluses of 100–150 mg intravenously every 15 minutes for 1 hour followed by a continuous infusion of 1–3 mg/kg/h. Other measures to prevent increases in intracerebral pressure include: minimizing disturbance; controlling agitation; elevating the head 20–30° above the horizontal; provide moderate hyperventilation to a partial carbon dioxide pressure of 25–30 mmHg; and phenytoin use for subclinical seizures detectable by electroencephalography.

Coagulopathy

The coagulation abnormalities noted in acute liver failure include decreased levels of factors II, V, VII, IX and X resulting in prolonged prothrombin time and partial thromboplastin time. The coagulation studies are closely and serially monitored as a prognostic indicator. Patients with coagulopathy in the setting of fulminant hepatic failure are at increased risk for bleeding from the gastrointestinal tract and arteriovenous access sites. Therefore, use of fresh frozen plasma to correct coagulopathy is only indicated for a bleeding complication or prior to invasive procedures. Thrombocytopenia is commonly associated with fulminant hepatic failure as a result of bone marrow suppression and disseminated intravascular coagulation. Platelet counts should be monitored closely. Platelet transfusion is indicated if the platelets count drops below 50 000/μL in a patient with a bleeding complication.

Renal failure

Renal failure complicates 50% of cases with fulminant hepatic failure and indicates a poor prognosis. Renal failure is typically oliguric as a result of functional hepatorenal syndrome. Although, rarely patients may progress to acute tubular necrosis depending on the severity and duration of renal insult. Nephrotoxic drugs, such as aminoglycosides, nonsteroidal antiinflammatory agents, or contrast agents, should be avoided. Circulatory shock should be aggressively treated with intravenous colloids to maintain intravascular oncotic pressures and prevent lactic acidosis. Dopamine may be needed to maintain blood pressure. The indications for hemodialysis or continuous arteriovenous hemofiltration include severe metabolic acidosis, hyperkalemia or fluid overload.

Hypoglycemia

Hypoglycemia in the setting of fulminant hepatic failure is not uncommon and is caused by impaired hepatic glucose production, impaired hepatic gluconeogenesis and elevated serum insulin levels. Patients with fulminant hepatic failure should be placed on continuous intravenous infusion of 10% dextrose. Infusion of hypertonic glucose may be needed to maintain blood glucose levels between 60–200 mg/dL. Caloric intake should be maintained at 35–50 kcal/kg to meet resting metabolic need. Blood glucose levels should be monitored every 4 hours following the onset of hepatic encephalopathy.

Infection

The risk of bacterial and fungal infections is significantly higher in patients with fulminant hepatic failure. Sepsis is one of the leading contraindication for liver transplantation in the setting of fulminant hepatic failure. Bacteremia is a common problem in patients with altered mental status and indwelling catheters. Up to 80% of patients with fulminant hepatic failure have clinical evidence of an underlying infection. The most common sites of infection are respiratory and urinary tract systems. The most prevalent infectious organisms include gram-positive streptococci, *Staphylococcus aureus*, and gram-negative organisms. Approximately one-third of patients with fulminant hepatic failure develop fungal infections and *Candida albicans* is the most common etiology. Broad-spectrum, intravenous antibiotic and antifungal therapy should be initiated based on presumed or documented infection. Surveillance cultures should be performed as well. Prophylactic, empiric, parenteral, broad-spectrum antibiotics in combination with enteral amphotericin B and clotrimazole may reduce the risk of infection to 20%. Prophylactic antifungal agents are more commonly used in grade 3 and grade 4 hepatic encephalopathy due to a significantly higher risk of fungal infections.

Treatment

Patients with acute liver failure should be immediately admitted to an intensive care unit for supportive care. Pulmonary artery monitoring is warranted in patients with hemodynamic instability. In patients with grade 3 or grade 4 hepatic encephalopathy, mechanical

Table 25.5 Criteria for liver transplantation in fulminant hepatic failure.

Criteria of King's College, London[1]
Acetaminophen patients
  pH <7.30, or
  Prothrombin time 6.5 (INR)[2] and serum
    creatinine >3.4 mg/dL
Nonacetaminophen patients
  Prothrombin time 6.5 (INR), or
  Any 3 of the following variables:
    Etiology: non-A, non-B hepatitis or drug reaction
    Age <10 and >40 years
    Duration of jaundice before encephalopathy >7 days
    Serum bilirubin >17.6 mg/dL
    Prothrombin time >3.5 (INR)

Criteria of Hospital Paul-Brousse, Villejuif[3]
Hepatic encephalopathy, and:
  Factor V level <20% in patient younger than 30 years
    of age, or
  Factor V level <30% in patients 30 years of age or older

---

[1]Data from ref. 6.
[2]INR, international normalized ratio.
[3]Data from ref. 16.
Reproduced from ref. 1.

ventilation and intracerebral pressure monitoring should be considered. The etiology of fulminant hepatic failure should be determined and specific antidote therapy should be immediately initiated. Fulminant hepatic failure associated with acetaminophen and mushroom poisoning may benefit from prompt N-acetylcysteine treatment, particularly in patients with suicide attempt who present early after ingestion of a large quantity of acetaminophen. Acid suppression therapy is used routinely to prevent stress-induced ulceration and gastrointestinal bleeding. Subsequently, the need and candidacy for liver transplantation should be evaluated.

Patients with fulminant hepatic failure should be transferred to a liver transplant center for further evaluation and management (Tables 25.4 and 25.5). Liver transplantation is a proven therapy for patients with fulminant hepatic failure. In a retrospective study from the US of 295 patients with acute liver failure, 41% underwent liver transplantation, 25% recovered with supportive therapy and 34% did not survive. The 1-year survival rate following liver transplantation

was 76%. The predictors of improved survival following liver transplantation for fulminant hepatic failure included improvements in surgical procedures, more effective immunosuppressive drugs, and a multidisciplinary approach to the intensive care management. Marginal donors can be considered. Liver transplantation can be performed across ABO blood groups. Some factors that prevent a successful liver transplant include lack of access to a transplant center, inadequate psychosocial support system and donor shortage.

Patients have also undergone auxiliary heterotropic liver transplantation in emergent situations with comparable results, although this approach is rarely used in routine practice. In patients who demonstrate recovery of native liver posttransplant, immunosuppression can be discontinued. The heterotopic graft undergoes rejection and atrophy following withdrawal of immunosuppression. Living donor liver transplantation using a donor right lobe to an adult recipient and donor left lobe or left lateral segment to a child recipient has been performed in patients with fulminant hepatic failure as a result of the organ shortage, but ethical issues surrounding informed consent are challenging. Extracorporeal human donor graft has been used for a few days if the organ is not suitable. The methods of temporary liver support include various hepatic assist or support devices; these approaches remain experimental and should only be used in the context of a clinical trial. Research is ongoing to develop transgenic pig livers that may be used in future to provide extracorporeal organ as a bridge to liver transplantation, but this approach is not likely to be available in the near future. Charcoal hemoperfusion demonstrated benefit in an uncontrolled pilot trial, but a follow-up controlled trial showed no improvement in survival rates. The use of corticosteroids, insulin, glucagon, prostaglandin analogues, repeated exchange transfusions, plasmapheresis, total body washout, and hemoperfusion through isolated primate livers remains experimental with no proven clinical benefit in patients with fulminant hepatic failure.

Prognosis

The prognostic indicators of acute liver failure were studied by O'Grady and colleagues in London at the King's College Hospital Acute Liver Failure Unit [15].

The observations made by these experts demonstrate a gradual improvement in survival over a 15-year period. The survival benefit is clearly associated with improvement in supportive care in the setting of the intensive care unit and has no relationship with specific therapy. The overall mortality declined from 80% in 1973 to less than 50% in 1988. The etiology of acute liver failure is a major determinant of likelihood of recovery with supportive management and without the need for liver transplantation. Patients with acetaminophen hepatotoxicity and fulminant hepatitis A demonstrated much the best survival rates, whereas patients with non-A, non-B hepatitis or idiosyncratic drug reactions having the worst survival rates. Other predictors of prognosis in patients with fulminant hepatic failure include stage of hepatic encephalopathy and factor V levels. The grade of hepatic encephalopathy is an important predictor of outcome, with poor survival rates associated with grade 3 and grade 4 hepatic encephalopathy. Bernuau and colleagues have reported that factor V levels of less than 20% in patients younger than 30 years of age or less than 30% in older patients predict poor survival rate in the setting of viral hepatitis-related fulminant hepatic failure [16]. It is important to closely monitor serial changes in the prognostic predictors and overall clinical status. It is crucial to establish the need for liver transplantation prior to the onset of grade 4 hepatic encephalopathy, cerebral edema and multiorgan failure (Table 25.5). In the era of donor shortage and increasing demand for liver transplantation, prudent utilization of liver transplantation in the setting of acute liver failure is necessary.

References

1. Keeffe EB. Acute liver failure. In: McQuaid KR, Friedman SL, Grendell JH, eds. Current Diagnosis and Treatment in Gastroenterology, 2nd edition. New York: Lange Medical Books/McGraw-Hill, 2003: 536–45.
2. Riordan SM, Williams R. Fulminant hepatic failure. Clin Liver Dis 2000; 4:25–45.
3. Hoofnagle JH, Carithers RL Jr, Shapiro C, et al. Fulminant hepatic failure: summary of a workshop. Hepatology 1995; 21:240–52.
4. Trey C, Davidson LS. The management of fulminant hepatic failure. In: Popper H, Schaffner F, eds. Progress in Liver Disease. New York: Grune & Stratton, 1970: 282–98.
5. Bernuau J, Rueff B, Benhamou J-P. Fulminant and subfulminant liver failure: definitions and causes. Semin Liver Dis 1986; 6:97–106.
6. O'Grady JG, Schalm SW, Williams R. Acute liver failure: redefining the syndromes. Lancet 1993; 342:273–5.
7. Lee WL. Acute liver failure. N Engl J Med 1993; 329:1862–72.
8. Davern TJ, James LP, Hinson J, et al. Acute Liver Failure Study Group. Measurement of serum acetaminophen-protein adducts in patients with acute liver failure. Gastroenterology 2006; 130:687–94.
9. Shakil AO, Kramer D, Mazariegos GV, et al. Acute liver failure: clinical features, outcome analysis, and applicability of prognostic criteria. Liver Transpl 2000; 6:163–9.
10. Ostapowicz G, Fontana RJ, Schiodt FV, et al. Results of a prospective study of acute liver failure at 17 tertiary care centers in the United States. Ann Intern Med 2002; 137:947–54.
11. Teo EK, Ostapowicz GA, Hussain M, et al. Hepatitis B infection in patients with acute liver failure in the United States. Hepatology 2001; 33:972–6.
12. Umemura T, Tanaka E, Lee WM, et al. The role of SEN virus infection in various liver diseases from different geographic regions (Abstract). Hepatology 2002; 36:646A.
13. Keeffe EB. Acute hepatitis A and B in patients with chronic liver disease: prevention with vaccination. Am J Med 2005; 118:21S–27S.
14. Bernal W, Wendon J. Liver transplantation in adults with acute liver failure. J Hepatol 2004; 40:192–7.
15. O'Grady JG, Alexander GJM, Hayllar KM, et al. Early indicators of prognosis in fulminant hepatic failure. Gastroenterology 1989; 97:439–45.
16. Bernuau J, Samuel D, Durand F, et al. Criteria for emergency liver transplantation in patients with acute viral hepatitis and factor V below 50% of normal: a prospective study. Hepatology 1991; 14:49A (Abstract).
17. Gimson AES et al. Clinical and prognostic differences in fulminant hepatitis type A, B, and non-A, non-B. Gut 1983; 24:1194.
18. Muñoz SJ. Difficult management problems in fulminant hepatic failure. Semin Liv Dis 1993; 13:395.

26 Management of Ascites and Spontaneous Bacterial Peritonitis

Andrés Cárdenas, Pere Ginès

Ascites is a common presenting sign in patients with various gastroenterological disorders. The most common cause of ascites is portal hypertension secondary to cirrhosis, which accounts for over 80% of patients with ascites [1]. Malignancy, congestive heart failure, tuberculosis, peritoneal diseases and other causes are the etiology of ascites in approximately 20% of cases. The development of ascites is a major complication of cirrhosis associated with an impaired quality of life and decreased survival. Nearly 60% of patients with compensated cirrhosis develop ascites within a period of 10 years after diagnosis of the disease [2]. The development of ascites in cirrhosis is associated with a probability of survival of 85% at 1 year and 56% at 5 years [3]. Patients with cirrhosis and ascites are at risk of developing complications associated with a poor prognosis such as dilutional hyponatremia, refractory ascites, spontaneous bacterial peritonitis (SBP) and/or hepatorenal syndrome (HRS) and as a result should always be considered for liver transplantation [4]. This chapter will discuss the management of ascites and SBP in the setting of cirrhosis.

Pathophysiology of ascites in cirrhosis

Patients with advanced cirrhosis and portal hypertension develop an inability to maintain extracellular fluid volume within normal limits, which leads to the accumulation of fluid in the peritoneal and/or pleural cavities and interstitial tissue [5–7]. The main cause of fluid accumulation is an abnormal increase in renal sodium reabsorption. Patients with cirrhosis develop arterial splanchnic vasodilation likely secondary to the release of local vasodilator factors such as nitric oxide, glucagon or prostacyclin with a subsequent decrease in effective arterial blood volume [6,7]. The accumulation of fluid and the abnormalities in renal function are the consequence of the homeostatic activation of vasoconstrictor and antinatriuretic factors triggered to compensate for a relative arterial underfilling. A detailed review of the pathogenesis of ascites in cirrhosis is beyond the scope of this chapter and can be found elsewhere [6,7].

Clinical presentation and diagnosis

Clinical features

The main clinical symptom of patients with ascites is abdominal distension often accompanied by lower extremity edema. Some patients presenting with tense ascites have difficulty breathing and limited physical activity. In cases where ascites occurs de novo, it usually develops slowly over the course of several weeks or months. Worsening liver disease, portal vein thrombosis, organic renal failure and development of hepatocellular carcinoma with tumor invasion of the portal vein may also precipitate the development of ascites. In severe alcoholic hepatitis, ascites may appear rapidly but in most cases there is resolution following therapy and abstinence. Dyspnea may also occur as a consequence of accompanying pleural effusions.

Gastrointestinal Emergencies, 2nd edition. Edited by Tony Tham, John Collins and Roy Soetikno. © 2009 by Blackwell Publishing, ISBN: 978-1-4051-4634-0.

Patients with spontaneous bacterial peritonitis (SBP) can present with fever, chills, abdominal pain, hepatic encephalopathy, and rebound abdominal tenderness. However, in some cases patients with SBP may be asymptomatic or present with very few symptoms.

Other common manifestations of patients with ascites include fatigue, weakness, malnutrition and jaundice. Abdominal hernias due to increased intraabdominal pressure may occur in patients with cirrhosis and long-standing ascites [8]. Umbilical hernias may increase in size in untreated ascites and sometimes cause significant complications such as rupture and infection due to previous ulcer formation on the surface and delayed wound healing. Inguinal hernias can also be problematic in patients with ascites. Painful gynecomastia may occur in patients with cirrhosis and ascites either due to estrogen excess in cirrhotic patients or the estrogenic effects of spironolactone, a diuretic commonly used in these patients.

It is considered that patients must have approximately 1.5 liters of fluid for ascites to be detected reliably by physical examination [9]. The current classification of ascites defined by the International Ascites Club divides patients into three groups [10]. Patients with grade 1 ascites are those in whom ascites is detected only by ultrasonography. Patients with grade 2 ascites are those in whom ascites causes moderate distension of the abdomen associated with mild or moderate discomfort. Patients with grade 3 ascites have large amounts of ascitic fluid causing marked abdominal distension and associated with significant discomfort. Patients with refractory ascites are those that do not respond to high doses of diuretics or develop side effects that preclude their use.

Evaluation

The evaluation of a cirrhotic patient either in the emergency room or in the hospital ward must include standard hematology, electrolyte, renal (serum creatinine and blood urea nitrogen), coagulation (prothombin time or international normalized ratio) and liver tests (aminotransferases, bilirubin, albumin, total protein, alkaline phosphatase, serum alpha-fetoprotein) [11]. An abdominal ultrasonography to rule out hepatocellular carcinoma and evaluate the patency of the portal venous system should be performed [11,12]. In addition, an upper gastrointestinal endoscopy to assess the presence and characteristics of esophageal and gastric varices

Table 26.1 Initial evaluation of patients with cirrhosis and ascites.

Checklist
1. Admission to the hospital: patients presenting with the first episode of ascites, those with known ascites and fever, abdominal pain, gastrointestinal bleeding, hepatic encephalopathy, hypotension or renal failure
2. Monitor arterial pressure, pulse, intake and outtake, urine volume and daily weight
3. Standard hematology, coagulation, liver tests and alpha-fetoprotein
4. Abdominal ultrasonography and Doppler flow (including the kidneys)
5. Upper gastrointestinal endoscopy to assess the presence of esophageal and gastric varices
6. Evaluation of ascitic fluid Total protein and albumin measurement Cell count Culture in blood culture bottles
7. Evaluation of renal function* 24-h urine sodium Serum electrolytes, serum blood urea nitrogen and serum creatinine Urine sediment and protein excretion

*Renal function should initially be assessed with the patient maintained on a low–sodium diet without diuretic therapy.

is recommended [11]. In patients with renal failure (serum creatinine greater than 1.5 mg/dL), urine sediment and 24-hour urine protein should be assessed and the kidneys examined by ultrasonography. Evaluation of circulatory function should include measurement of arterial pressure and heart rate. A checklist of tests that need to be performed in patients with cirrhosis and ascites is described in Table 26.1.

Ascitic fluid analysis

The technique for performing paracentesis has been described elsewhere [13,14]. The risk of bleeding in cirrhotic patients when performing a paracentesis is extremely low; the frequency of severe hemorrhage after a tap is approximately 0.20% and a lethal outcome occurs in less than 0.01% of cases [15]. Most clinical trials in patients with cirrhosis and ascites have excluded patients with an elevated prothrombin time greater than 21 seconds or international normalized ratio (INR) greater than 1.6 or platelet count below 50 000 per μL. Therefore the risk of bleeding complications in patients with more severe coagulopathy is unknown and deserves investigation. Nonetheless consensus meetings, guidelines and expert opinion consider that the abnormal coagulation profile of the cirrhotic patient (mild prolonged prothrombin time and low platelets with a value >50 000 per μL) is not an absolute contraindication for paracentesis and the routine administration of platelets or fresh frozen plasma as prophylaxis for bleeding is not recommended [12–14, 16,17]. In a recent survey of the use of coagulation products in performing a paracentesis in patients with cirrhosis among practitioners, 50% indicated that they either never used prophylaxis or only used it if the INR of the patient was >2.5 [17]. In patients with severe thrombocytopenia with a platelet count <40 000 per μL some authors recommend the administration of platelets, although the risk of bleeding in this situation has not been specifically assessed [16]. Patients with suspected disseminated intravascular coagulopathy should not undergo a paracentesis [12].

A diagnostic paracentesis (30 mL of fluid) is required in all patients presenting with their first episode of ascites and in those requiring hospitalization with any evidence of clinical deterioration such as fever, abdominal pain, gastrointestinal bleeding, hepatic encephalopathy, hypotension or renal failure. The ascitic fluid in cirrhotic patients is mostly transparent and yellow or amber in color. Necessary tests in the ascitic fluid include cell count, albumin, total protein and cultures in blood culture bottles (10 mL of fluid injected at the bedside) [10–12,16]. Glucose, lactate dehydrogense, amylase, bilirubin, triglyceride, tuberculosis smear and cytological analysis of the fluid are optional and may provide important information in the differential diagnosis of ascites in selected cases.

Patients with cirrhosis and ascites for the most part have a low total ascitic fluid protein concentration of less than 30 g/L, the vast majority have a protein concentration in ascitic fluid lower than 15 g/L. A low protein concentration in ascitic fluid (<10–15 g/L) is associated with an increased risk of SBP [18,19]. Patients with low ascitic fluid protein should be given prophylaxis with oral quinolones to reduce the risk of SBP and HRS (see later). The difference between

serum albumin concentration and ascites albumin concentration (serum–ascites albumin gradient) in patients with cirrhosis and ascites is usually greater than 11 g/L, values lower than 11 g/L suggest a cause of ascites other than cirrhosis [12].

The cell count is the most helpful test in determining bacterial infection. In most cases the ascitic fluid white blood cell count is less than 500/mm^3 with a predominance of mononuclear cells (>75%) and a low number of neutrophils. An increased number of white blood cells with predominance of neutrophils indicates peritoneal infection. The diagnosis of SBP is made when the fluid sample has >250/mm neutrophils [20]. Reagent strips may be useful for the rapid diagnosis of peritoneal fluid infection in the emergency department where a prompt diagnosis may enable the physician to begin therapy right after the tap [21,22]. The strips might be useful in diagnosing peritoneal infection, but since they do not provide a cell count number or differential, it is prudent to also obtain a concomitant cell count and differential with cultures if they are going to be used. Bloody ascites (>50 000 red blood cells/mm^3) which may occur due to a traumatic tap or underlying hepatocellular carcinoma may lead to a higher neutrophil count in the absence of infection, in this case a correction factor of 1 neutrophil per 250 red blood cells is recommended [20].

The distinction of secondary bacterial peritonitis (peritoneal infection arising from gut perforation) from SBP is critical as mortality in the former is extremely high without surgical intervention. On the other hand, mortality is near 80% if a patient with advanced liver disease and SBP is subjected to an unnecessary exploratory laparotomy [23]. Patients with secondary bacterial peritonitis usually have a clinical picture of severe abdominal pain, high fever and a rigid abdomen and therefore an abdominal CT scan or ultrasonography should be performed. A multimicrobial positive ascitic fluid culture or a reduction in ascitic fluid neutrophil count of less than 25% of the pretreatment value after two days of antibiotic treatment suggests failure to respond to therapy and should raise the suspicion of secondary peritonitis. Patients with secondary bacterial peritonitis from gastrointestinal perforation can also have an elevation of the ascitic fluid total protein to levels >10 g/L, glucose <50 mg/dL, and LDH >225 mU/mL

[24]. Also an ascitic fluid carcinoembryonic antigen >5 ng/mL or an ascitic fluid alkaline phosphatase >240 units/L have been proposed as accurate markers in detecting gut perforation into the ascitic fluid [25].

Treatment of ascites

Evaluation for liver transplantation

Figure 26.1 outlines the different treatment modalities applicable to patients with cirrhosis and ascites. After the initial evaluation described above, the most important aspect of the management of all patients with cirrhosis and ascites is an evaluation for liver transplantation. Most patients with cirrhosis and ascites have advanced liver disease with high Child–Pugh scores. Patients with an elevated serum bilirubin level, an elevated prothrombin time and a low serum albumin level have an impaired liver function that is associated with a poor prognosis without liver transplantation. Other important factors indicating a poor prognosis in cirrhosis with ascites are those related to renal and circulatory function. These include dilutional hyponatremia (serum sodium <130 mEq/L), low arterial blood pressure, serum creatinine >1.2 mg/dL, and intense sodium retention (urine sodium less than 10 mEq/day) [26]. Patients with any of these manifestations should be given priority for liver transplantation as they have a poor outcome since medical therapy of these conditions is not curative of the underlying cause. Allocation for liver transplantation in some countries is based on the model for end-stage

liver disease (MELD) score that includes serum bilirubin, serum creatinine and the INR as variables [27]. This scoring system is objective, includes a parameter of renal function, and predicts survival in cirrhotics. In patients with cirrhosis and ascites the MELD score is also predictive of survival and might be a reliable parameter that helps calculate risk in these patients once they present with their first episode of ascites.

Sodium restriction and nutritional recommendations

A reduction in sodium intake alone achieves a negative sodium balance in approximately 10% of patients. A low sodium diet with 90 mmol/day is recommended because a more severe restriction is usually unpalatable [10–12]. Patients with dilutional hyponatremia (serum sodium level <130 mEq/L) need fluid restriction of 1–1.5 liters per day. An evaluation by a nutritionist is recommended for appropriate education regarding an appropriate caloric and salt intake. Improvement of the nutritional status is extremely important because patients with advanced liver disease have decreased intake and absorption of nutrients, increased energy expenditure and altered fuel metabolism with an accelerated starvation metabolism [28,29]. Nutritional therapy in cirrhotic patients can improve nutritional status, reduce infection rates and decrease perioperative morbidity [28,29]. It is also recommended that nutritional therapy be instituted for long periods of time or until patients reach liver transplantation. The goal is for nutritional supplementation to correct the underlying

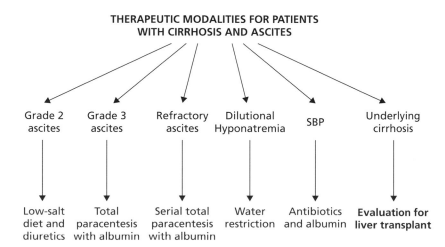

Figure 26.1 Treatment modalities for patients with ascites and cirrhosis.

protein energy malnutrition. Enteral nutrition in cirrhotic patients with ascites may improve liver function and hepatic encephalopathy [28–31]. There is data that suggests that enteral feeding in decompensated cirrhosis is more effective than a conventional diet in improving liver function and survival [31].

Uncomplicated ascites

Patients with *grade 1 ascites* do not require any specific treatment. Patients with *grade 2 ascites* should be treated with a low-sodium diet and diuretics [11]. The best initial regimen for reducing ascites is spironolactone (initial doses 50 to 100 mg/day), a drug that inhibits sodium reabsorption by binding to the mineralocorticoid receptor in the renal collecting tubules, thus blocking the effects of aldosterone. Furosemide (initial doses 20 to 40 mg/day) is useful in patients with concomitant peripheral edema or anasarca. Spironolactone alone may be used up to a dose of 400 mg/day and furosemide subsequently added up to 160 mg/day in progressively increasing doses [16,32]. In patients who do not respond, compliance with the low-sodium diet and the diuretics should be confirmed, afterwards the dose may be increased every 5–7 days. Spironolactone may cause painful gynecomastia in some patients and oral tamoxifen (20 mg twice daily) has been used in the management of this complication with some success [33]. Muscle cramps due to diuretic therapy may require a reduction in diuretic dosage. Quinidine (quinidine sulfate, 400 mg/day) [34] and intravenous albumin administration (25 g/week) [35] have been reported to reduce the frequency and intensity of muscle cramps in cirrhotic patients with ascites treated with diuretics, but more information is needed. The goal of treatment is to produce an average weight loss of 0.5 kg/day in patients without edema and 1 kg/day in those with peripheral edema.

Therapeutic paracentesis is the treatment of choice in the management of *grade 3 ascites* [10–13,16,36]. Complete removal of ascites in one tap with intravenous albumin (8 g per liter tapped) has been shown to be a fast and effective measure in controlling tense ascites and associated with a lower number of complications than conventional diuretic therapy [36]. A post-paracentesis circulatory dysfunction may develop after a large tap; this is a circulatory derangement that is accompanied by activation of the renin-angiotensin system that occurs few days after the procedure [36,37].

Table 26.2 Management practice points in patients with ascites and cirrhosis (all patients must be evaluated for liver transplantation).

A. Treatment strategy for patients with cirrhosis and grade 2 ascites
- Start with a low-sodium diet (90 mmol/day) and spironolactone (50–100 mg/day) to reach goal of weight loss: 500 g/day. If needed, doses to be increased every 7 days up to 400 mg/day of spironolactone. Furosemide can be added at a staring dose of 40 mg/day and subsequently increased to 160 mg/day in patients with peripheral edema and anasarca.

B. Treatment strategy for patients with cirrhosis and grade 3 ascites or refractory ascites
- Total paracentesis plus intravenous albumin (8 g per liter of ascites removed) followed by a low-sodium diet (90 mmol/day) and diuretics if patient tolerated them beforehand.
- Total paracentesis plus intravenous albumin can be performed as needed. Consider use of TIPS in patients with very frequent recurrent ascites and preserved hepatic function, aged <70 years, and no hepatic encephalopathy.

This disorder, although silent, may be associated with hyponatremia, renal impairment and decreased survival. It may be effectively prevented with the administration of plasma expanders [38,39]. When less than 5 L of ascites are removed, artificial plasma expanders, saline and albumin are equally effective [39–41]. However, if more than 5 L are removed, albumin is recommended [39–41]. Since in virtually all patients after a paracentesis ascites will recur, they need to be started or continued on spironolactone in order to prevent a positive sodium balance and recurrence of ascites [42]. Recommendations for the management of ascites are summarized in Table 26.2.

Refractory ascites

The definition and diagnostic criteria of refractory ascites are listed in Table 26.3 [43]. The vast majority of patients with refractory ascites have very intense sodium retention and a severely impaired capacity to excrete solute-free water, the latter resulting in dilutional hyponatremia [43]. Moreover, most patients have a reduction in renal plasma flow and glomerular

Table 26.3 Definition and diagnostic criteria for refractory ascites in cirrhosis.

Diuretic-resistant ascites: Ascites that cannot be mobilized or the early recurrence of which cannot be prevented because of a lack of response to sodium restriction and diuretic treatment

Diuretic-intractable ascites: Ascites that cannot be mobilized or the early recurrence of which cannot be prevented because of the development of diuretic-induced complications that preclude the use of an effective diuretic dosage

Requisites:
1. Treatment duration: Patients must be on intensive diuretic therapy (spironolactone 400 mg/d and furosemide 160 mg/d) for at least 1 week and on a salt-restricted diet of less than 90 mmol/day.
2. Lack of response: Mean weight loss of <0.8 kg over 4 days and urinary sodium output less than the sodium intake.
3. Early ascites recurrence: Reappearance of grade 2 or 3 ascites within 4 weeks of initial mobilization.
4. Diuretic-induced complications: Diuretic-induced hepatic encephalopathy is the development of encephalopathy in the absence of any other precipitating factor. Diuretic-induced renal impairment is an increase of serum creatinine by >100% to a value >2 mg/dL in patients with ascites responding to treatment. Diuretic-induced hyponatremia is defined as a decrease of serum sodium by >10 mmol/L to a serum sodium of <125 mmol/L. Diuretic induced hypo- or hyperkalemia is defined as a change in serum potassium to <3 mmol/L or >6 mmol/L despite appropriate measures.

*Modified with permission from ref 10 (Moore KP, Wong F, Ginès P, et al. The management of ascites in cirrhosis: report on the consensus conference of the International Ascites Club. Hepatology 2003; 38:258–66)

filtration rate. The difference with nonrefractory ascites patients is that, in these, sodium excretion may be increased with the use of diuretics, whereas in refractory ascites, sodium retention cannot be treated with diuretics either because patients do not respond to high doses or they develop side effects that preclude their use.

Current treatment strategies include repeated therapeutic paracentesis plus intravenous albumin or the use of a transjugular intrahepatic portosystemic shunt (TIPS). TIPS is a nonsurgical method of portal decompression that consists of the insertion of an intrahepatic stent between one hepatic vein and the portal vein using a transjugular approach [44]. Reduction in portal pressure is accompanied by a resolution of ascites in most patients. This method may be associated with several side effects such as the development of hepatic encephalopathy and obstruction of the prosthesis.

Therapeutic paracentesis is the most accepted initial therapy for refractory ascites. Patients generally require a tap every 2 to 4 weeks which can be performed in an outpatient setting. This approach is therefore easy to perform and relatively inexpensive [45]. Uncovered TIPS are very effective in relieving ascites, but frequently complicated by obstruction of the prosthesis (70% in 1 year) [44]. Polytetrafluoroethylene-covered

prostheses seem to improve TIPS patency and decrease the number of clinical relapses and reinterventions without increasing the risk of encephalopathy [46]. Randomized clinical trials comparing TIPS vs. repeated paracentesis demonstrate that TIPS controls ascites effectively and is associated with a lower rate of ascites recurrence [45,47–50]. In addition patients with ascites who undergo TIPS improve their nutritional status as measured by resting energy expenditure, total body nitrogen, body fat and food intake [51]. Hepatic encephalopathy occurs in approximately 30–50% of patients [45,48,49]. Two studies showed a survival benefit with TIPS [48,50], but two other studies demonstrated no difference in survival [45,49]. Several meta-analyses of these randomized controlled studies conclude that TIPS is better at controlling ascites but survival is not different [52–54]. For the above reasons large-volume paracentesis appears to be the initial treatment of choice in patients with refractory ascites [55]. TIPS placement may be reserved for patients with very rapid recurrence of ascites and preserved liver function (bilirubin <5 mg/dL, Child–Pugh score <12, MELD score <14), aged below 70, without hepatic encephalopathy or cardiopulmonary disease [54,55]. Recommendations for the management of refractory ascites are summarized in Table 26.2.

Treatment and prophylaxis of spontaneous bacterial peritonitis

SBP is a common and severe complication of cirrhotic patients with ascites characterized by a monomicrobial infection of ascitic fluid in the absence of any intraabdominal source of infection [20,56]. The prevalence of SBP in hospitalized cirrhotic patients ranges between 10% and 30% [56]. Gram-negative bacteria are responsible for nearly 80% of cases, with *Escherichia coli* accounting for most of them. Aerobic gram-positive bacteria, mostly *Streptococcus viridans*, *Staphylococcus aureus* and *Enterococcus fecalis*, are isolated in approximately 20% of cases [57]. The pathogenesis of SBP involves passage of bacteria from the intestinal lumen to the systemic circulation through translocation of bacteria to mesenteric lymph nodes, bacteremia secondary to the impairment of the reticuloendothelial system phagocytic activity, and infection due to poor opsonization and defective bactericidal activity of ascitic fluid [58].

The clinical spectrum of SBP is variable and ranges from an asymptomatic presentation to a full-blown picture of peritonitis, therefore the diagnosis relies on a high index of suspicion and prompt examination of the ascitic fluid. Additionally patients with cirrhosis and sepsis-related infections including SBP may develop adrenal insufficiency in 50–70% of cases [59,60]. The development of adrenal insufficiency is associated with hemodynamic instability and increased mortality (80% in those with adrenal insufficiency vs. 37% without adrenal insufficiency) [59]. Furthermore in cirrhotic patients with adrenal insufficiency (diagnosed by the short corticotropin test within the first 24 hours of admission) and septic shock administration of intravenous hydrocortisone (50 mg every 6 hours) helps with the resolution of shock and improves survival in those with advanced Child C cirrhosis [60]. An important clinical feature of SBP is the development of renal failure during the infection as it develops in 30 to 40% of patients with SBP, and is a major cause of death [61,62]. The risk may be decreased with infusion of intravenous albumin [62].

Therapy and prognosis

Antibiotic therapy should be initiated in patients with a neutrophil count in ascitic fluid greater than $250/mm^3$ before microbiologic results are obtained [20]. Empiric antibiotic therapy with an intravenous third-generation cephalosporin (cefotaxime 2 g every 8–12 hours or ceftriaxone 1 g/24 hours) for 5 days is required after diagnosis is confirmed [20,56]. Therapy modification depends on results from cultures. Assessment of response to therapy includes frequent clinical evaluation and repeat diagnostic paracentesis 2–3 days after beginning antibiotics. In case of treatment failure (worsening infection or no decrease in PMN count), antibiotic therapy should be revised and appropriately changed. SBP resolves in over 90% of cases if treated with the above regimens [20]. However, hospital mortality remains between 10% and 30%, because most of these patients have advanced liver failure and complications such as gastrointestinal bleeding, renal failure and hepatic encephalopathy. The most important predictor of survival in patients with SBP is the development of renal failure during the infection [61]. Renal failure is triggered by an impairment of circulatory function with activation of vasoconstrictor systems. The administration of albumin at a dose of 1.5 g/kg at the diagnosis of the infection and 1 g/kg 48 hours later prevents renal failure and improves survival in patients with SBP [62]. Recommendations for the management of SBP are summarized in Table 26.4.

Prophylaxis

Unfortunately life expectancy after an episode of SBP is short, with a 1-year probability of survival of 30–50% if antibiotic prophylaxis is not given [56,63]. Conditions associated with an increased risk of SBP include: gastrointestinal bleeding, low protein concentration in ascitic fluid, advanced liver failure (high serum bilirubin and/or markedly prolonged prothrombin time) and past history of SBP. Because most episodes of SBP are caused by gram-negative bacteria present in the normal intestinal flora, oral quinolones such as norfloxacin or ciprofloxacin have been used as prophylactic agents. The efficacy of this approach has been demonstrated in patients with gastrointestinal hemorrhage [64–66] and patients who have recovered from the first SBP episode [67] and has been recommended by a panel of experts in an International Consensus Conference on SBP [20].

In patients with gastrointestinal hemorrhage, the short-term administration of norfloxacin or intravenous ceftriaxone reduces the incidence of SBP or bacteremia as compared with patients not receiving prophylactic antibiotics [64–66,68,69]. In patients with advanced liver disease who are actively bleeding,

Table 26.4 Recommendations for the management and prevention of spontaneous bacterial peritonitis.

Therapy
1. After diagnosis of peritonitis has been made (>250 neutrophils/mm^3 in ascitic fluid), start with third-generation cephalosporins (e.g. cefotaxime 2 g/8–12 h iv or ceftriaxone 1 g/24 h iv)
2. Infuse albumin (1.5 g/kg at diagnosis of the infection and 1 g/kg 48 hours later)
3. Maintain antibiotic therapy for at least 5 days or until disappearance of signs of infection. Patients should be evaluated daily to assess signs of infection. A follow-up paracentesis helps evaluate response to therapy
4. After resolution of infection, start long-term oral norfloxacin 400 mg/day

Prevention
1. Patients with gastrointestinal hemorrhage:
   Norfloxacin 400 mg/12 h orally or per gastric tube for 7 days in patients with preserved liver function and not actively bleeding
   Intravenous ceftriaxone 1 g/day for 7 days in patients with advanced liver failure and/or actively bleeding
2. Patients with ascites with a previous episode of SBP
   Norfloxacin 400 mg/day indefinitely
   Evaluation for liver transplantation
3. Patients with ascites and advanced liver disease* without a previous episode of SBP and low ascitic fluid protein concentration (<15 g/liter):
   Norfloxacin 400 mg/day indefinitely

*Serum bilirubin >3 mg/dL, Child–Pugh score >10, dilutional hyponatremia (serum sodium <130 mEq/L) and/or renal impairment.

intravenous ceftriaxone is preferred [68]. Previous metaanalyses indicate that antibiotic prophylaxis in patients with gastrointestinal bleeding not only prevents infection but also improve survival [64,66]. Long-term norfloxacin administration is effective in the prevention of SBP recurrence (secondary prophylaxis) [67]. Antibiotic prophylaxis also appears to be effective in the prevention of SBP (primary prophylaxis) in patients with low ascitic fluid protein (<15 g/L), who are at high risk of developing the first episode of SBP. Primary prophylaxis with norfloxacin reduces the incidence of SBP, delays the development of HRS and improves survival in patients with advanced cirrhosis [70].

References

1. Càrdenas A, Ginés P, Arroyo V. Ascites. In: Weinstein W, Hawkey CJ, Bosch J, eds. Clinical Gastroenterology and Hepatology. Elsevier Science, 2005: 101–4.
2. Ginés P, Quintero E, Arroyo V, et al. Compensated cirrhosis: natural history and prognostic factors. Hepatology 1987; 7:122–8.
3. Planas R, Montoliu S, Ballesté B, et al. Natural history of patients hospitalized for management of cirrhotic ascites. Clin Gastroenterol Hepatol 2006; 4:1385–94.
4. Murray KL, Carithers RL. AASLD practice guidelines: evaluation of the patient for liver transplantation. Hepatology 2005; 41:1407–32.
5. Schrier RW, Arroyo V, Bernardi M, et al. Peripheral arterial vasodilation hypothesis: a proposal for the initiation of renal sodium and water retention in cirrhosis. Hepatology 1988; 8:1151–7.
6. Cárdenas A, Arroyo V. Mechanisms of water and sodium retention in cirrhosis and the pathogenesis of ascites. Best Pract Res Clin Endocrinol Metab 2003; 17:607–22.
7. Schrier RW. Water and sodium retention in edematous disorders: role of vasopressin and aldosterone. Am J Med 2006; 119(7 Suppl 1):S47–53.
8. Belghiti J, Durand F. Abdominal wall hernias in the setting of cirrhosis. Semin Liver Dis 1997; 17:219–26.
9. Cattau EL Jr, Benjamin SB, Knuff TE, Castell DO. The accuracy of the physical exam in the diagnosis of suspected ascites. JAMA 1982; 247:1164–6.
10. Moore KP, Wong F, Ginès P, et al. The management of ascites in cirrhosis: report on the consensus conference of the International Ascites Club. Hepatology 2003; 38:258–66.
11. Ginès P, Cárdenas, A, Arroyo V, Rodés J. Management of cirrhosis and ascites. N Engl J Med 2004; 350:1646–54.
12. Runyon B. Management of adult patients with ascites due to cirrhosis. Hepatology 2004; 39:841–56.
13. Cárdenas A, Guevara M, Ginés P. Paracentesis. In: Weinstein W, Hawkey CJ, Bosch J, eds. Clinical

Gastroenterology and Hepatology. Elsevier Science, 2005: 1097–100.

14. Thomsen TW, Shaffer RW, White B, Setnik GS. Videos in clinical medicine. Paracentesis. N Engl J Med 2006; 355:e21.

15. Pache I, Bilodeau M. Severe haemorrhage following abdominal paracentesis for ascites in patients with liver disease. Aliment Pharmacol Ther 2005; 21:525–9.

16. Moore KP. Aithal GP. Guidelines on the management of ascites in cirrhosis. Gut 2006; 55 Suppl 6:vi1–vi12.

17. Caldwell S, Hoffmann M, Lisman B, et al. Coagulation disorders and hemostasis in liver disease: pathophysiology and critical assessment of current management. Hepatology 2006; 44: 1039–46.

18. Runyon BA. Low-protein-concentration ascitic fluid is predisposed to spontaneous bacterial peritonitis Gastroenterology 1986; 91:1343–6.

19. Llach J, Rimola A, Navasa M, et al. Incidence and predictive factors of first episode of spontaneous bacterial peritonitis in cirrhosis with ascites: relevance of ascitic fluid protein concentration. Hepatology 1992; 16:742–47.

20. Rimola A, Garcia-Tsao G, Navasa M, et al. Diagnosis, treatment and prophylaxis of spontaneous bacterial peritonitis: a consensus document. International Ascites Club. J Hepatol 2000; 32:142–53.

21. Castellote J, López C, Gornals J, et al. Rapid diagnosis of spontaneous bacterial peritonitis by use of reagent strips. Hepatology 2003; 37: 893–96.

22. Sapey T, Mena E, Fort E, et al. Rapid diagnosis of spontaneous bacterial peritonitis with leukocyte esterase reagent strips in a European and in an American center. J Gastroenterol Hepatol 2005;20:187–92.

23. Garrison RN, Cryer HM, Howard DA, Polk HC Jr. Clarification of risk factors for abdominal operations in patients with hepatic cirrhosis. Ann Surg 1984; 199:648–55.

24. Runyon BA, Hoefs JC. Ascitic fluid analysis in the differentiation of spontaneous bacterial peritonitis from gastrointestinal tract perforation into ascitic fluid. Hepatology 1984; 4:447–50.

25. Wu SS, Lin OS, Chen Y-Y, et al. Ascitic fluid carcinoembryonic antigen and alkaline phosphatase levels for the differentiation of primary from secondary bacterial peritonitis with intestinal perforation. J Hepatol 2001; 34:215–21.

26. Llach J, Ginès P, Arroyo V, et al. Prognostic value of arterial pressure, endogenous vasoactive systems, and renal function in cirrhotic patients admitted to the hospital for the treatment of ascites. Gastroenterology 1988; 94:482–7.

27. Kamath P, Wiesner R, Malinchoc M, et al. A model to predict survival in patients with end-stage liver disease. Hepatology 2001; 33:464–70.

28. Henkel AS, Buchman AL. Nutritional support in patients with chronic liver disease. Nat Clin Pract Gastroenterol Hepatol 2006; 3:202–9.

29. McCullough AJ. Nutrition and malnutrition in liver disease. In: Wolfe MM, Davis GL, Farraye F, Giannella RA, Malagelada JR, Steer ML, eds. Therapy of Digestive Disorders, 2nd edition. WB Saunders, 2006: 67–83.

30. Kearns PJ, Young H, Garcia G, et al. Accelerated improvement of alcoholic liver disease with enteral nutrition. Gastroenterology 1992; 102:200–5.

31. Cabrè E, Gonzalez-Hux F, Abad-Lacruz A, et al. Effect of total enteral nutrition on the short-term outcome of severely malnourished cirrhotics: a randomized controlled trial. Gastroenterology 1990; 98:715–20.

32. Santos J, Planas R, Pardo A et al. Spironolactone alone or in combination with furosemide in the treatment of moderate ascites in nonazotemic cirrhosis: a randomized comparative study of efficacy and safety. J Hepatol 2003; 39:187–92.

33. Li CP, Lee FY, Hwang SJ, et al. Treatment of mastalgia with tamoxifen in male patients with liver cirrhosis: a randomized crossover study. Am J Gastroenterol 2000; 95:1051–5.

34. Lee FY, Lee SD, Tsai YT, et al. A randomized controlled trial of quinidine in the treatment of cirrhotic patients with muscle cramps. J Hepatol 1991; 12:236–40.

35. Angeli P, Albino G, Carraro P, et al. Cirrhosis and muscle cramps: evidence of a causal relationship. Hepatology 1996; 23:264–73.

36. Ginès P, Arroyo V, Quintero E, et al. Comparison of paracentesis and diuretics in the treatment of cirrhotics with tense ascites: results of a randomized study. Gastroenterology 1987; 93:234–41.

37. Ruiz-del-Arbol L, Monescillo A, Jiménez W, et al. Paracentesis-induced circulatory dysfunction: mechanism and effect on hepatic hemodynamics in cirrhosis. Gastroenterology 1997; 113:579–86.

38. Ginès P, Tito L, Arroyo V, et al. Randomized comparative study of therapeutic paracentesis with and without intravenous albumin in cirrhosis. Gastroenterology 1988; 94:1493–502.

39. Ginès A, Fernández-Esparrach G, Monescillo A, et al. Randomized trial comparing albumin, dextran 70, and polygeline in cirrhotic patients with ascites treated by paracentesis. Gastroenterology 1996; 111:1002–10.

40. Moreau R, Valla DC, Durand-Zaleski I, et al. Comparison of outcome in patients with cirrhosis and ascites following treatment with albumin or a synthetic colloid: a randomised controlled pilot trail. Liver Int 2006; 26:46–54.

41. Sola-Vera J, Minana J, Ricart E, et al. Randomized trial comparing albumin and saline in the prevention of paracentesis-induced circulatory dysfunction in cirrhotic patients with ascites. Hepatology 2003; 37:1147–53.

42. Fernández-Esparrach G, Guevara M, Sort P, et al. Diuretic requirements after therapeutic paracentesis in non-azotemic patients with cirrhosis: a randomized double-blind trial of spironolactone versus placebo. J Hepatol 1997; 26:614–20.

43. Arroyo V, Ginès P, Gerbes A, et al. Definition and diagnostic criteria of refractory ascites and hepatorenal syndrome in cirrhosis. Hepatology 1996; 23:164–76.

44. Boyer TD, Haskal Z. The role of transjugular intrahepatic portosystemic shunt in the management of portal hypertension. Hepatology 2005; 41:386–400.

45. Ginès P, Uriz J, Calahorra B, et al. Transjugular intrahepatic portosystemic shunting versus paracentesis plus albumin for refractory ascites in cirrhosis. Gastroenterology 2002; 123:1839–47.

46. Bureau C, García-Pagan JC, Otal P, et al. Improved clinical outcome using polytetrafluoroethylene-coated stents for TIPS: results of a randomized study. Gastroenterology 2004; 126:469–75.

47. Lebrec D, Giuily N, Hadengue A, et al. Transjugular intrahepatic portosystemic shunts: comparison with paracentesis in patients with cirrhosis and refractory ascites: a randomized trial. J Hepatol 1996; 25:135–44.

48. Rossle M, Ochs A, Gulberg V, et al. A comparison of paracentesis and transjugular intrahepatic portosystemic shunting in patients with ascites. N Engl J Med 2000; 342:1701–7.

49. Sanyal A, Genning C, Reddy RK, et al. The North American Study for Treatment of Refractory Ascites. Gastroenterology 2003; 124:634–41.

50. Salerno F, Merli M, Riggio O, et al. Randomized controlled study of TIPS versus paracentesis plus albumin in cirrhosis with severe ascites. Hepatology 2004; 40:629–35.

51. Allard JP, Chau J, Sandokji K, Blendis LM, Wong F. Effects of ascites resolution after successful TIPS on nutrition in cirrhotic patients with refractory ascites. Am J Gastroenterol 2001; 96:2442–7.

52. Delterne P, Mathurin P, Dharancy S, et al. Transjugular intrahepatic portosystemic shunt in refractory ascites: a meta-analysis. Liver Int 2005; 25:349–56.

53. Albillos A, Banares R, Gonzales M, et al. A meta-analysis of transjugular intrahepatic portosystemic shunt versus paracentesis for refractory ascites. J Hepatol 2005; 43:990–6.

54. Dámico G, Luca A, Morabito A, et al. Uncovered transjugular intrahepatic portosystemic shunt for refractory ascites: a meta-analysis. Gastroenterology 2005; 129:1282–93.

55. Cárdenas A, Ginès P. Management of refractory ascites. Clin Gastroenterol Hepatol 2005; 3:1187–91.

56. Garcia-Tsao G. Bacterial infections in cirrhosis: treatment and prophylaxis. J Hepatol 2005; 42 Suppl(1):S85–92.

57. Fernández J, Navasa M, Gómez J, et al. Bacterial infections in cirrhosis: epidemiological changes with invasive procedures and norfloxacin prophylaxis. Hepatology 2002; 35:140–8.

58. Wiest R, Garcia-Tsao R. Bacterial translocation (BT) in cirrhosis. Hepatology 2005; 41:422–33.

59. Tsai MH, Peng YS, Chen YC, et al. Adrenal insufficiency in patients with cirrhosis, severe sepsis and septic shock. Hepatology 2006; 43:673–81.

60. Fernández J, Escorsell A, Zabalza M, et al. Adrenal insufficiency in patients with cirrhosis and septic shock: effect of treatment with hydrocortisone on survival. Hepatology 2006: 44:1288–95.

61. Follo A, Llovet JM, Navasa M, et al. Renal impairment after spontaneous bacterial peritonitis in cirrhosis: incidence, clinical course, predictive factors and prognosis. Hepatology 1994; 20:495–501.

62. Sort P, Navasa M, Arroyo V, et al. Effect of intravenous albumin on renal impairment and mortality in patients with cirrhosis and spontaneous bacterial peritonitis. N Engl J Med 1999; 341:403–9.

63. Tito L, Rimola A, Ginès P, et al. Recurrence of spontaneous bacterial peritonitis in cirrhosis: frequency and predictive factors. Hepatology 1988; 8:27–31.

64. Bernard B, Grangé JD, Nguyen K, et al. Antibiotics prophylaxis in cirrhotic patients with gastrointestinal bleeding: a meta-analysis. Hepatology 1999; 29:1655–61.

65. Soriano G, Guarner C, Tomás A, et al. Norfloxacin prevents bacterial infection in cirrhotics with gastrointestinal hemorrhage. Gastroenterology 1992; 103:1267–72.

66. Soares-Weiser K, Brezis M, Tur-Kaspa R, Leibovici L. Antibiotic prophylaxis for cirrhotic patients with gastrointestinal bleeding. Cochrane Database Syst Rev. 2002; (2):CD002907.

67. Ginès P, Rimola A, Planas R, et al. Norfloxacin prevents spontaneous bacterial peritonitis recurrence in cirrhosis: results of a double blind, placebo-controlled trial. Hepatology 1990; 12:716–24.

68. Rimola A, Bory F, Terés J, et al. Oral, nonabsorbable antibiotics prevent infection in cirrhotics with gastrointestinal hemorrhage. Hepatology 1995; 5:463–7.

69. Fernández J, Ruiz del Arbol L, Gomez C, et al. Norfloxacin versus ceftriaxone in the prophylaxis of infections in patients with advanced cirrhosis and hemorrhage. Gastroenterology 2006; 131:1049–56.

70. Fernández J, Navasa M, Planas R, et al. Primary prophylaxis of spontaneous bacterial peritonitis delays hepatorenal syndrome and improves survival in cirrhosis. Gastroenterology. 2007; 133:818–24.

27 Alcoholic Hepatitis

David Patch

Introduction

While many patients presenting with alcoholic liver disease will have cirrhosis, as many as 60% will have evidence of an alcohol-related hepatitis [1]. For the clinician, the critical point is that alcoholic hepatitis is potentially reversible both clinically and histologically, and those patients who survive the inpatient period, and remain abstinent, may have a dramatic recovery in liver function. However, the short-term mortality of alcoholic hepatitis is particularly high among those with indicators of severe disease: patients with a Maddrey score of $\geq$ 32 have a 28-day mortality of 30–40% [1], and the 28-day mortality of patients with a Glasgow alcoholic hepatitis score $\geq$ 9 is 60% [2] (see below). Partly as a consequence, trials have tended to focus on this early period of the patient's care, as it has been assumed this is where there would be greatest impact. However, any such discussion has to be put in the overall context of the patient: the acute management of alcoholic hepatitis cannot be divorced from the prevention of further harmful drinking, and the latter will have an equal if not greater impact on the longer-term mortality and morbidity. The sobering evidence for this is provided by a recent epidemiological paper that failed to identify any improvement in the mortality of patients with cirrhosis in the Oxford area of the UK [3].

Pathogenesis

Ethanol is metabolized in the liver via two pathways: alcohol dehydrogenase and cytochrome P450 2E1. Both result in acetaldehyde formation which is highly reactive, and may modify microtubular function as well as form. Alcohol metabolism also puts the hepatocyte under significant oxidant stress, and a combination of these cellular insults is proposed to initiate an inflammatory response. This response involves an endotoxin-like cytokine cascade, characterized by neutrophil infiltration, high levels of NFKb, TNFα and IL8, and is modified between individuals by genetic polymorphisms identified in both CPP450 2E1 and acetaldehyde dehyrogenase, the hepatic enzyme responsible for the metabolism of acetaldehyde. While much of these proposed mechanisms are derived from animal models, and evidence for these mechanisms in humans is either absent or, at best, indirect, they have largely provided the rationale for the treatment modalities evaluated thus far. In particular, the four therapies, corticosteroids, pentoxifylline, enteral nutrition and anti-TNFα antibodies, are all directed at various components of the endotoxin-cytokine cascade.

Clinical features

When illness is severe, the patient will typically present with a history of long-term heavy alcohol use (40–80 units per week), and usually a preceding period of binging. Because the symptom onset may be relatively acute, the patient will often stop drinking just prior to admission, and indeed blame the continued deterioration in their clinical state on abstinence as opposed to the preceding alcohol use. Symptoms include anorexia, fever, malaise, malnutrition and the onset of jaundice/ascites. On examination, the patients are usually jaundiced with stigmata of chronic liver disease, and fever may be present which is rarely >38.5°C. The liver may be enlarged and tender. A bruit may

Gastrointestinal Emergencies, 2nd edition. Edited by Tony Tham, John Collins and Roy Soetikno. © 2009 by Blackwell Publishing, ISBN: 978-1-4051-4634-0.

be present. Ascites is common, and the presence of encephalopathy is associated with a poor prognosis.

Biochemical features

Typical features of severe acute alcoholic hepatitis include polymorph leukocytosis and prolonged prothrombin time. Mean corpuscular volume is often increased and marked thrombocytopenia attributable to a direct effect of alcohol on the bone marrow is also recognized.

The aspartate transaminase (AST) and alanine transaminase (ALT) are usually only mildly elevated (levels typically remain below 400 U/L (higher levels would suggest additional or other pathology such as viral hepatitis or drug toxicity), and the AST is usually greater than ALT. The serum bilirubin is elevated and can exceed 750 µmol/L (44 mg/dL). Gamma glutamyl transferase and serum immunoglobulin A concentrations are also often increased. Serum ferritin may be very high (above 1000 µg/L) even in the absence of hemochromatosis. The patient's condition, both clinical and biochemical, may deteriorate following admission and alcohol withdrawal, suggesting continued inflammatory hepatic insult.

Investigations

All patients with suspected alcoholic hepatitis should have a full blood count, clotting studies, renal and liver function tests, serum magnesium and phosphate. Other causes of liver disease should be excluded by appropriate blood tests, e.g. autoimmune liver disease (chronic active hepatitis, PBC, etc.), HCV, HBV, genetic hemochromatosis (ferritin and % iron saturation may be misleading in patients ingesting large quantities of alcohol or with acute illness), Wilson disease and alpha-1-antitrypsin disease. Structural disease should be excluded with ultrasound or CT scan. Fatty infiltration of the liver is common, and may be focal, mimicking space-occupying lesions.

A definitive diagnosis requires histology, indeed clinical trials where this has not been routinely obtained have been criticized, and a biopsy adds both therapeutic and prognostic information. The key pathological features are ballooned hepatocytes, with or without

Mallory hyaline, neutrophil infiltration and pericellular fibrosis. Of these patients 50% will have cirrhosis. However, by the very nature of the disease, clotting is abnormal, ascites is frequently present and the platelet count is low. Hence a percutaneous approach is contraindicated and a liver biopsy can usually only be safely obtained via the transjugular route, and while this is a straightforward procedure it is not commonly available. It is reasonable therefore to diagnose and treat patients on clinical grounds but to seek histological confirmation where possible, and in particular in patients where there are inconsistencies in clinical course.

Prognostic factors

Death usually results from hepatorenal failure, uncontrollable sepsis or variceal hemorrhage. These events can occur throughout the inpatient stay and in the author's opinion are often consequences of a poor response to predictable changes.

There are three scoring systems that may be applied to patients presenting with acute alcoholic hepatitis. The most recognized is the *modified Maddrey's discriminate function*. Serum bilirubin, the prolongation of prothrombin time (PT) and the presence of hepatic encephalopathy and renal impairment have been shown to be independent predictors of short-term survival in patients presenting acutely. Two of these laboratory indices have been combined to derive a Maddrey discriminant function (df) = (bilirubin (µmol/L)/17 or bilirubin in mg/dl + 4.6 × [PT prolongation]). A value of 32 or greater has been shown in several prospective studies to predict a 28-day mortality of around 35% [4]. As a consequence most treatment trials have focused on patients with a Maddrey df more than 32 and/or encephalopathy and have examined short-term (usually 1 month) mortality only. Patients with less severe disease appear to have a good short-term prognosis even when jaundiced [4]. Accordingly, in these patients, and in severe patients surviving their initial presentation, treatment is focused on achieving abstinence, which has been convincingly shown to improve long-term outcome [5], with liver transplantation reserved for patients who fail to improve after a period of abstinence.

More recent prognostic indices include *MELD* (Model for End stage Liver Disease) and *Glasgow alcoholic hepatitis score*. The *MELD score* is calculated from the

Table 27.1 The Glasgow alcoholic hepatitis score.

	Score given		
	1	2	3
Age	<50	≥ 50	—
WCC (10⁹/L)	<15	≥ 15	—
Urea (mmol/L)	<5	≥ 5	—
PT ratio	<1.5	1.5–2.0	>2.0
Bilirubin µmol/L	<125	125–250	>250
(mg/dL)	(<7.4)	(7.4–15)	(>15)

PT, prothrombin time; WCC, white cell count

formula MELD = $3.8 \times \log_e$(bilirubin [mg/dL]) + $1.2 \times \log_e$(INR) + $9.6 \times \log_e$(creatinine [mg/dL]). Recent studies have suggested that a score of >20 is a better predictor of mortality in acute alcoholic hepatitis than the Maddrey scoring system. While useful for comparison of patients, the MELD is impractical for day-to-day use in a clinical setting.

The *Glasgow alcoholic hepatitis score* is a simpler and more accurate means of predicting mortality compared to the MELD [4]. A score of >9 at day 1 was associated with a 28-day mortality of 46% and at day 7 with a 28-day survival of 47%. The Glasgow scoring system (see Table 27.1) is based on the following intuitively logical factors: age, markers of renal and liver function, as well as sepsis/inflammation.

Management

General

Patients with severe alcoholic hepatitis should be considered as being nutritionally deficient, immunosuppressed and with critical renal impairment. Thus baseline interventions should include aggressive fluid resuscitation, intravenous B vitamin supplementation and gastric acid suppression, early use of antibiotics following a full septic screen (including diagnostic ascitic tap) when there is clinical suspicion of sepsis and *early* use of vasoactive agents such as glypressin if hepatorenal syndrome is developing. The focus should *not* be on the management of ascites when present since this can be tapped for comfort, but instead on preservation of renal function and awareness of events that can occur in this fragile group of patients. Diuretics should only be used when the renal function is stable and normal. Alcohol withdrawal should be managed with oral benzodiazepines and these should be titrated according to the severity of withdrawal, and the possible presence of encephalopathy. While there are no guidelines on who to refer to specialist liver units, it is the author's opinion that those in whom it is the first presentation, and the young, should be considered for maximal support, and hence should be discussed with the regional liver unit.

This chapter does not deal with the (perhaps more difficult) topic of maintaining abstinence. It does however seem obvious that having struggled to get a patient through a severe attack of alcoholic hepatitis, to then discharge them without any provision for outpatient care is both illogical and poor medicine.

Specific
Steroids

Steroid therapy has been the most intensively studied therapy in alcoholic hepatitis and is aimed at suppressing or 'switching off' the florid inflammatory response observed in liver biopsies from patients with severe acute alcoholic hepatitis. The mechanism of this effect is, at least in part, through the inhibition of NFkB transcriptional activity, with the transcription of many inflammatory cytokines, chemokines and adhesion molecules dependent on this ubiquitous signaling cascade. There have been 14 published studies of steroid therapy for alcoholic hepatitis since 1971 and the majority have found no overall benefit from steroid treatment. These have been subjected to a number of systematic reviews and metaanalyses [6], most recently and comprehensively in 1995 [7]. This latter, and widely quoted metaanalysis, demonstrated that although there was a trend of benefit with steroids, the results were not statistically significant ($p = 0.2$). The problem of trial design is exemplified by the largest placebo controlled study, which treated 90 patients with mild and severe alcoholic hepatitis, and found no benefit with prednisolone compared with a similar placebo-treated group [8]. This study was hampered by the inclusion of patients with both moderate and severe alcoholic hepatitis, as well as end-stage alcoholic liver disease. There has been only one randomized clinical trial in which all patients had a pathological diagnosis of alcoholic hepatitis histologically proven using transjugular biopsy where necessary.

This trial has been the subject of two reports [9,10], the second including an open treatment prednisolone group ($n = 61$), in addition to the placebo ($n = 29$) and randomized prednisolone ($n = 32$) groups. The overall survival at 6 months in the two treated groups was 73% and 84%, compared with 41% in the placebo group ($p = 0.02$). However by 2 years the mortality in all three groups was identical. Thus, in this study, prednisolone was associated with a short-term improvement in mortality in patients with histologically proven alcoholic hepatitis.

Rather than performing a further conventional metaanalysis, the authors of the last three large randomized controlled trials have recently pooled their individual patient data, only including patients with encephalopathy and/or a df greater than 32 [11]. This study showed that steroids improved survival versus placebo (85% versus 65%), with placebo treatment, increasing age and creatinine independent predictors of mortality on multivariate analysis. A weakness of this study is that two of the three original trials included gastrointestinal bleeding as a contraindication, while one did not, and only one trial required a liver biopsy for diagnosis. Nonetheless, the large numbers (102 on placebo, 113 on steroids) make this the most robust metaanalysis to date.

Further analysis of the steroid trial data has identified a group who appear to show a good response to steroids, identified by an early change in bilirubin levels (ECBL) at 7 days, and defined as a bilirubin at day 7 following initiation of steroids lower than the bilirubin on the first day of treatment [12]. It has been suggested from this data that patients who do not have an ECBL should therefore stop steroids. It is the author's opinion that this is an overinterpretation of the trial data. Not having an ECBL only identifies a poor prognosis – it does not indicate that steroids should be ceased because of lack of efficacy.

Pentoxyphylline

Following the identification of high levels of tumor necrosis factor (TNF) in patients with acute alcoholic hepatitis, pentoxifylline (PTX; an inhibitor of TNF synthesis) was compared with placebo in a randomized placebo-controlled trial [15]. 100 patients were enrolled, all with severe disease as evidenced by a Maddrey df of >32. PTX was administered for 3 weeks, at a dose of 400 mg three times a day. In the PTX group 12/49

(24.5%) died compared to 24/52 (46.1%) in the placebo group during the index hospitalization ($p = 0.037$). The principal benefit for the agent appeared to be a reduction in the development of hepatorenal syndrome. Unlike steroids, PTX could be administered following recent gastrointestinal bleeding and during evidence of sepsis. The trial was criticized however for the absence of a steroid arm.

Nutritional therapy

Because of the evidence of malnutrition in many patients with alcoholic hepatitis, as well as the association between mortality and nutritional status, this has been an area of considerable research. While there have been a number of small trials, the two main studies were both done by the same group. In the first, enteral tube feeding of an energy-dense formula supplying >2000 kcal/day was compared with a standard oral diet [14]. The tube feed was perhaps unusual in that it contained whole protein plus a combination of maltodextrin, branched-chain amino acids as well as medium and long-chain triglycerides. The in-hospital mortality was 12% in the tube-fed patients, compared to 47% in the oral diet group. Only 37 (admittedly malnourished and sick) patients were randomized. Nonetheless, this prompted a further study comparing enteral feeding to steroids. A total of 71 patients were randomized, and while there was no difference in mortality during the 28 days duration of the trial, deaths occurred earlier in the steroid-treated patients and the mortality rate was lower in the enterally fed group in the year following treatment [15]. The overall mortality rate at one year was 61% in the steroid-treated group and 38% in the enteral group ($p = 0.26$).

One of the benefits of nasogastric tube feeding is a reliable source of hydration, and its ease of use should make this a more popular therapy. The presence of varices is not a contraindication to nasogastric tube placement (though softer, fine-bore tubes are recommended) and the use of bridles tends to stop even the most determined of individuals from removing the tube.

Anti-TNF antibodies

Early enthusiasm for the potential of these (expensive) drugs was fueled by initial reports of improved liver function tests in patients with alcoholic hepatitis, either when used alone or in combination with steroids [16,17]. However, this was rapidly tempered by the early cessation of a randomized trial of infliximab in conjunction with steroids, principally because of sepsis [18]. This is perhaps not surprising, since sepsis is such a common event in patients with advanced liver disease, and has been a well-described complication of anti-TNF therapy. While the trial has been criticized on the grounds of excessive dosing, and the choice of antibody, it should also be borne in mind that TNFα is required for hepatocellular regeneration [19], and as in many of the sepsis studies, blocking one part of the various cascades runs the risk of 'shooting the messenger'.

Molecular absorbent recirculating system

The molecular absorbent recirculating system (MARS) involves hemofiltration against an albumin gradient, aiming to remove metabolites. Despite initial enthusiasm [20], it is highly expensive therapy, its efficacy is unclear [21] and its use is not recommended outside of the trial scenario.

Liver transplantation

The low organ donation rates in the UK means it is ethically questionable to consider liver transplantation in this high-risk group of patients, with a well-documented poor outcome. The UK guidelines recommend abstinence for at least 6 months prior to transplantation in patients with alcoholic liver disease, which effectively excludes patients with acute alcoholic hepatitis [22].

Other therapies

Other therapies that have been tried and not shown efficacy include antioxidants [23], propylthiouracil [24] and anabolic steroids [25].

Conclusion

Acute alcoholic hepatitis is an increasing burden for the attending clinician. There can at times be a sense of therapeutic nihilism with a difficult group of patients. However, it is also true that with attentive medical care, excellent results can be achieved. While the data is unsatisfactory, steroids, pentoxiphylline and nutritional support have been shown to improve survival. One could use all three modalities, but this also needs to be combined with close attention to prevention of sepsis, withdrawal, and fluid/electrolyte balance, as well as provision of alcohol services once the patient has been discharged.

References

1. Maddrey WC, Boitnott JK, Bedine MS, Weber FL, Jr., Mezey E, White RI, Jr. Corticosteroid therapy of alcoholic hepatitis. Gastroenterology 1978; 75(2):193–9.

2. Forrest EH, Evans CD, Stewart S, Phillips M, Oo YH, McAvoy NC et al. Analysis of factors predictive of mortality in alcoholic hepatitis and derivation and validation of the Glasgow alcoholic hepatitis score. Gut 2005; 54(8):1174–9.

3. Roberts SE, Goldacre MJ, Yeates D. Trends in mortality after hospital admission for liver cirrhosis in an English population from 1968 to 1999. Gut 2005; 54:1615–21.

4. Goldberg S, Mendenhall C, Anderson S, Garcia-Pont P, Kiernan T, Seeff L et al. VA Cooperative Study on Alcoholic Hepatitis. IV. The significance of clinically mild alcoholic hepatitis – describing the population with minimal hyperbilirubinemia. Am J Gastroenterol 1986; 81(11):1029–34.

5. Alexander JF, Lischner MW, Galambos JT. Natural history of alcoholic hepatitis. II. The long-term prognosis. Am J Gastroenterol 1971; 56(6):515–25.

6. Imperiale TF, McCullough AJ. Do corticosteroids reduce mortality from alcoholic hepatitis? A meta-analysis of the randomized trials. Ann Intern Med 1990; 113(4):299–307.

7. Christensen E, Gluud C. Glucocorticoids are ineffective in alcoholic hepatitis: a meta-analysis adjusting for confounding variables. Gut 1995; 37(1):113–18.

8. Mendenhall CL, Anderson S, Garcia-Pont P, Goldberg S, Kiernan T, Seeff LB et al. Short-term and long-term survival in patients with alcoholic hepatitis treated with oxandrolone and prednisolone. N Engl J Med 1984; 311(23):1464–70.

9. Ramond MJ, Poynard T, Rueff B, Mathurin P, Theodore C, Chaput JC et al. A randomized trial of prednisolone in patients with severe alcoholic hepatitis. N Engl J Med 1992; 326(8):507–12.

10. Mathurin P, Duchatelle V, Ramond MJ, Degott C, Bedossa P, Erlinger S et al. Survival and prognostic factors in patients with severe alcoholic hepatitis treated with prednisolone. Gastroenterology 1996; 110(6):1847–53.

11. Mathurin P, Mendenhall CL, Carithers RL, Jr., Ramond MJ, Maddrey WC, Garstide P et al. Corticosteroids

improve short-term survival in patients with severe alcoholic hepatitis (AH): individual data analysis of the last three randomized placebo-controlled double-blind trials of corticosteroids in severe AH. J Hepatol 2002;36(4):480–7.

12. Mathurin P, Abdelnour M, Ramond MJ, Carbonell N, Fartoux L, Serfaty L et al. Early change in bilirubin levels is an important prognostic factor in severe alcoholic hepatitis treated with prednisolone. Hepatology 2003; 38(6):1363–9.

13. Akriviadis E, Botla R, Briggs W, Han S, Reynolds T, Shakil O. Pentoxifylline improves short-term survival in severe acute alcoholic hepatitis: a double-blind, placebo-controlled trial. Gastroenterology 2000;119(6):1637–48.

14. Cabre E, Gonzalez-Huix F, Abad-Lacruz A, et al. Effect of total enteral nutrition on the short-term outcome of severely malnourished cirrhotics: a randomized controlled trial. Gastroenterology 1990; 98:715–20.

15. Cabre E, Rodriguez-Iglesias P, Caballeria J, et al. Short- and long-term outcome of severe alcohol induced hepatitis treated with steroids or enteral nutrition: a multicentre randomised trial. Hepatology 2000; 32:36–42.

16. Spahr L, Rubbia-Brandt L, Frossard JL, Giostra E, Rougemont AL, Pugin J et al. Combination of steroids with infliximab or placebo in severe alcoholic hepatitis: a randomized controlled pilot study. J Hepatol 2002; 37(4):448–55.

17. Menon KV, Stadheim L, Kamath PS, Wiesner RH, Gores GJ, Peine CJ et al. A pilot study of the safety and tolerability of etanercept in patients with alcoholic hepatitis. Am J Gastroenterol 2004; 99(2):255–60.

18. Naveau S, Chollet-Martin S, Dharancy S, Mathurin P, Jouet P, Piquet MA et al. A double-blind randomized controlled trial of infliximab associated with prednisolone in acute alcoholic hepatitis. Hepatology 2004; 39(5):1390–7.

19. Akerman P, Cote P, Yang SQ, McClain C, Nelson S, Bagby G et al. Antibodies to tumor necrosis factor-alpha inhibit liver regeneration after partial hepatectomy. Am J Physiol 1992; 263:G579–G585.

20. Jalan R, Sen S, Steiner C, Kapoor D, Alisa A, Williams R. Extracorporeal liver support with molecular adsorbents recirculating system in patients with severe acute alcoholic hepatitis. J Hepatol 2003; 38(1):24–31.

21. Wai CT, Lim SG, Aung MO, Lee YM, Sutedja DS, Dan YY et al. MARS: a futile tool in centres without active liver transplant support. Liver Int 2007; 27:69–75.

22. O'Grady JG, Devlin J. Indications for referral and assessment in adult liver transplantation: a clinical guideline. Gut 1999; 45: suppl 6.

23. Phillips M, Curtis H, Portmann B, Donaldson N, Bomford A, O'Grady J. Antioxidants versus corticosteroids in the treatment of severe alcoholic hepatitis: a randomised clinical trial. J Hepatol 2006; 44(4):784–90.

24. Halle P, Pare P, Kaptein E, Kanel G, Redeker AG, Reynolds TB. Double-blind, controlled trial of propylthiouracil in patients with severe acute alcoholic hepatitis. Gastroenterology 1982; 82(5 Pt 1):925–31.

25. Rambaldi A, Iaquinto G, Gluud C. Anabolic-androgenic steroids for alcoholic liver disease: a Cochrane review. Am J Gastroenterol 2002; 97(7):1674–81.

28 Acute Appendicitis

John Moorehead, Ian McAllister

Introduction

The presentation of appendicitis is variable and although it may occur at any age the condition has a peak incidence in young adults with a second peak around the seventh decade of life. It remains the most common intraabdominal surgical emergency with a lifetime risk of 8.6% risk for males and 6.7% for females [1], although over the last decade there has been a 12–19% decline in admission rates for acute appendicitis in the UK [2]. The current mortality rate of appendicitis is well under 1%. The small group of patients who do not survive are often very young or elderly with a perforated appendix and peritonitis.

The mainstay of diagnosis of acute appendicitis remains accurate history and physical examination. The typical clinical findings are outlined below; however, a wide range of conditions, involving a variety of organ systems, present in a similar fashion occasionally making accurate diagnosis difficult [3] (Table 28.1).

The main aim of early diagnosis in this condition is to avoid the complication of a perforated appendix with the subsequent development of an abscess or widespread peritonitis.

Etiology

Acute appendicitis is probably triggered by obstruction of the appendix lumen. Common obstructing agents include fecoliths, lymphoid hyperplasia, pinworms and

Table 28.1 Differential diagnosis of acute appendicitis

Site of pathology	Diagnosis
Gynecological	Pelvic inflammatory disease
	Ectopic pregnancy
	Ovarian cyst (rupture/torsion)
	Tubuloovarian abscess
	Endometriosis
Gastrointestinal	Crohn's disease
	Ileal perforation
	Meckel's diverticulum
	Small bowel neoplasm
	Gastroenteritis
	Intestinal obstruction
	Omental torsion
	Pancreatitis
	Cholecystitis
	Peptic ulcer
	Diverticulitis
Genitourinary	Urinary tract infection
	Renal calculus
	Pyelonephritis
	Testicular torsion
Other	Infective (TB/*Yersinia*)
	Pulmonary
	Systemic (diabetes, porphyria)
	Mesenteric adenitis
	Nonspecific abdominal pain

neoplasms of the cecum. Others have suggested that a low-fiber diet may increase the risk [4]. Reports of appendicitis clusters within populations raise the possibility of an infective origin, some authors suggesting that infection with *Yersinia* may be a significant etiological factor [5].

Gastrointestinal Emergencies, 2nd edition. Edited by Tony Tham, John Collins and Roy Soetikno. © 2009 by Blackwell Publishing, ISBN: 978-1-4051-4634-0.

The appendix is the commonest site for carcinoid tumors in the gastrointestinal tract. They are usually less than 1 cm in size and found at the appendix tip but are of low malignant potential with lymph node metastases identified in only 3% of cases. Carcinoid is identified as the etiological factor in only 1.5% of patients with acute appendicitis but approximately half of all appendiceal carcinoids will cause luminal obstruction and progress to appendicitis.

Typically luminal obstruction leads to ischemia in combination with bacterial infection and mucosal inflammation. As the disease progresses full thickness inflammation may involve other structures such as the omentum or adjacent small bowel, producing an inflammatory phlegmon. Gangrene of the appendix wall may intervene leading to perforation with the potential for a localized purulent collection or generalized peritonitis.

History

The clinical presentation of appendicitis is unpredictable with the classical history of central abdominal pain localizing to the right iliac fossa evident in only 50% of cases. The symptoms will usually have developed within the preceding 24–36 hours and can often be associated with anorexia, nausea, vomiting and dysuria. A careful review of the patient's gynecological, urological and respiratory systems should also be obtained.

Examination

Typical findings on examination include low-grade pyrexia, right iliac fossa tenderness, with associated peritonism demonstrated by abdominal guarding and percussion rebound. A Rovsing sign (pain in the right iliac fossa elicited with palpation of left) and Dunphy sign (increased pain with coughing) are also good indicators of peritoneal irritation and are suggestive of acute appendicitis. The psoas sign of forced right hip extension against resistance produces pelvic pain in the presence of an inflamed retroperitoneal appendix. A digital rectal examination is of little value unless the appendix lies within the pelvis, and does not confer any additional diagnostic information, particularly when the abdominal findings are suggestive [6].

Unusual presentations

In cases of retrocecal appendix the classical shift of pain from the centre to the right maybe absent, abdominal tenderness may be minimal and the signs of peritonism may be deficient.

With a pelvic appendix the pain could be evident on the left side, again with minimal abdominal findings. The patient may describe the urge to urinate or defecate and rectal tenderness is often present.

The diagnosis of appendicitis in the elderly is often not considered and can be difficult as the symptoms and signs are often subtle; this can delay diagnosis and subsequent management which can be significant in a group of patients with other comorbidity who can ill afford perforation or abscess formation.

The existence of chronic or grumbling appendicitis is still controversial but it is accepted that recurrent episodes of luminal obstruction with spontaneous resolution may well result in an appendix which is chronically inflamed or fibrotic. In a patient with significant symptoms appendicectomy often results in cure and a histologically abnormal appendix. However, it must be emphasized that true chronic appendicitis is rare and therefore other significant diagnoses should be ruled out and the possibility of nonspecific chronic abdominal pain considered before embarking on surgical intervention.

Investigation

Laboratory markers of an inflammatory response such as an increased white cell count, with a shift towards polymorponuclear cells, and C-reactive protein elevation have a high discriminatory power in the diagnosis of acute appendicitis. Appendicitis would be an unlikely diagnosis if both these inflammatory markers were normal [7].

A number of clinical scoring systems have been developed to improve the diagnosis of acute appendicitis. The Alvarado score is the most well known; relying on eight variables to predict the likelihood of appendicitis [21]. The variables include symptoms such as nausea/vomiting, migratory pain and anorexia, signs including localized right iliac fossa tenderness, rebound tenderness and pyrexia, and laboratory tests such as leukocytosis with a left shift. Some reports suggest that the use of such scores are helpful in reducing negative appendicectomy rates but they are seldom used in routine clinical practice and are not superior to assessment by a senior clinician.

The value of transabdominal ultrasound in the diagnosis of acute appendicitis remains unclear, with good results reported from single-centre studies (sensitivity 82%) compared to disappointing multi-centre results (sensitivity 38%) [8]. Graded compression ultrasonography has been recommended by the American College of Radiology as a useful screening tool in the diagnosis of appendicitis, citing a sensitivity of 95% but a specificity of only 52% [9]. Ultrasound may also have benefits in identifying other causes for right iliac fossa pain such as ovarian cysts, renal tract pathology or gallstones.

Computed tomography is probably more accurate in diagnosing acute appendicitis in adults and adolescents, with a sensitivity of 94% and a specificity of 95%.

The rate of negative appendicectomy should be as low as possible; the rates quoted in the literature are variable ranging from 5% to 40%. However, it is worth noting that the negative appendicectomy rates and rates of perforated appendix have remained unchanged despite the increased use of both these imaging modalities [10].

The highest incidence of false positive diagnosis is in women of child-bearing age when the diagnosis is often pelvic inflammatory disease or other gynecological conditions. With this in mind radiological imaging in patients with suspected appendicitis should be reserved for those where diagnostic doubt remains.

Management

When the diagnosis of appendicitis is suspected the patient should be fluid resuscitated and given analgesia. Evidence suggests that administration of opioids does not mask the clinical findings and therefore should not be withheld [11].

Appendicectomy remains the treatment of choice, however in the patient with a significant operative risk without peritonitis, management with intravenous antibiotics such as metronidazole and a cephalosporin may be considered (Figure 28.1). Resolution should occur within 24 hours but this approach should be tempered by the notion that there is a significant risk of recurrent symptoms within the next 12 months [12].

Open appendicectomy

A standard appendicectomy is performed through a gridiron or Lanz incision in the right iliac fossa. The appendix stump should be short, simply ligated and not buried [13]. Care should be taken to aspirate all free fluid from the pelvis and paracolic gutter although formal peritoneal lavage is often not necessary. A single dose of prophylactic antibiotic such as metronidazole administered intravenously or per rectum 2 hours before surgery is effective in reducing the incidence of postoperative wound infection [14] in simple appendicitis. Initially the organisms are usually anaerobes

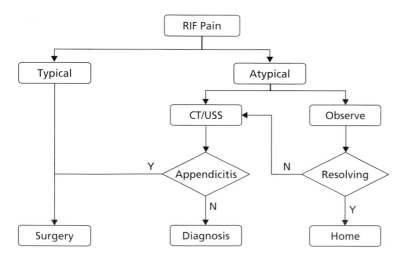

Figure 28.1 Algorithm for management of right iliac fossa pain.
RIF = right iliac fossa, CT = computerized tomography scan, USS = ultrasound scan.

such as *Bacteroides*, later there is a more mixed picture involving the usual aerobic enteric bacteria.

If the appendix has perforated and there is significant peritoneal contamination then copious lavage is advised and then most surgeons would advocate a treatment course of broad-spectrum antibiotics for 5 days or until the patient is apyrexic and the inflammatory markers have normalized. Early postoperative feeding, mobilization and deep venous thrombosis prophylaxis should ensure a rapid recovery and prompt discharge.

Laparoscopic appendicectomy

Studies have demonstrated improved postoperative pain, faster recovery and reduced wound infection rate in patients undergoing laparoscopic appendicectomy. Laparoscopic procedures generally take longer, require the presence of a senior surgeon with the appropriate skills and there have been reports of increased rates of intraabdominal collections postoperatively [15].

In the clinical settings where surgical expertise and affordable equipment are available, laparoscopic appendicectomy seems to have advantages over the open approach [16].

Controversy exists as how best to manage the problem of the grossly normal appendix at laparoscopy. Some would argue that if other significant pathology has been identified such as pelvic inflammatory disease then the appendix should be left intact. Others always advocate excision, suggest that removal of the appendix adds little to the surgical insult, and that there may be significant histological evidence of inflammation despite a normal gross appearance.

Management of complicated appendicitis

Appendix mass

Occasionally patients present with a longer history of abdominal pain and on examination a palpable mass is found in the right lower quadrant. This may represent an appendix mass fashioned by the adherence of omentum and small bowel to an acutely inflamed appendix creating an inflammatory phlegmon. The diagnosis is best made with CT scan but a barium enema or colonoscopy may be required to exclude a cecal carcinoma or a Crohn's mass. This finding is best managed initially, nonoperatively with intravenous antibiotics such as metronidazole and a cephalosporin.

The majority of patients respond to this approach; however, a small number will come to early surgery which is hazardous at this stage, resulting in higher rates of enteric injury, fistula formation and right hemicolectomy. Traditionally, following successful resolution, these patients would then have proceeded to interval appendicectomy at 6 weeks but this may be unnecessary as it has been shown that only 9% will go on to develop recurrent symptoms [17]. A balance must therefore be struck between the risks of recurrent appendicitis compared to the risk of interval appendicectomy. A reasonable compromise may be to perform interval appendicectomy in the young who have a low operative risk but a higher lifetime risk of recurrence.

Appendix abscess

A localized abscess collection may result from a perforated appendix and often the patient displays systemic signs of sepsis. Drainage of the abscess is often required and is usually best performed with a radiologically placed percutaneous drain [18]. Following resolution of the abscess the situation is similar to that of a conservatively managed appendix abscess with the decision for an interval appendicectomy based on a balance of risk.

Postoperative complications

The rate of superficial wound infection following appendicectomy is 15%, with the majority responding to antibiotics.

Intraabdominal collections occasionally develop after appendicectomy. The patient may describe abdominal pain, swinging temperature or diarrhea in the case of a pelvic collection. Most cases will settle with antibiotics alone, others may require percutaneous drainage. Infertility following appendicectomy has been reported at around 5% [19] although a more recent study suggests that the risk has been overstated [20].

References

1. Addiss DG, Shaffer N, Fowler BS, Tauxe RV. The epidemiology of appendicitis and appendectomy in the United States. Am J Epidemiol 1990; 132(5):910–25.

2. Kang JY, Hoare J, Majeed A, Williamson RC, Maxwell JD. Decline in admission rates for acute appendicitis in england. Br J Surg 2003; 90(12):1586–92.

3. Graffeo CS, Counselman FL. Appendicitis. Emerg Med Clin North Am 1996; 14(4):653–71.

4. Black J. Acute appendicitis in Japanese soldiers in Burma: support for the 'fibre' theory. Gut 2002; 51(2):297.

5. Andersson R, Hugander A, Thulin A, Nystrom PO, Olaison G. Clusters of acute appendicitis: further evidence for an infectious aetiology. Int J Epidemiol 1995; 24(4):829–33.

6. Dixon JM, Elton RA, Rainey JB, Macleod DA. Rectal examination in patients with pain in the right lower quadrant of the abdomen. BMJ 1991; 302 (6773):386–8.

7. Andersson RE. Meta-analysis of the clinical and laboratory diagnosis of appendicitis. Br J Surg 2004; 91(1):28–37.

8. Obermaier R, Benz S, Asgharnia M, Kirchner R, Hopt UT. Value of ultrasound in the diagnosis of acute appendicitis: interesting aspects. Eur J Med Res 2003; 8(10):451–6.

9. Lee JH, Jeong YK, Hwang JC, Ham SY, Yang SO. Graded compression sonography with adjuvant use of a posterior manual compression technique in the sonographic diagnosis of acute appendicitis. Am J Roentgenol 2002; 178(4):863–8.

10. Flum DR, Morris A, Koepsell T, Dellinger EP. Has misdiagnosis of appendicitis decreased over time? A population-based analysis. JAMA 2001; 286(14):1748–53.

11. Attard AR, Corlett MJ, Kidner NJ, Leslie AP, Fraser IA. Safety of early pain relief for acute abdominal pain. BMJ 1992; 305(6853):554–6.

12. Eriksson S, Granstrom L. Randomized controlled trial of appendicectomy versus antibiotic therapy for acute appendicitis. Br J Surg 1995; 82(2):166–9.

13. Engstrom L, Fenyo G. Appendicectomy: assessment of stump invagination versus simple ligation. A prospective, randomized trial. Br J Surg 1985; 72(12): 971–2.

14. Andersen BR, Kallehave FL, Andersen HK. Antibiotics versus placebo for prevention of postoperative infection after appendicectomy. Cochrane Database Syst Rev 2003; (2):CD001439.

15. Golub R, Siddiqui F, Pohl D. Laparoscopic versus open appendectomy: a metaanalysis. J Am Coll Surg 1998; 186(5):545–53.

16. Sauerland S, Lefering R, Neugebauer EA. Laparoscopic versus open surgery for suspected appendicitis. Cochrane Database Syst Rev 2004; (4):CD001546.

17. Bagi P, Dueholm S. Nonoperative management of the ultrasonically evaluated appendiceal mass. Surgery 1987; 101(5):602–5.

18. Hurme T, Nylamo E. Conservative versus operative treatment of appendicular abscess: experience of 147 consecutive patients. Ann Chir Gynaecol 1995; 84(1):33–6.

19. Mueller BA, Daling JR, Moore DE, Weiss NS, Spadoni LR, Stadel BV, et al. Appendectomy and the risk of tubal infertility. N Engl J Med 1986; 315(24):1506–8.

20. Andersson R, Lambe M, Bergstrom R. Fertility patterns after appendicectomy: historical cohort study. BMJ 1999; 318(7189):963–7.

21. Alvarado A. A practical score for the early diagnosis of acute appendicitis. Ann Emer Med 1986; 315:557–64.

29 Ischemic Bowel

Shai Friedland, Roy Soetikno

Introduction

Intestinal ischemia occurs when perfusion to the bowel is inadequate to meet metabolic demands. Ischemia can be classified as acute or chronic, and it can occur in response to arterial or venous insults. In acute mesenteric ischemia, all or part of the small bowel is affected. In addition, the right colon can be involved since its blood supply is also derived from the superior mesenteric artery (SMA). Acute mesenteric ischemia is a clinical emergency with a mortality rate of over 60%; a high index of suspicion is required for early detection before bowel necrosis occurs. In contrast, the more common syndrome of ischemic colitis often has a milder clinical course characterized by transient bloody diarrhea and mild lower abdominal pain. Chronic mesenteric ischemia, also called intestinal angina, is relatively rare and is characterized by abdominal pain following meals and weight loss. It can develop into an emergency if bowel viability is compromised by further deterioration in the blood supply.

Diagnosis of intestinal ischemia can be challenging; clinical suspicion and eliciting an adequate history from the patient play a more significant role than in many other gastrointestinal emergencies. Multidetector CT angiography is now commonly performed as the initial noninvasive test for acute and chronic mesenteric ischemia. In patients who are diagnosed prior to bowel infarction, percutaneous treatment using angiography is often possible. Colonoscopy is often performed to diagnose ischemic

colitis and in some cases to assess viability of the colon when there is doubt.

Acute mesenteric ischemia

Etiology

Superior mesenteric artery embolus is present in 50% of cases with sudden catastrophic abdominal pain out of proportion to physical findings. Atrial fibrillation is a common risk factor.

Nonocclusive mesenteric ischemia (25%) is a splanchnic vasoconstriction in response to preceding cardiovascular event, and may persist after the precipitating event has been corrected. SMA thrombosis (10%) is typically in an area of severe baseline atherosclerosis. Patients may have chronic mesenteric ischemia before thrombosis occurs. Mesenteric venous thrombosis (10%) may have a more subacute course. Patients often have risk factors such as hypercoagulable state or inflammation from other abdominal disorders.

Presentation

The patient may complain of severe, acute abdominal pain, sometimes accompanied by forceful bowel evacuation. The abdomen is initially often soft and nontender but increasing abdominal tenderness, rebound and guarding develop as bowel infarcts. Occult blood in the stool is common but maroon stool is less common. Leukocytosis, elevated amylase, elevated lactate, metabolic acidosis are increasingly common as bowel infarcts.

Evaluation

Multidetector CT angiography may detect embolic occlusion of the SMA just beyond the origin of the middle colic artery. Proximal SMA occlusion is typically

Gastrointestinal Emergencies, 2nd edition. Edited by Tony Tham, John Collins and Roy Soetikno. © 2009 by Blackwell Publishing, ISBN: 978-1-4051-4634-0.

seen with thrombosis, and collaterals are visualized in patients with preceding chronic symptoms. Superior mesenteric vein and portal vein thrombosis may be detected on CT. Nonocclusive ischemia may be difficult to detect. Other findings on CT include bowel wall thickening, abnormal bowel wall enhancement and intramural or venous gas.

Magnetic resonance angiography is less commonly used than CT as it is typically less readily available and has lower spatial resolution in comparison. Advantages include absence of radiation (children) and no iodinated contrast (renal failure). Angiography is now more commonly performed for treatment following a positive CT.

Management

The patient should be resuscitated and broad-spectrum antibiotics administered.

Angiography can permit papaverine infusion for treatment of vasoconstriction. Thrombolytics, angioplasty and stenting are used increasingly although there is some controversy as to their preferred role. Surgery provides the definitive assessment of viability and the decision can be made between resection of necrotic bowel, embolectomy or revascularization.

Ischemic colitis

Etiology

This condition is usually due to nonocclusive ischemia. A precipitating event such as hypotension or arrhythmia may or may not be identified. Other causes include coagulopathy, emboli, vasculitis, abdominal aortic aneurysm surgery, cocaine or amphetamine abuse and volvulus. Involvement of the ascending colon should raise suspicion of small bowel involvement (acute mesenteric ischemia). The splenic flexure and rectosigmoid are 'watershed' areas which are commonly involved, but all other regions of colon and rectum can be involved.

Presentation

The patient will usually complain of sudden mild left lower quadrant abdominal pain. There may an urge for urgent defecation with bloody diarrhea. On examination there will be mild to moderate abdominal tenderness over the involved area. Many cases resolve spontaneously however, and some patients do not seek medical attention. Increasing tenderness, guarding, fever and ileus occur with infarction and colonic strictures may occur with healing.

Evaluation

Colon blood flow has often normalized by the time that symptoms occur.

Computed tomography and plain radiography may show colon wall thickening or thumbprinting due to edema of the bowel wall. Colonoscopy may show submucosal hemorrhage, ulcers, or gangrenous bowel in severe cases.

Management

Resuscitation and broad-spectrum antibiotics are the initial emergency steps in management. Peritoneal signs suggest the need for emergency laparotomy and colon resection. Recurrent sepsis, bloody diarrhea and chronic diarrhea with protein loss occur with segmental ulcerating colitis. This is a chronic form of ischemic colitis and is sometimes mistaken for inflammatory bowel disease. Surgery is often required. Symptomatic strictures may occur following healing. While some may resolve spontaneously, surgical resection may be required.

Chronic mesenteric ischemia

Etiology

This condition is usually due to atherosclerosis of mesenteric arteries and rarely due to vasculitis. Abdominal pain typically occurs within 30 minutes of eating. This is likely due to reduced small intestine blood flow as blood preferentially flows to the stomach.

Severe stenosis or occlusion of two or three of the main splanchnic arteries (celiac, superior mesenteric and inferior mesenteric) is typical. Some patients with occlusion of all three arteries are asymptomatic due to collaterals.

Presentation

Abdominal pain within 30 minutes of meals that resolves within 3 hours. Severity of pain is mild initially, but becomes severe within months. As pain worsens, patients develop a fear of eating, and weight loss occurs. Pain may become continuous as infarction occurs.

Evaluation

Computed tomographic angiography: is useful to assess the splanchnic vessels for calcified plaques, stenosis, or occlusion. It has higher spatial and temporal resolution than MR angiography.

Duplex ultrasound is favored in some centers to demonstrate elevated peak systolic velocity in the celiac and superior mesenteric arteries as an indication of significant stenosis. Newer techniques include specialized MR sequences for evaluating blood flow after meals and endoscopic oximetry.

Management

Surgical revascularization may be attempted in suitable cases. Percutaneous techniques, including stenting, are used increasingly and are favored for patients considered too high risk for surgery. These techniques have been associated with high recurrence rates in the past, but improvements in initial treatment and successful percutaneous treatment of restenosis makes this approach increasingly attractive.

Further reading

Chang RW, Chang JB, Longo WE. Update in management of mesenteric ischemia. World J Gastroenterol 2006; 12:3243–7.

Friedland S, Benaron D, Coogan S, Sze DY, Soetikno R. Diagnosis of chronic mesenteric ischemia by visible light spectroscopy during endoscopy. Gastrointest Endosc 2007; 65:294–300.

Shih MP, Hagspiel KD. CTA and MRA in mesenteric ischemia. Am J Radiol 2007; 188:452–61.

Silva JA, White CJ, Collins TJ, et al. Endovascular therapy for chronic mesenteric ischemia. J Am Coll Cardiol 2006; 47:944–50.

Sreenarasimhaiah J. Diagnosis and management of ischemic colitis. Curr Gastroenterol Rep 2005; 7:421–6.

Ujiki M, Kibbe MR. Mesenteric ischemia. Perspect Vasc Surg Endovasc Ther 2005; 17:309–18.

Acute Severe Ulcerative Colitis

Subrata Ghosh

Introduction

Acute severe ulcerative colitis is a medical emergency. Recognition of severe ulcerative colitis is based on a comprehensive clinical assessment. The Truelove and Witts criteria [1] still remain useful in characterizing the severity of this condition (Table 30.1). These patients require hospitalization and urgent management. Acute severe ulcerative colitis may be further subclassified into severe colitis and fulminant colitis. The latter is associated with abdominal distension, tenderness on palpation and colonic dilatation on plain abdominal radiograph. Most patients will give a history of the gradual onset of diarrhea with the passage of blood and mucus. There may be severe abdominal cramps and tenesmus. Constitutional symptoms may include severe malaise, fever, joint and muscle pain and marked weight loss. In some cases the onset may be abrupt over 24–48 hours. There is often a history of ulcerative colitis.

Clinical examination should include rectal examination and flexible sigmoidoscopy which can usually be carried out on the unprepared colon. This must be followed by abdominal radiography, stool culture, *Clostridium difficile* toxin assay and blood tests including hemoglobin, white cell count, platelet count, C-reactive protein, erythrocyte sedimentation rate and albumin concentration. A number of intestinal diseases which mimic acute severe ulcerative colitis should be excluded by initial history and investigations (Table 30.2).

Gastrointestinal Emergencies, 2nd edition. Edited by Tony Tham, John Collins and Roy Soetikno. © 2009 by Blackwell Publishing, ISBN: 978-1-4051-4634-0.

Table 30.1 Truelove and Witts classification of ulcerative colitis.

Mild	Moderate	Severe
<5 bowel motions/day	Intermediate between mild and severe	≥6 bowel motions/day
Blood in stool +		Blood in stool +++
No fever		Temperature >37.5°C
No tachycardia		Pulse >90 beats/minute
Hemoglobin ≥10 g/dL		Hemoglobin <10 g/dL
ESR<30 mm/1st hour		ESR >30 mm/1st hour

Table 30.2 Diseases mimicking severe ulcerative colitis.

Acute infectious gastroenteritis: outbreak related to contaminated food or drinks, recent travel
Radiation proctopathy : history of pelvic radiotherapy
Pseudo-membranous colitis (*C. difficile*): history of antibiotic exposure
Sexually transmitted infections: history of anal sex
Amoebiasis: recent travel to endemic areas

Acute severe Crohn's colitis

This condition is less common than ulcerative colitis but may present as severe or fulminant colitis which is difficult to distinguish clinically and is an important differential diagnosis. Approximately 65% of Crohn's disease patients have either colonic involvement alone or ileocecal disease. There may be a previous clinical history of Crohn's disease with small bowel involvement and previous surgical procedures. Perianal disease will point to a diagnosis of Crohn's disease. Initial clinical assessment is identical for these patients, with the exception that there may be concomitant small bowel disease which has to be considered as a potential cause of internal fistulization or abdominal sepsis with abscess formation. If Crohn's colitis is suspected and accompanied by fever, abdominal tenderness or the presence of a mass on palpation, an abdominal CT or MRI may be indicated to assist the surgeon in planning management. Active sepsis should also induce caution in commencing immunosuppression before it is controlled with antibiotic therapy (see below).

Principles of management

Acute severe ulcerative colitis patients require hospitalization and close monitoring. Some patients at presentation may appear to be less ill than the Truelove and Witts criteria suggest. Therefore it is important to monitor the patient in a gastroenterology (not a general) ward with an accurate record of stool frequency, blood in stool, temperature, pulse rate and abdominal tenderness. Infection must be eliminated by stool culture but commencement of treatment should not wait until the stool culture reports become available. The management of severe ulcerative colitis patients is a team effort between gastroenterologists, surgeons, inflammatory bowel disease nurses, dieticians and clinical psychologists. In a patient admitted with acute severe ulcerative colitis and dilatation of the colon, joint assessment by a gastroenterologist and a colorectal surgeon is required urgently. In all other patients admitted with acute severe colitis, a colorectal surgical assessment will be required within 24 hours.

Initial therapy

The standard initial therapy of acute severe ulcerative colitis consists of intravenous corticosteroids [2], fluid and electrolyte replacement with special attention to potassium. Blood transfusion may be required to maintain a hemoglobin concentration above 10 g/L and subcutaneous heparin should be started to prevent thromboembolic complications. Intravenous corticosteroids generally chosen include hydrocortisone 100 mg

Table 30.3 Monitoring regimen in acute severe ulcerative colitis.

Detecting impending complications
Daily abdominal radiographs till the patient improves
Watch for colonic dilatation
Watch for colonic perforation (often silent)
Watch for small intestinal dilatation
Assessing course of disease
Stool frequency
Blood in stool
Pulse rate
Temperature
C-reactive protein (CRP)
Albumin
Hemoglobin
Flexible sigmoidoscopy to look for deep ulcerations

four times a day or methylprednisolone 60 mg/daily by continuous infusion. Addition of rectal therapy has no clear advantages and is generally poorly tolerated by patients in the acute severe phase. Antibiotics are not necessary unless infection is considered a strong differential diagnosis from history (Table 30.2).

Monitoring of such patients needs to be intensive and should be directed at detecting impending complications which may necessitate urgent colectomy (Table 30.3). Abdominal radiography accurately denotes extent of disease, but colonoscopy to assess extent is unnecessary. The majority of patients with acute severe ulcerative colitis suffer from extensive colitis. Nutritional support is important and most patients can be encouraged to have an adequate oral intake. Rarely, patients may require supportive parenteral nutrition. Codeine and loperamide should not be used and nonsteroidal antiinflammatory drugs avoided.

Overall, patients hospitalized for acute severe colitis and treated with intravenous steroids may have a colectomy rate between 29% and 46% over the next 90 days. The colectomy rates vary between countries, indicating different thresholds for offering surgery.

Managing intravenous steroid refractory acute severe colitis

Close monitoring should lead to early recognition of those patients who fail to respond to intraveous steroids. Such recognition may be aided by formal rules, but clinical judgment is paramount based on the monitoring parameters noted in Table 30.3. The two commonly used rules which are very similar to each other are:

1. Fulminant colitis (Sweden) index: Number of daily bowel movements + (0.14 × C-reactive protein mg/L). A value ≥8 predicts colectomy with 75% sensitivity and specificity. This index was recently used in a salvage therapy trial discussed below [4].

2. Travis index: At day 3 after commencement of intravenous steroids, a stool frequency of more than 8 per day or C-reactive protein concentration of >45mg/L is 85% predictive of colectomy and therefore may be used to seek surgical team involvement and consider start of salvage therapy with infliximab or ciclosporin [5].

Some patients respond initially to intravenous steroids but continue to have symptoms. These patients should be offered salvage therapy 5–7 days after initiation of intravenous corticosteroids as the colectomy rate is high in this group. This latter group may also benefit from a careful flexible sigmoidoscopy, as demonstration of deep ulceration indicates a poor prognosis and consideration of salvage therapy or surgery (Plate 30.1). Overall, a high proportion of patients failing intravenous steroids will undergo colectomy – 67% underwent colectomy within 90 days without salvage therapy in a study reported recently.

It is important in acute severe colitis refractory to intravenous steroids to exclude coinfections with cytomegalovirus (CMV) and *Clostridium difficile* as treatment of these infections with ganciclovir or metronidazole may rescue the patient from possible colectomy (Table 30.4). Such infections are uncommon but important to detect.

Two principal medical salvage therapies are currently available, ciclosporin and infliximab.

Ciclosporin

Ciclosporin, a cyclic peptide of 11 amino acids, acts by binding to cyclophilin and thereby inhibiting calcineurin. Inhibition of calcineurin prevents transcription of interleukin-2 (IL-2) and activation of T-lymphocytes. With the demonstration that treatment with 2mg/kg of ciclosporin is as effective as the conventional 4mg/kg with fewer occurrence of some side effects such as hypertension [6], the lower dose is now accepted as standard therapy in most hospitals. The dose is not generally adjusted according to serum ciclosporin levels, unless serum levels are in toxic range. Once the patient

has responded and is feeling better, the intravenous preparation may be replaced by oral micro-emulsion ciclosporin 5mg/kg. It is no longer necessary to exclude patients with low plasma cholesterol due to risk of seizures, as the intravenous preparation does not contain the incriminating chromophore. Ciclosporin may also be used as monotherapy in place of intravenous steroids [7], but this is hardly ever considered in practice, unless steroid therapy is contraindicated. In a patient who responds to ciclosporin, the drug is continued as oral therapy for 3–4 months, while corticosteroids are tapered and discontinued and azathioprine 2.5mg/kg or 6-mercaptopurine 1.5mg/kg is introduced at the time of discharge as long-term maintenance therapy. Such patients are quite severely immunosuppressed and therefore a high vigilance for opportunistic infections and prophylaxis for *Pneumocystis carinii* with cotrimoxazole is necessary. Ciclosporin is associated with a number of serious adverse events including an appreciable mortality (Table 30.5) and therefore the use of ciclosporin as rescue therapy is limited in acute severe colitis – both surgery and infliximab are considered as potentially more attractive options by both physicians and patients. In patients rescued by ciclosporin, 58% eventually have a colectomy over the next 7 years, not surprising as ciclosporin is not considered a long-term therapy due to its adverse effect profile on long-term use. A number of predictive factors for response to ciclosporin have been proposed based on simple clinical criteria such as fever, tachycardia, C-reactive protein > 45mg/l and the presence of severe endoscopic lesions [8]. In patients with acute severe Crohn's colitis there is

Table 30.4 Principles of salvage therapy in intravenous steroid-refractory patients.

Monitor very carefully
Pulse rate
Temperature
Hemoglobin and albumin
CRP
AXR
In case of nonresponse
Repeat stool cultures, *C difficile*
Cytomegalovirus (in tissue and blood)
Colonoscopy
If a patient deteriorates on salvage therapy, move to immediate colectomy

no evidence that ciclosporin is effective and treatment failure after commencing ciclosporin may be an indication that this condition is in fact causing the patient's illness. In these cases infliximab or other biological agents are indicated (see below as for ulcerative colitis).

Infliximab

The chimeric anti-TNF antibody infliximab was used in intravenous steroid refractory ulcerative colitis in a pivotal Scandinavian study in which a single 5 mg/kg infusion of infliximab was used [4]. The trial design is shown in Fig. 30.1. Patients unresponsive to IV corticosteroids at day 3 were randomized to additional single dose of 5 mg/kg of infliximab or placebo. Patients who were not considered unresponsive at day 3 but remained symptomatic at day 5–7 were also randomized to a single 5 mg/kg dose of infliximab or placebo. Overall, 29% of patients underwent colectomy in the infliximab arm compared with 67% in the placebo arm (Fig. 30.2). In a recent Italian study, patients who had received multiple doses of infliximab had

better outcome than those receiving a single dose of infliximab in a group of intravenous steroid resistant acute severe colitis patients [9]. Keeping this in mind, it may be wise to administer infliximab at 0, 2, 6 weeks and thereafter every 8 weeks till the patient is in remission. Subsequently, in those patients who are azathioprine/6-mercaptopurine naïve, this drug may be used as long-term therapy and infliximab discontinued. In patients who developed acute severe intravneous steroid resistant colitis while on azathioprine or 6-mercaptopurine, infliximab should preferably be continued long term. The use of infliximab may be associated with opportunistic infections but, in the Swedish randomized controlled trial, adverse effects were similar in those receiving infliximab or placebo.

Though patients failing ciclosporin may respond to infliximab, repeated salvage therapy generally results in unacceptable delay to surgery and profound immunosuppression. Therefore only one form of salvage therapy should be decided upon after discussion with the

Table 30.5 Incidence of adverse events associated with ciclosporin.

Tremor/paresthesia	9%
Hypertrichosis	6%
Gingival hyperplasia	6%
Renal insufficiency	6%
Seizures	1%
Anaphylaxis	0.3%
Hypertension	7%
Opportunistic infections	3%

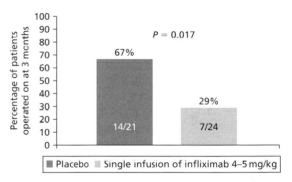

Figure 30.2 90 day colectomy rate in infliximab arm compared to placebo arm in IV steroid refractory ulcerative colitis (4).

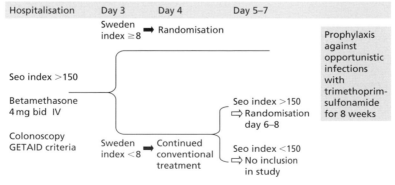

Figure 30.1 Scandinavian randomised controlled trial of infliximab in acute severe ulcerative colitis (4).

patient, and failure of such therapy should lead to surgery. A patient developing acute severe colitis while on therapy with oral corticosteroids should be admitted but may proceed straight to second-line salvage therapy.

Other therapies
Visilizumab
Humanized IgG2 antibody against CD3 lymphocytes have undergone preliminary trials in intravenous steroid refractory ulcerative colitis [10]. Though initially promising, subsequent phase II studies were prematurely terminated due to lack of efficacy. Anti-CD3 antibodies also have a propensity to cause an acute cytokine release syndrome, which may be minimized by hydration and premedication with acetaminophen (paracetamol) and antihistamines.

Daclizumab
Monoclonal humanized antibody to interleukin-2 receptor (CD25, IL-2R) was considered an attractive potential therapy for ulcerative colitis as the mechanism of action is similar to ciclosporin. However, a randomized controlled trial in 159 patients with moderate active ulcerative colitis showed no evidence of efficacy [11] and therefore it is unlikely that this antibody will have any place in the treatment of severe steroid-refractory ulcerative colitis.

Basiliximab
Monoclonal chimeric antibody to interleukin-2 receptor (CD25, IL-2R) has been shown to act as a steroid sensitizing agent but an uncontrolled trial failed to demonstrate promising efficacy in steroid-refractory severe ulcerative colitis – 4 out of 7 treated patients underwent colectomy [12]. Therefore anti-CD25 monoclonal antibodies cannot be considered effective salvage therapy in severe steroid-refractory ulcerative colitis.

Tacrolimus
A randomized controlled trial of oral tacrolimus in acute moderate-severe steroid-refractory ulcerative colitis has been reported [13]. Encouraging results were obtained in patients treated with a high trough level of tacrolimus (10–15 ng/mL), but the necessity of frequent measurements of trough levels, toxicities and lack of clear evidence of efficacy in hospitalized acute severe colitis makes tacrolimus a generally unattractive choice for the majority of such patients.

Leukocyte apheresis
Commercial columns to remove different white cell populations from circulation via an extracorporeal circuit have been used extensively in Japan and some Scandinavian countries, but randomized controlled trials in true acute severe hospitalized patients are lacking. Only scant anecdotal data exists in the context of response in steroid-refractory acute severe colitis [14] and this intervention is generally not used in most centers.

General management
Prophylaxis of thromboembolic complications
Patients with acute severe colitis are very ill, often confined to bed, dehydrated and have a hypercoagulable state. Active inflammation may play a direct role in producing a thrombophilic state [15] and all patients should receive prophylactic heparin. Administration of heparin is safe and does not increase the incidence of colonic bleeding [16]. Either unfractionated and low molecular weight heparin may be used for prevention of venous thrombosis at least as long as the patient is on intravenous steroids or is confined to bed.

Management of nutritional status
Bowel rest via total parenteral nutrition has no therapeutic benefit in reducing the inflammation in acute severe ulcerative colitis. However, a number of patients are admitted with very poor nutritional status and are too ill to have adequate oral nutritional intake. A dietician should always be involved in managing such patients, and parenteral nutrition (along with oral nutrition) should be considered on nutritional grounds if oral intake is persistently inadequate, so that emergency surgery in a nutritionally debilitated patient can be avoided.

Management of fluid and electrolyte disturbances
Many of these patients are dehydrated and hypokalemic especially after high doses of steroids and careful monitoring and replacement are necessary. If the patient is unable to drink adequately, intravenous fluids will be required.

Blood transfusion
Blood transfusion and iron replacement should be considered in patients in order to maintain a hemoglobin

concentration above 10 g/dL. This is important in terms of keeping a patient in a fit state for surgery if medical management fails.

Surgery

A well-timed operation is an invaluable part of appropriate management of acute severe ulcerative colitis and can be life-saving. With the availability of more salvage therapy choices, it is important that these are offered early to patients failing steroid therapy; therefore, in most instances, surgery will be offered after failure of second-line salvage therapy with infliximab or ciclosporin. An exception may be patients presenting with fulminant colitis who may be ill enough to undergo surgery if they do not rapidly improve after intravenous corticosteroids. Severe hemorrhage, perforation or toxic megacolon developing on treatment are indications for emergency surgery.

Surgery should be discussed with all patients admitted with acute severe ulcerative colitis as one of the possible options. Colorectal surgeon, gastroenterologist, stoma therapist and inflammatory bowel disease specialist nurse will all play a role in discussing surgery as one of the therapeutic options if intravenous steroid therapy fails. The opportunity to discuss the implications of surgery with a patient who has undergone colectomy in the past is often considered useful by the patient. Some of the potential complications and drawbacks of surgery also require balanced discussion and deliberation (Table 30.6). It is therefore inappropriate to present colectomy as a cure of ulcerative colitis to the patient.

In patients with acute severe colitis, surgery has to be a staged process. Subtotal colectomy with ileostomy is performed initially, increasingly laparoscopy-assisted in specialized centers. After 3–6 months with the patient in much better health, completion proctectomy with ileal pouch anal anastomosis (IPAA) is performed. Use of salvage therapy such as infliximab [4] or ciclosporin [6] in the setting of acute severe colitis does not appear to increase the risks of complications after colectomy. In a minority of patients with poor anal sphincter function, a permanent ileostomy may be preferable to avoid disabling incontinence. Careful psychological support and counseling throughout the process are invaluable, especially in patients who lose their colon after only a short spell of illness.

Table 30.6 Potential problems and complications after ileal pouch anal anastomosis.

Sepsis
Small intestinal obstruction
Urinary retention
Pouchitis
Fecundity and impotence
Other forms of pouch dysfunction
Incontinence
Pouch failure

Conclusion

Acute severe ulcerative colitis is a medical emergency. All patients require hospitalization and precise management, otherwise mortality rates will increase. With optimum medical and surgical management, however, the mortality rate should approximate zero. Two golden rules are important in management:

Rule 1

In hospitalized patients with acute severe ulcerative colitis on intravenous corticosteroids, worsening of disease on *any day*, or lack of response by day 3, should result in consideration of salvage therapy or surgery.

Rule 2

In intravenous steroid-refractory acute severe ulcerative colitis on second-line therapy (infliximab or ciclosporin) significant worsening of clinical status on any day compared with previous day should lead to consideration of surgery.

A management algorithm to summarize the approach discussed in this chapter is illustrated in Fig. 30.3. Intravenous steroids remain first-line therapy, but infliximab appears a more acceptable salvage therapy than ciclosporin though results of randomized trials are awaited.

All patients require assessment by a senior gastroenterologist twice daily to analyze potentially confusing features such as a decrease in stool frequency heralding worsening colonic status. In addition, patients require surgical assessment on a daily basis until the patient is considered to be no longer at a risk for colectomy. With

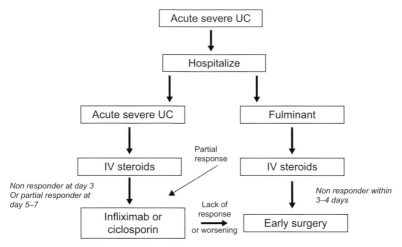

Figure 30.3 A management algorithm for short term management of acute severe colitis.

precise medical and surgical management, caring for acute severe ulcerative colitis patients can be extremely gratifying. Decisions have to be taken quickly and correctly, so that a patient is never put in a life-threatening situation after admission.

References

1. Truelove SC, Witts LJ. Cortisone in ulcerative colitis: final report on a therapeutic trial. Br Med J 1955; ii:1041–8.
2. Truelove SC, Jewell DP. Intensive intravenous regimen for severe attacks of ulcerative colitis. Lancet 1974; i:1067–70.
3. Gustavsson A, Halfvarson J, Magnuson A, Sandberg-Gertzen H, Tysk C, Jarnerot G. Long-term colectomy rate after intensive intravenous corticosteroid therapy for ulcerative colitis prior to the immunosuppressive treatment era. Am J Gastroenterol 2007; 102:2513–19.
4. Jarnerot G, Hertervig E, Friis-Liby I, Blomquist L, Karlen P, Granno C, et al. Infliximab as rescue therapy in severe to moderately severe ulcerative colitis: a randomized, placebo-controlled study. Gastroenterology 2005; 128:1805–11.
5. Travis SPL, Farrant JM, Ricketts C. Predicting outcome in severe ulcerative colitis. Gut 1996; 38:905–10.
6. Van Assche G, D'Haens G, Noman M. Randomised, double blind comparison of 4mg/kg vs 2mg/kg intravenous cyclosporine in severe ulcerative colitis. Gastroenterology 2003; 125:1025–31.

7. D'Haens G, Lemmens L, Geboes K. Intravenous cyclosporine versus intravenous corticosteroids as a single therapy for severe attacks of ulcerative colitis. Gastroenterology 2001; 120:1323–9.
8. Cacheux W, Selsik P, Lemann M, Marteau P, Nion-Larmurier I, Afchain P, et al. Predictive factors of response to cyclosporine in steroid-refractory ulcerative colitis. Am J Gastroenterol 2007 Nov 28 (epub ahead of print).
9. Kohn A, Daperno M, Armuzzi A, Capello M, Biancone L, Orlando A. Infliximab in severe ulcerative colitis: short-term results of different infusion regimens and long-term follow-up. Aliment Pharmacol Ther 2007; 26:747–56.
10. Plevy S, Salzberg B, Van Assche G, Regueiro M, Hommes D, Sandborn W. A phase I study of visilizumab, a humanized anti-CD3 monoclonal antibody, in severe steroid-refractory ulcerative colitis. Gastroenterology 2007; 133:1414–22.
11. Van Assche G, Sandborn WJ, Feagan BG, Salzberg BA, Silvers D, Monroe PS. Daclizumab, a humanised monoclonal antibody to the interleukin 2 receptor (CD25), for the treatment of moderately to severely active ulcerative colitis: a randomised, double blind, placebo controlled, dose ranging trial. Gut 2006; 55:1568–74.
12. Creed TJ, Probert CS, Norman MN, Moorghen M, Shepherd NA, Hearing SD. Basiliximab for the treatment of steroid-resistant ulcerative colitis: further experience in moderate and severe disease. Aliment Pharmacol Ther 2006; 23:1435–42.
13. Ogata H, Matsui T, Nakamura M, Ida M, Takazoe M, Suzuki Y, Hibi T. A randomised dose finding study of

oral tacrolimus (FK506) therapy in refractory ulcerative colitis. Gut 2006; 56:1255–62.

14. Hanai H, Watanabe F, Saniabadi AR, Matsushitai I, Takeuchi K, Ida T. Therapeutic efficacy of granulocyte and monocyte adsorption apheresis in severe active ulcerative colitis. Dig Dis Sci 2002; 47:2349–53.

15. Danese S, Papa A, Saibeni S, Repici A, Malesci A, Vecchi M. Inflammation and coagulation in inflammatory bowel disease: the clot thickens. Am J Gastroenterol 2007; 102:174–86.

16. Shen J, Ran ZH, Tong JL, Xiao SD. Meta-analysis: the utility and safety of heparin in the treatment of active ulcerative colitis. Aliment Pharmacol Ther 2007; 26:653–63.

31 Gastrointestinal Infections

Graham Morrison, John S. Collins

Gastrointestinal infections are a major cause of mortality and morbidity worldwide. The vast majority of these are due to gastroenteritis/infectious diarrhea which will be the focus of this chapter. The approach to diarrhea and its definition has already been discussed.

While the mortality rate in developed countries has improved infectious diarrhea continues to affect 1 in 5 people per year [1]. There are an estimated 1.8 billion episodes of childhood diarrhea per year in the developing world, where diarrheal disease is responsible for approximately 3 million deaths each year among children under 5 years of age [2]. In both the developed and developing world the young, elderly and immunocompromised are at particular risk.

Gastroenteritis

This is by far the commonest manifestation of gastrointestinal infection. It presents with diarrhea which may be accompanied by nausea, vomiting and abdominal pain. Onset is often abrupt and can range from mild illness to life-threatening sepsis. It is most problematic in high-risk groups (Table 31.1). Most cases do not need hospital admission and can be managed in the community. The pathogen involved is often not isolated but this rarely has an impact upon treatment as most episodes are self-limiting.

Causes

A variety of viral, bacterial and parasitic pathogens can be implicated (Table 31.2). Viral infections cause the majority of gastroenteritis in developed countries, especially among children. Pathogens are isolated in

Table 31.1 High-risk groups for infectious diarrhea.

Factor	Patients at risk
Age	Infants/Children
	Elderly
Immunodeficiency	HIV/AIDS
	Malignancy
	Chemotherapy/Drugs
	Genetic disease
	Malnutrition
Low gastric acidity	Elderly
	Achlorhydria
	Medications
	Total gastrectomy
Altered gut flora	Antibiotics
Increased exposure	Travelers
	Contaminated food or water

fewer than 50% of cases. Of those identified the most common are: viral 40–50%, particularly rotavirus and norovirus; *Campylobacter* 20%; *Salmonella* 15%; others 15% (see below).

History and examination

The history of infectious diarrhea can provide important clues to the infecting organism and etiology of infection. Relevant history includes foreign travel, contact with carriers (human and animal), contaminated food (unpasteurized dairy produce, uncooked food, seafood and unwashed or unpeeled fruit), antibiotics, comorbidities and relevant immune status. Clinically three syndromes are seen:
- Acute watery diarrhea, usually resolving within 5–10 days
- Bloody diarrhea
- Persistent diarrhea (>14 days) with or without malabsorption.

Gastrointestinal Emergencies, 2nd edition. Edited by Tony Tham, John Collins and Roy Soetikno. © 2009 by Blackwell Publishing, ISBN: 978-1-4051-4634-0.

Table 31.2 Laboratory isolates for gastroenteritis, England and Wales, January–June 2006 [3].

Infecting organism	Number of isolates
Campylobacter	17,791
Rotavirus	11,887
Non-typhoidal salmonellosis	3,644
Norovirus	2,990
Giardia	1,068
Cryptosporidium	976
Escherichia coli O157:H7	296
Shigella sonnei	293

Figures from Health Protection Agency 2006

Table 31.3 Indications for further investigation.

Indications for further investigations
Prolonged symptoms
Severe disease
Atypical features
Multiple (>1) people affected
Bloody diarrhea
Elderly
Residential or institutional outbreak
Public health reasons

Although useful there is considerable overlap making prediction of the pathogen involved unreliable. Crampy abdominal pain, diarrhea, mucus and pyrexia are common presenting symptoms. Nausea, vomiting, arthralgia, fatigue and headache may also occur and may precede diarrhea. Most bacterial and viral illnesses resolve within 5–10 days. Parasitic infections tend to be more insidious, as do those in immunocompromised patients.

Examination findings tend to be nonspecific. Abdominal tenderness and fever are common. Tachycardia and hypotension may occur in severe cases. Peritonism may occur and suggests perforation. Examination findings are rarely useful in distinguishing infectious diarrhea from inflammatory bowel disease. The presence of a self-limiting illness without relapse or identification of the organism are the only reliable indicators of an infectious cause.

Investigations

Mild self-limiting illness requires no formal investigation unless a more serious condition is suspected. Supportive measures will usually suffice in these cases. Patients who should be investigated are shown in Table 31.3.

Generally it is best to start with the simplest, least invasive test and work upwards as required to more invasive testing. General examination and routine blood tests should be done first before proceeding onto looking for specific pathogen.

Stool microscopy and culture

This is the first-line investigation. It is simple, relatively cheap and can provide an early diagnosis. Three samples are usually examined under the light microscope for parasites by an experienced observer. Samples are then cultured for bacterial pathogens. Microscopy is used for diagnosis of *G. lamblia, E. histolytica, Cryptosporidium* and *Cyclospora* species. Rapid enzyme immunoassays are used for detection of *Clostridium difficile* toxins, *Campylobacter*, enterohemorrhagic *E. coli* and *Shigella*.

Electron microscopy

Useful in diagnosis of viral infection but rarely required. Large outbreaks in institutions or culture negative outbreaks are the main use.

Serological diagnosis

Antibody testing is useful in a limited number of infections. It is particularly useful in amebiasis where antibodies are present in 80–90% of patients. Others include *Yersinia, Strongyloides* and schistosomiasis.

Abdominal imaging

A plain radiograph is useful in severely unwell patients to exclude colonic dilatation and perforation. It can be used to assess the severity and extent of infectious colitis.

Endoscopy

Lower gastrointestinal endoscopy is useful when symptoms persist despite negative cultures. The main indication is to distinguish between infectious colitis and inflammatory bowel disease. Biopsies can be unreliable but may show features in keeping with inflammatory bowel disease and can identify cytomegalovirus, *E. histolytica* and the ova of *Schistosoma* spp. [2]. Pseudomembranes are typical of *C. difficile*. Upper gastrointestinal endoscopy can be useful in patients with persistent diarrhea. Duodenal biopsies may show villous atrophy in keeping with intestinal protozoa and may even reveal the presence of cysts or trophozoites. Giardiasis and *Strongyloides* can be diagnosed on aspiration of duodenal fluid.

General management

Supportive care is the mainstay of treatment. Mild self-limiting cases can be managed by encouraging oral intake of fluids and electrolytes. In most cases this will be sufficient unless the patient is vomiting or very unwell. Contact precautions should be strictly adhered to and oral intake of both fluids and food should be encouraged.

Maintenance of hydration is critical in management. This is preferably achieved via the oral route with solutions containing water, salt and sugar [4]. Oral rehydration solutions are designed to meet this need and have revolutionized the treatment of infectious diarrhea. They are underused in treatment, especially in the developed world [5]. Several preparations are available and are shown in Table 31.4.

Most patients can be managed with oral rehydration solutions that can be given via nasogastric tube if required. Patients who are vomiting, unable to tolerate oral fluids or have severe dehydration should receive intravenous fluids until the diarrhea has settled.

Antibiotics are usually reserved for patients who are severely unwell with evidence of systemic upset. They may also be considered for prolonged disease or certain virulent pathogens (see specific conditions below). Antibiotics for specific infections are discussed later and outlined in Table 31.6. If empirical antibiotics are required ciprofloxacin 500 mg twice daily for 5–7 days is a reasonable choice.

Antimotility drugs are best avoided but may be used for symptomatic relief in those without fever or bloody stools. Loperamide is most frequently used, 4 mg initially followed by 2 mg after each unformed stool to a maximum of 16 mg/24 hours. Antimotility drugs are best avoided in children.

Recently there has been interest in antisecretory drugs and in particular the development of an enkephalinase inhibitor, racecadotril, which potentiates enkephalins in the intestine and increases absorptive activity [6]. These drugs and others remain mainly in the research domain at present but hold promise for the future.

Specific infections

Viral

Viral pathogens cause the majority of childhood gastroenteritis and a significant proportion of adult cases. The commonest agents are rotavirus, norovirus, enteric adenovirus and astrovirus. Rotavirus and norovirus are the commonest and most medically important and will be discussed here.

In recent times norovirus has presented significant problems in the hospital and institutional setting leading to large-scale outbreaks and public health initiatives to reduce infection.

The management of viral cases is supportive with the general measures described above. Other measures will depend on the setting in which the infection occurs, for example institutional outbreaks will require appropriate infection control measures. Enteric precautions should be taken and include hand washing, barrier use and the wearing of gloves. These simple measures can lead to a significant reduction in diarrheal risk [7]. If an outbreak is suspected the public health authority should be involved to identify a source and take appropriate measures.

Rotavirus

This is primarily an infection of children and most will have been infected by age 5 [8]. It is a significant health burden causing over 100 million diarrhea episodes

Table 31.4 Oral rehydration solutions.

| | mmol/L | | | |
	Na+	K+	CL−	CHO
Dioralyte (powder) (Aventis Pharma)	60	20	60	90 (Glucose)
Electrolade (Baxter)	50	20	40	111 (Glucose)
Rapolyte (Provalis)	60	20	50	110 (Glucose)
Dioralyte Relief (Aventis Pharma)	60	20	50	30 g (Rice Starch)
WHO Forulation Oral Rehydration Salts	75	20	65	75 (Glucose)

Note: WHO solution above is revised 2002 solution containing less Na.

each year and 600000 deaths in children younger than 5 years worldwide [9], almost all of which are in the developing world. It is uncommon in adults and usually presents with fever, watery diarrhea and vomiting. The virus is highly infectious and can occur as outbreaks.

Diagnosis can usually be made on clinical grounds but stool analysis for viral antigens is possible. Treatment is supportive and the infection usually resolves within 5 days. A vaccine against rotavirus has been developed and is available in some countries.

Norovirus

Norovirus is a common cause of nonbacterial gastroenteritis and can be responsible for epidemic outbreaks throughout a variety of settings [10]. Large-scale outbreaks in hospitals and institutions have increased public awareness of these infections. The virus is readily transmitted via food with uncooked food and shellfish being a particular risk. The illness normally lasts around 24–48 hours and usually presents with acute onset diarrhea and vomiting. Elderly patients are most prone to severe disease.

Diagnosis is usually on clinical grounds but specific viral diagnosis can be achieved by reverse transcriptase PCR on stool samples which has superseded electron microscopy [11].

Again the virus is highly infectious and strict contact precautions should be followed as well as general supportive care and adequate hydration.

The other viral pathogens are managed as outlined above. Of special note are cytomegalovirus and herpes simplex virus. These are discussed later in the chapter.

Bacterial

Bacterial infection can cause severe and even life-threatening gastroenteritis.

Campylobacter

Campylobacter (*C. jejuni* and *C. coli*) is an important cause of diarrhea worldwide and one of the commonest causes of bacterial gastroenteritis [12]. It is a zoonosis and transmitted via poultry, pigs, cattle, water, unpasteurized milk and pets. The organism is very sensitive to cooling and drying and large foodborne outbreaks do not usually occur (compare with *Salmonella*).

The incubation period ranges from 3 to 5 days with a prodrome of fever and malaise that is commonly followed by mild diarrhea. Vomiting is unusual but enterocolitis with abdominal pain and severe bloody diarrhea with an acute abdomen can occur.

Arthritis (2%), pancreatitis and septicemia can rarely occur. The diagnosis is usually made on stool culture and ciprofloxacin (750 mg twice daily for 5 days) or erythromycin (500 mg four times a day for 5 days) can be used for severe cases.

Of note the organism can be excreted for up to 5 weeks after infection but no treatment is required unless severe signs are present.

Salmonella

Salmonella can cause a variety of infections in humans that are commonly described as typhoidal and non-typhoidal. These include classical typhoid fever, gastroenteritis, bacteremia and metastatic infection such as osteomyelitis and abscesses. Non-typhoidal disease tends to be a domestic illness while typhoidal tends to be acquired abroad.

Nontyphoidal salmonella (*S. enteritidis* and *S. typhimurium*) is the commonest cause of food poisoning in the UK [3,13]. It is a zoonosis with a large reservoir in the animal population with poultry, raw eggs, meat and unpasteurized milk often being implicated [14]. Gastroenteritis is the commonest presentation. The incubation period is 12–36 hours after which diarrhea, vomiting, abdominal pain and fever occur. Severe infection can cause enterocolitis, which may mimic ulcerative colitis, and can lead to septicemia and death.

Diagnosis is made on stool culture and most cases will settle on supportive therapy. Severe cases and high-risk patients should be treated with ciprofloxacin (750 mg twice daily for 7 days), although multiresistant organisms are now emerging. The feces may be positive for weeks after infection and rarely a chronic carrier state may occur. Treatment for this is not usually required unless a specific indication is present, e.g. immunocompromised individuals. Chronic carriers can be treated with 4–6 weeks of antibiotics. Food handlers should be advised to remain at home during the illness and public health advice should be sought.

Typhoidal salmonella (*S. typhi* and *S. paratyphi*) causes a systemic febrile illness in which diarrhea is less prevalent [15]. In contrast to above *S. typhi* has no animal host and causes disease in humans only. Spread is via contact with those infected or indirectly via contaminated water and food. Infection usually follows an insidious onset with headache, dry cough, malaise and anorexia. This is followed by a bacteremic phase in the first 7–10 days with abdominal pain and fever during which time blood cultures are usually positive. Rose spots, a relative bradycardia and hepatosplenomegaly may occur by the second week. Without treatment this may progress to meningitis, pneumonia, osteomyelitis and intestinal hemorrhage. Recovery starts in the fourth week but mortality remains high without treatment and up to 10% of patients will relapse and around 2–4% of affected individuals will become chronic carriers (commoner in those with cholelithiasis or biliary tract disease).

Diagnosis may be made on cultures from blood, stool, urine and bone marrow as well as the clinical picture. Supportive treatment and hydration is essential and antibiotic therapy should be instigated. Ciprofloxacin, chloramphenicol or cotrimoxazole (usually for 2 weeks) are suitable choices. Chronic carriage may be treated with longer courses of antibiotics with consideration to cholecystectomy. Of note a vaccine for typhoid is available and should be recommended to those travelling to high-risk areas [16].

Shigella

Shigella (*S. sonnei*, *S. flexneri* and others) is the classic cause of colonic or dysenteric diarrhea and transmission is by person-to-person spread and contaminated food and water. It remains a major problem in institutions and the developing world. The infecting dose is low, making transmission easy. Incubation is 2–3 days followed by small bowel invasion and watery diarrhea that then progresses to the colonic phase with bloody diarrhea. Most cases tend to be mild and self-limiting. However, severe disease with fever, malaise and abdominal pain may occur [17]. Toxic megacolon is a rare complication and a reactive arthritis may also occur.

Diagnosis is by stool culture. The majority of cases settle with supportive measures but severe cases may be treated with ciprofloxacin (500 mg twice daily for 3 days) or cotrimoxazole (3-day course).

Escherichia coli

Escherichia coli are common organisms and occur naturally in the human gastrointestinal tract. They can, however, become pathogenic and are a frequent cause of diarrhea [18]. The type of clinical syndrome produced generally classifies them. The three main types to consider are enterotoxigenic *E. coli* (ETEC), enteroinvasive (EIEC) and enterohemorrhagic *E. coli* (EHEC). Two other varieties enteropathogenic (EPEC) and enteroaggregative (EAEC) also occur less commonly in children and the immunocompromised.

ETEC

Common in the developing world, this organism causes watery diarrhea in children and travelers and is a major cause of traveler's diarrhea [19]. The organism is acquired via contaminated food and water with rapid onset of watery diarrhea, nausea and crampy abdominal pain. Vomiting may also occur. The classical case is the traveler moving from an area of good to poor hygiene with subsequent gastroenteritis. Diagnosis can be made on stool culture. Supportive therapy is usually sufficient as the disease is self-limiting in the majority of cases. Severe cases can be treated with ciprofloxacin and advice regarding meticulous attention to food and water consumption should be given to travelers.

EIEC

Enteroinvasive *E. coli* are similar and closely related to *Shigella* spp. and cause a disease similar to bacillary dysentery. Diagnosis is by stool culture and management is as above.

EHEC

Enterohemorrhagic *E. coli* was first described in 1982 after an outbreak in the US [20]. They are responsible for large outbreaks of hemorrhagic colitis around the world and act via production of shiga toxins that play a major role in pathogenesis and development of complications. The main serotype, 0157:H7, is responsible for the majority of outbreaks [21].

EHEC is acquired via undercooked beef, meat, milk and contaminated water. After a short incubation (12–24 hours) it causes diarrhea that is frequently bloody with associated abdominal pain and nausea. This may progress to septicemia and multiorgan failure. Thrombotic thrombocytopenic purpura (TTP) and hemolytic uremic syndrome (HUS) are recognized complications and are more common in children [22,23].

Treatment is mainly supportive. Antibiotics have been suggested as a trigger for release of shiga toxin and possible precipitant of hemolytic uremic syndrome but evidence for this remains controversial [24].

Yersinia

Yersinia (*Y. enterocolitica* and *Y. pseudotuberculosis*) infection is common in developed countries with *Y. enterocolitica* being common in the US and *Y. pseudotuberculosis* in Europe. Infection is associated with waterborne or foodborne outbreaks. Presentation ranges from mild watery diarrhea to prolonged diarrhea, dysentery and terminal ileitis that may be indistinguishable from Crohn's disease.

Diagnosis is usually on stool culture or serology in delayed presentation. The illness is often self-limiting but ciprofloxacin (500 mg twice daily for 5 days) may be used for severe cases.

Bacillus cereus

Bacillus is usually contracted via infected food; boiled and fried rice are commonly implicated. The incubation period is a matter of hours before abrupt onset of diarrhea and vomiting. The organism can be cultured from stool but recovery is usually rapid and anything more than supportive care is rarely required.

Vibrios (V. cholerae)

Cholera is a disease of the tropics, particularly Africa and Asia. It is an important cause of diarrhea in travelers returning from endemic areas. It is a disease of poverty and poor sanitation and remains a significant cause of morbidity and mortality worldwide [25]. It is a waterborne disease and transmission is via the fecal-oral route. Contaminated water is the major carrier of the disease and once ingested the organisms grow on the epithelia of the small bowel where they produce enterotoxin that leads to a massive secretory diarrhea.

Incubation is 1–5 days and clinical infection is heralded by the abrupt onset of painless diarrhea sometimes referred to as "rice-water stools".

Fluid and electrolyte losses may be massive and can lead rapidly to death from dehydration [26].

Diagnosis is made by direct stool microscopy for organisms but can often be made on clinical grounds. The cornerstone of treatment is aimed at replacing fluid and electrolytes. Oral rehydration solutions have revolutionized this. Tetracycline (500 mg three times daily for 3 days) or ciprofloxacin (500 mg twice daily for 3 days) can be used to shorten the period of diarrhea and excretion as well as to aid recovery.

Vaccination is available but currently suboptimal, with new vaccines currently under development.

Clostridium difficile

This is one of the most common nosocomial infections and has become a major problem in hospital practice. *Clostridium difficile*-associated disease (CDAD) is a common cause of morbidity and mortality among hospitalized patients [27], and is on the increase in both the inpatient and outpatient setting.

The organism exerts its effect via toxin production (A and B) that leads to secretory diarrhea and colonic inflammation. Different strains have varying toxigenicity and some patients will be colonized and become asymptomatic carriers of the organism (approx 2% of the population). Those who are colonized or infected shed the organism and transmission is most often by contaminated hands and equipment.

Risk factors for infection include: old age; debilitation; concomitant illness; gastrointestinal surgery; antibiotic use (all but especially penicillins, clindamycin and cephalosporins); gastric acid suppression; enteral feeding; and NSAID use.

Colonized individuals are at particular risk of CDAD after treatment with antibiotics.

Clinical infection ranges from an asymptomatic carrier state to acute, persistent or recurrent diarrhea. Pseudomembranous colitis and death may occur. In those who develop diarrhea, symptoms usually begin soon after colonization, with the incubation period normally less than 1 week. Diarrhea is typically loose or watery and while mucus may be present overt blood is rare. Diarrhea may be minimal in severe disease and ileus, toxic dilatation and pseudomemebranous colitis may develop.

Diagnosis is made by demonstration of toxins in stool samples and occasionally endoscopy. Stool toxin may be positive for up to 6 weeks after treatment. General management involves introduction of infection control policies and correction of any of the above risk factors if possible. Supportive treatment is coupled with specific antibiotic therapy. First-line therapy is with oral metronidazole (400 mg three times daily for 10–14 days). Vancomycin (250 mg four times daily for 14 days) is second-line therapy (see below).

Relapse may occur in up to one third of patients [28, 29] and should be managed as above with Metronidazole or vancomycin while other causes of diarrhea should also be considered. An approach to recurrent infection is shown in Table 31.5.

Table 31.5 Approach to recurrent *Clostridium difficile* infection.

First relapse	Second relapse	Further relapse
Confirm diagnosis and exclude others. 14-day course of metronidazole or vancomycin as outlined above.	Confirm diagnosis and exclude others. Discuss with microbiology. Vancomycin taper 125 mg q.d.s. for 7 days 125 md t.d.s. for 7 days 125 mg b.d. for 7 days 125 mg o.d. for 7 days (other regimes available)	Discuss with microbiology Several possibilities: 1. Microorganisms with vancomycin or metronidazole 2. Vancomycin plus cholestyramine 3. Vancomycin plus rifampicin 4. Intravenous immunoglobulin

Source: *Sleisenger & Fordtran's Gastrointestinal and Liver Disease*. 7th edition: volume two.

Treatment of colonized individuals remains unclear, as does the use of probiotics in the management of CDAD. Severe disease can be difficult to manage and toxic dilatation may rarely require surgical intervention and resection.

Parasites/Protozoa
Giardiasis
Giardia lamblia is a protozoan parasite and is the most common protozoal infection of the gastrointestinal tract [30]. It causes sporadic, epidemic and endemic diarrheal illness throughout the world and is most common in areas of poor sanitation. It is particularly common in travelers. Cysts (the infectious form) are passed into water supplies by the human host and are then ingested via contaminated food or water. Trophozoites then multiply in the small bowel causing clinical disease and release of further cysts and so on [31]. Most cases are either asymptomatic or have self-limiting diarrhea and gastrointestinal disturbance. Infection can lead to chronic diarrhea, malabsorption and growth retardation in children.

Diagnosis is by the identification of trophozoites or cysts on stool examination and three samples may be required. Rarely duodenal fluid aspiration may be required and giardiasis is a cause of villous atrophy.

Tindazole 2 g in a single dose or metronidazole 750 mg three times daily for 3 days are the treatments of choice. Patients with symptoms, children and those at risk of spreading infection should be treated. Relapse can be treated with a longer course of antibiotics or a second line agent such mepacrine (alone or in combination with above).

Amebiasis
Entamoeba histolytica is another protozoan parasite also occurring worldwide but is more common in developing countries with poor sanitation and lower socioeconomic conditions. Infection is usually seen in migrants from endemic areas as well as travelers to these areas. It is a significant health problem with an estimated 40 000 deaths per year [32] and significant complications [33]. As with *Giardia* it is the cysts that are infectious and the trophozoites that cause clinical disease. Cysts are ingested via contaminated food or water.

Most infections are asymptomatic. Of those that develop clinical amebiasis two forms are recognized:
1. Amebic dysentery, which occurs over several weeks and can range from diarrhea through to bloody stools, weight loss and fever. Uncommonly a fulminant colitis with toxic megacolon (mimicking ulcerative colitis) can occur with a high mortality.
2. Nondysenteric which is less common and consists of diarrhea, abdominal pain and weight loss. This form may persist for years and can be confused with Crohn's disease. Localized colonic infection leading to an ameboma can occur, as can strictures, abscesses and fistulae.

Amebic liver abscesses may also occur and are heralded by right upper quadrant pain and fever. Metastatic spread can develop and rupture can lead to peritonitis.

Diagnosis is made by antigen testing of stool and serum. Serology can also be used but remains positive for years after infection. Stool microscopy is often used but is less sensitive and unable to exclude non-pathogenic strains.

Treatment should be given to all patients to avoid risk of invasive disease. Metronidazole (750 mg three times daily for 5 days) will eliminate trophozoites and should be followed by either paromyocin (25 mg/kg/day in three divided doses for 7 days) or diloxanide (500 mg three times daily for 10 days) to eradicate luminal parasites. Follow-up stool examination is required to ensure eradication.

Cryptosporidiosis

Cryptosporidium species are intracellular protozoa, which are associated with gastrointestinal and biliary tract disease [34]. It is a common pathogen in humans and an important cause of persistent diarrhea in the developing world. Children, the immunocompromised and those from areas of poor sanitation and lower socio-economic standing are at particular risk. Clinical disease can range from asymptomatic infection to mild diarrhea or a severe enteric illness with biliary involvement. Transmission is by person-to-person spread and via infected food and water.

Immunocompetent patients typically develop diarrhea, malaise and occasionally abdominal pain that usually resolve in 10–14 days without treatment. Oocyst (infectious) excretion can continue for prolonged periods after clinical infection has resolved. Immunocompromised patients tend to have more prolonged and severe illness. AIDS patients are particularly at risk and can develop prolonged, large volume diarrhea and wasting. Cholecysytitis, cholangitis, hepatitis and pancreatitis may occur.

Diagnosis is based on identification of oocysts in stool, tissue or aspirates from the gastrointestinal or biliary tract. Treatment depends upon the immune status of the infected patient. Healthy individuals will usually recover spontaneously. For HIV-infected patients the initiation of HAART is the crucial step in therapy. This may lead to resolution of infection but often antibiotics are required. Co-trimoxazole (960 mg twice daily for 3 weeks) or metronidazole (750 mg three times daily for 5 days) are suitable choices.

Cyclospora

This parasite is an increasingly recognized cause of diarrhea. It occurs most often in foreign travelers and in patients with AIDS. Large outbreaks can occur and transmission is via contaminated food and water. Diarrhea and malaise are the most frequent symptoms and, while disease may be short and self-limiting, prolonged illness commonly occurs.

Diagnosis is made on stool microscopy and treatment is with double strength co-trimoxazole (800 mg/160 mg twice daily) for 1 week.

Other important gastrointestinal conditions

Tuberculosis (TB)

Intestinal tuberculosis is relatively uncommon in the developed world but increasing as the incidence of TB rises throughout the world. This is due to immigration from high-risk areas and the problems posed by increasing HIV. The commonest site affected is the ileocecal region but the peritoneum and perianal area may also be affected. Clinical presentation is often vague and nonspecific and can lead to delay in diagnosis. Abdominal pain, anorexia, fever, sweats, weight loss and altered bowel habit are the commonest symptoms. A right lower quadrant mass may be present. Ascites, obstruction and perforation may occur.

Diagnosis is usually made in the clinical setting of known TB or in high-risk individuals, e.g. immunocompromised, immigrants, intravenous drug abusers or immunosuppressive therapy. CT scanning and small bowel radiology are useful but colonoscopy and biopsy for histology and PCR will usually provide a definitive diagnosis. Fine needle biopsy or guided biopsy may occasionally be required. Differential diagnoses include Crohn's, cancer, lymphoma, *Yersinia* and actinomycosis.

Treatment is as for pulmonary TB.

Schistosomiasis

This is a waterborne fluke infection found in the tropics and subtropics where it is endemic. Of the three species that cause disease *Schistosoma mansoni* affects the large bowel. Infection is acquired via skin penetration by the organism following fresh water exposure in an endemic area. Chronic disease is rare in travelers as time is required for the worm burden to develop. Travelers may develop dermatitis or an acute illness (Katayama fever) with fever, rigors, bloody diarrhea and hepatosplenomegaly. If not treated eggs may migrate to the liver causing hepatitis followed by periportal fibrosis that can lead to portal hypertension and its complications.

Table 31.6 Antibiotic treatments for infectious diarrhea.

Organism	1st Line	Alternative	Efficacy
Campylobacter	Erythromycin 250 mg–500 mg q.d.s. 1 week	Ciprofloxacin 500 mg b.d. 5 Days	Severe disease
Salmonella	Ciprofloxacin 500 mg b.d. 10–14 Days 3rd Gen cephalosporin	Cotrimoxazole Amoxycillin	Usually severe disease only
E. Coli	Ciprofloxacin 500 mg b.d.	Ciprofloxacin as single dose dose	Yes
ETEC	3–5 Days		
EIES	As for *Shigella*		
EHEC	Controversal given risk of HUS		
Shigella	Ciprofloxacin 500 mg b.d Cotrimoxazole	Other 3rd generation cephalosporin Nalidixic acid 1g q.d.s. 5 Days	Yes for dysentric shigellosis
Yersinia	Ciprofloxacin 500 mg b.d. 5–7 Days	Tetracycline 250 mg q.d.s. 7–10 Days	Doubtful unless septicaemic
Clostridium difficile	Metronidazole 400 g t.d.s. 7 Days	Vancomycin 125 g q.d.s 7–10 Days	Yes
Vibrio cholera	Ciprofloxacin 1g Single dose or Tetracycline 500 mg q.d.s 5 Days	Cotrimoxazole Doxycycline	Yes
Gardia	Tinidazole 2g stat or Metronidazole 750 mg t.d.s 3 Days	Mepacrine 100 mg t.d.s 1 Week	Yes
Entamoeba Histolytica	Metronidazole 750 mg t.d.s 5 Days	Diloxanide furoate 500 mg t.d.s 10 Days	Yes

The diagnosis is made by identifying the schistosome ova in feces and this may require repeat samples. Serology can be useful in the symptomatic traveler but indicates previous exposure only.

Treatment is with praziquantel (40 mg/kg as a single dose) but is best managed by infectious diseases or those with experience of the condition.

Infection in the immunocompromised

Opportunistic gastrointestinal infections may occur in the immunocompromised. HIV infection is the commonest cause worldwide with chemotherapy and the use of other immune suppressing drugs being common in the developed world. Several infections that are more common in the immunocompromised have already been discussed above. Some other important pathogens are outlined below.

Candida

Oral and esophageal candidiasis are common illnesses. They present with a painful mouth, odynophagia and occasionally dysphagia. Diagnosis is clinically on sight of characteristic white oral plaques and may be confirmed by culture of a swab or biopsy.

Treatment is with nystatin (1 mg four times daily) or fluconazole (50 mg o.d. for 2 weeks). Prophylactic treatment should be given in the setting of AIDS after the first infection.

Cytomegalovirus

Cytomegalovuris (CMV) rarely causes significant disease in the immunocompetent. Most of those infected have no symptoms or a mild mononucleosis syndrome that settles spontaneously. CMV colitis may occur but is rare in healthy subjects.

Immunocompromised patients are at risk of significant CMV gastrointestinal infection. Before the introduction of highly active antiretroviral therapy (HAART) for HIV it was commonly seen among AIDS sufferers, where it carried a poor prognosis. CMV can affect any part of the gastrointestinal tract but is seen most often in the esophagus and colon. CMV esophagitis causes nausea and odynophagia. Multiple discrete ulcers are usually seen at endoscopy. CMV colitis is the commonest gastrointestinal manifestation and mimics the presentation of ulcerative colitis. Fever, abdominal pain, anorexia, weight loss and watery diarrhea are common [35]. Widespread inflammation, ulceration and even perforation can occur and can be life-threatening.

Diagnosis is usually suspected in those known to be at risk and in whom other causes of symptoms have been excluded. Endoscopy and biopsy provide a definitive answer with the presence of inclusion bodies on histology.

Treatment involves anti-CMV treatment such as ganciclovir or foscarnet as well as initiation of HAART if appropriate.

In general these patients should have input from specialists in gastroenterology, infectious diseases and genitourinary medicine.

Herpes simplex virus

Herpes simplex (HSV 1) is rarely a clinical problem in the healthy patient. In the setting of immunosuppression, however, the virus can cause considerable illness and patients infected with HIV who have low CD4 counts are at particular risk. Gastrointestinal infection in these patients can produce esophagitis, hepatitis and colitis. Esophagitis may be severe and should be suspected in susceptible patients with odynophagia or dysphagia.

Diagnosis may be made by viral culture, serology or identification on histology. Treatment is with acyclovir (400 mg three times daily for 7 days).

Useful information and links

Common causes of food poisoning (UK)
Salmonella 70–80%
Clostridium spp. 15–20%
Staphylococcus aureus 2–5%
www.hpa.org.uk
www.cdc.gov
www.who.int.en/
www.cks.library.nhs.uk/gastroenteritis

References

1. Wheeler JG, Sethi D, Cowden JM, et al. Study of infectious intestinal disease in England: rates in the community, presenting to general practice, and reported to national surveillance. BMJ 1999; 318:1046–305.
2. Casburn-Jones AC, Farthing MJG. Management of infectious diarrhoea. Gut 2004; 53:296–305.
3. Health Protection Agency Annual Report 2006. www.hpa.org.uk
4. Avery ME, Snyder JD. Oral therapy for acute diarrhoea. N Engl J Med 1990; 323:891–4.
5. Santosham K, Keenan EM, Tulloch J, et al. Oral rehydration therapy for diarrhoea: an example of reverse transfer in technology. Paediatrics 1997; 100:E10
6. Turvill JL, Farthing MJG. Enkephalins and enkephalinase inhibitors in intestinal fluid and electrolyte transport. Eur J Gastroenterol Hepatolo 1997; 9:877–80.
7. Curtis V, Cairncross S. Effect of washing hands with soap on diarrhoea risk in the community: a systematic review. Lancet Infect Dis 2003; 3:275–81.
8. Soriano-Gabarro M, Mrukowicz J, et al. Burden of rotavirus disease in European Union countries. Paediatr Infect Dis 2006; 25:S7–S11.
9. Grimwood K, Buttery JP. Clinical update: rotavirus gastroenteritis and its prevention. Lancet 2007; 370:302–4.

10. Lopman B, Vennema H, Kohli E, et al. Increase in viral gastroenteritis outbreaks in Europe and epidemic spread of new Norovirus variant. Lancet 2004; 363:682–8.

11. Marshall JA. Bruggink LD. Laboratory diagnosis of Norovirus. Clin Lab 2006; 52:571–81.

12. Peterson MC. Clinical aspects of *Campylobacter jejuni* infection in adults. West J Med 1994; 161:148–52.

13. Adak GK, Long SM, O'Brien SJ. Trends in indigenous foodborne disease and deaths, England and Wales: 1992 to 2000. Gut 2002; 51(6):832–41.

14. Hohmann EL. Nontyphoidal salmonellosis. Clin Infect Dis 2001; 32:263–9.

15. Bhan MK, Bhatnagar S. Typhoid and paratyphoid fever. Lancet 2005; 366:749–62.

16. Steinberg EB, Bishop R, Haber P, et al. Typhoid fever in travellers: who should be targeted for prevention? Clin Infect Dis 2004; 39:186–91.

17. Shigella bacteraemia in adults: a report of five cases and review of the literature. Arch Intern Med 1987; 147(11):2034–7.

18. Nataro JP, Kaper JB. Diarrheagenic *Escherichia coli*. Clin Microbiol Rev 1998; 11:142–201.

19. Von Sonnenberg F, Tornieporth N, Waiyaki P, et al. Risk and aetiology of diarrhoea at various tourist destinations. Lancet 2000; 356:133–4.

20. Riley LW, Remis RS, Helgerson SD, et al. Haemorrhagic colitis associated with a rare *Escherichia coli* serotype. N Engl J Med 1983; 308:681–5.

21. Slutsker L, Ries AA, Greene KD, et al. *Escherichia coli* 0157:H7 diarrhoea in the United States: clinical and epidemiologic features. Ann Intern Med 1997; 126(7): 505–13.

22. Boyce TG, Swerdlow DL, Griffin PM. *Escherichia coli* 0157:H7 and the haemolytic-uraemic syndrome. N Engl J Med 1995; 333:364–8.

23. Razzaq S. Haemolytic uraemic syndrome: an emerging health risk. Am Fam Physician 2006; 74(6):991–6.

24. Safdar N, Said A, Gangon RE, Maki DG. Risk of haemolytic uraemic syndrome after antibiotic treatment of *Escherichia coli* 0157:H7 enteritis: a meta-analysis. JAMA 2002; 288(6):996–1001.

25. Griffith DC, Kelly-Hope LA, Miller MA. Review of reported cholera outbreaks worldwide, 1995–2005. Am J Trop Med Hyg 2006; 75(5):973–7.

26. Sack DA, Sack RB, Nair GB, Siddique AK. Cholera. Lancet 2004; 363:223–33.

27. Kyne L, Hamel MB, Polavaram R, Kelly CP. Health care costs and mortality associated with nosocomial diarrhoea due to *Clostridium difficile*. Clin Infect Dis 2002; 34:346–53.

28. Fekety R. Guidelines for the diagnosis and management of *Clostridium difficile* associated diarrhoea and colitis. American College of Gastroenterology, Practice Parameters Committee. Am J Gastroenterol 1997; 92:739–50.

29. Pepin J, Alary ME, Valiquette L, et al. Increasing risk of relapse after treatment of *Clostridium difficile* colitis in Quebec, Canada. Clin Infect Dis 2005; 40:1591–7.

30. Musher DM, Musher BL. Contagious acute gastrointestinal infections. N Engl J Med 2004; 351:2417–27.

31. Strickland GT: Giardiasis. In: Hunter GE, Strickland GT, eds. Hunter's Tropical Medicine. Saunders; 1991.

32. Li E, Stanley SL. Amoebiasis. Gastroenterol Clin North Am 1996; 25:471–2.

33. Haque R, Huston CD, Hughes M, et al. Amoebiasis. N Engl J Med 2003; 348:1565–73.

34. Chen XM, Keithly JS, Paya CV, LaRusso NF. Cryptosporidiosis. N Engl J Med 2002; 346:1723–31.

35. Dieterich DT, Rahmin M. Cytomegalovirus colitis in AIDS: presentation in 44 patients and a review of the literature. J Acquir Immune Defic Syndr 1991; 4 (supp 1):S29–35.

32 Diverticular Disease

Tonya Kaltenbach, Roy Soetikno

Introduction

Diverticular disease is common. Its prevalence increases with age, from less than 10% in persons younger than 40 years of age, to up to 66% in elderly patients over the age of 80 years. It has an estimated mortality rate of 2.5 per 100000 per year. Diverticulae are caused by alterations in colonic wall structure, colonic dysmotility and dietary fiber deficiencies. They typically occur between the taeniae coli due to weaknesses of the circular muscle layer at sites of penetration of the vasa recta. Most patients with diverticulosis are asymptomatic throughout their lifetime. About 20% of patients, however, may develop complications of diverticulosis such as diverticulitis with infection, abscess, fistula, obstruction and perforation; or diverticular bleeding.

Diverticulitis

Natural history

Acute diverticulitis is the most common clinical complication of diverticular disease. Hospitalization is required in less than 10% of diverticulitis attacks. With conservative management, 80% improve, and most patients have no future problems. Risk of recurrent symptoms, however, has been reported in up to 45% of patients. Recurrent attacks are less likely to respond to medical treatment and are associated with a high mortality rate. Elective resection is therefore considered after two attacks of uncomplicated diverticulitis.

Gastrointestinal Emergencies, 2nd edition. Edited by Tony Tham, John Collins and Roy Soetikno. © 2009 by Blackwell Publishing, ISBN: 978-1-4051-4634-0.

Presentation
- Visceral abdominal pain with tenderness localized to area of maximal inflammation
- Nausea, vomiting and altered bowel habits
- Rectal tenderness
- Fever
- Leukocytosis

Evaluation
- Complete blood count
- Radiographs
  - erect chest: assess for pneumoperitoneum
  - supine abdomen: assess for bowel dilation, ileus, pneumoperitoneum, obstruction or soft tissue densities to suggest an abscess
- Urinalysis: assess for colovesicular fistula
- CT (computed tomography) abdomen and pelvis with intravenous, oral and rectal contrast
  - pericolic fat infiltration
  - thickened fascia
    muscular hypertrophy
- Barium enema and endoscopy are generally avoided due to potential to exacerbate a perforation.

The diagnosis of diverticulitis should be suspected and made primarily on the basis of the history and physical examination. When the clinical picture is clear, additional tests are not necessary to make a diagnosis. In cases of uncertainty, a CT should be performed for confirmation.

Management
Outpatient
Patients with a mild presentation, ability to tolerate oral intake, low severity of illness and adequate support can be treated as an outpatient with:
- clear liquid diet
- broad-spectrum antibiotics for 7–10 days
  - amoxicillin-clavulanate or

– trimethoprim-sulfamethoxazole or
– fluoroquinolone + metronidazole

Symptomatic improvement should be appreciated within several days.

Hospitalized

Patients with a more severe attack of diverticulitis may require hospitalization with:

- analgesia
- bowel rest
- intravenous fluid
- broad-spectrum antibiotics for 7–10 days
  – anaerobes: metronidazole or clindamycin plus
  – gram negative rods: aminoglycoside or mono-bactam or third-generation cephalosporin

---

Complicated diverticulitis

Complications of diverticulitis include abscess, fistula, obstruction and perforation.

Abscess
Natural history

Abscesses complicate about 10% of acute diverticulitis episodes, and have an estimated 12% mortality.

Presentation

- Episodic fevers
- Weight loss
- Leukocytosis
- Pain localized to visceral and parietal innervation of the abscess wall
- Dysuria, urinary frequency, tenesmus, dyspareunia in pelvic collections

Evaluation

- Computed tomography

Management
Small pericolic

- Conservative
  – bowel rest
  – intravenous fluids
  – broad-spectrum antibiotics
- Intervention if not responsive to conservative
  – CT or ultrasound (US)-guided percutaneous drainage
    – surgical single-stage resection and anastomosis

Distant or unresolving abscesses

- Interventional
  – CT or US-guided percutaneous palliative drainage
  – surgical single-stage resection and anastomosis (eliminates need for two-stage surgical procedure with interval colostomy)

Fistula
Natural history

A fistula may form when a diverticular abscess extends into an adjacent organ. The most common diverticular fistula is colovesicular. Only about one-half of patients diagnosed with a diverticular fistula have a history of diverticulitis.

Presentation

- Symptoms suggestive of preceding abscess
  – abdominal pain
  – fever
  – weight loss
- Location of fistula
  – colovesicular: pneumaturia, fecaluria, urosepsis
  – colovaginal: perineum irritation, infections or feculent discharge
  – coloenteric: malabsorption and diarrhea from bacterial overgrowth
  – colocutaneous: abdominal wall irritation

Evaluation

The diagnostic yield of each modality varies widely.

- Colonoscopy
- Barium enema
- Fistulography
- Cystoscopy
- Computed tomography accurately predicts the presence of a fistula:
  – local colonic thickening adjacent to an area of thickened organ
  – associated diverticula
  – oral contrast material or air in the organ

Management

- Surgical single-stage fistula closure with resection of diseased colon and anastomosis and repair of contiguous organ.
- In those patients with severe co-morbid conditions, conservative therapy may be considered, eg prophylactic antibiotics for colovesical fistula.

Obstruction
Natural history
Intestinal obstruction is uncommon in diverticulitis, occurring in approximately 2% of patients. It may present in an episode of acute diverticulitis due to luminal narrowing caused by inflammation or compression by an abscess. Recurrent episodes of subclinical diverticulitis can result in progressive fibrosis and stricturing of the colonic wall without associated inflammation. Small bowel obstruction is usually the result of adhesions.

Presentation (see Chapter 19)
- Nausea
- Vomiting
- Weight loss
- Distention

Evaluation
- Fluid status
- Electrolytes
- Radiograph
- Endoscopy to assess stricture and exclude malignancy

Management
- Conservative
  - bowel rest
  - intravenous fluids
  - broad-spectrum antibiotics
- Intervention
  - endoscopic dilation
  - endoscopic stenting: palliative, or decompression prior to elective surgery
  - surgical resection

Perforation (see Chapter 19)
Natural history
Over 20% of patients hospitalized with diverticular disease have peritonitis due to a perforation. It is associated with a mortality rate as high as 35% and requires urgent surgical evaluation.

Presentation
- Severe acute abdominal pain
- Dehydration
- Fever
- Tachycardia
- Generalized tenderness with guarding
- Absent bowel sounds

Evaluation
- Complete blood count
- Serum electrolytes
- Arterial blood gas
- Radiograph
- Close surgical monitoring

Management
- Bowel rest
- Aggressive intravenous fluids
- Broad-spectrum antibiotics
- Surgery

Diverticular hemorrhage

Natural history
Diverticulosis remains the most frequent cause of lower gastrointestinal bleeding, and presents as acute, painless hematochezia, often in elderly patients with comorbid conditions including hypertension, ischemic heart disease, diabetes and who use oral anticoagulation or antiplatelet medication. Diverticulae are located in the colonic wall at the sites of penetrating nutrient vessels. Bleeding is arterial and can occur either at the dome or the neck of the diverticulum. It is important to recognize the various stigmata of diverticular bleeding including large and small vessel, adherent clot, flat pigmented spot and erosion.

Presentation
- Abrupt, voluminous, painless hematochezia

Evaluation
Stratification
Most acute diverticular bleeding is self-limiting. In general, patients with stable vital signs, no recent bloody effluent and no syncope have a low risk of continued bleeding and elective colonoscopy is appropriate. Urgent interventions should be targeted for patients with severe bleeding. Independent correlates of severe bleeding include:
- bleeding per rectum during the first 4 hours of evaluation
- vital sign instability
  - tachycardia (HR $\geq$100)
  - hypotension (SBP $\leq$115 mmHg)
- syncope
- nontender abdominal examination

- aspirin use
- ≥ 2 comorbid conditions.

Check Complete blood count

Assess Volume status

Exclude an upper gastrointestinal source

- Upper endoscopy
  - patients with a positive nasogastric aspirate
  - patients where a colonic source is not identified.

Management

Once the patient has been resuscitated, the severity of bleeding assessed, and an upper gastrointestinal source of bleeding excluded, urgent colonoscopy should be performed. In cases of continued bleeding not amenable to endoscopic therapy, angiography or surgery should be considered.

Colonoscopy

Available data suggest that endoscopic intervention for diverticular hemorrhage is safe and likely to be beneficial.

- Rapid purge preparation with polyethylene glycol-based solutions
  - Administer by a nasogastric tube or by drinking 1 L every 30–45 min
  - Median dose of 5.5 L (range 4–14 L) over 3–4 hours
  - Metoclopramide, 10 mg iv, before starting the purge to control nausea and promote gastric emptying
  - Nasogastric suction immediate prior to colonoscopy
  - Contraindications: bowel obstruction, gastroparesis
- Techniques
  - Mechanical methods are preferred. (a) Clip – marking for future localization; direct application to neck or dome; use of a cap may facilitate therapy. (b) Band ligation
  - Coagulation: generally avoided at the dome due to perforation concern
  - Injection: reported with limited success

Technetium scan

Literature dating since 1990 suggests that technetium scans are not particularly useful to confirm and localize the bleeding site in order to direct further angiographic or surgical intervention.

Angiography

Angiography techniques have been modified over time to use smaller catheters for coiling or gel foam embolization. Using this optimal embolization technique,

twelve published small studies have shown high rates of successful primary hemostasis in patients with active bleeding. Short-term, less than 1 week, rebleeding rates were, however, high, found to be about 25% with a mean of 10–53%; and data on long-term rebleeding rates is lacking. Ischemia was notably reported in close to 20% of patients despite using smaller catheter and more directed therapy.

Surgery

Whenever possible, it is preferable to perform surgery on an elective basis rather than emergently. Operative mortality is 10% even with accurate localization and up to 57% with blind subtotal colectomy.

Further reading

Elta GH. Urgent colonoscopy for acute lower-GI bleeding. Gastrointest Endosc 2004; 59:402–8.

Farrell JJ, Graeme-Cook F, Kelsey PB. Treatment of bleeding colonic diverticula by endoscopic band ligation: an in-vivo and ex-vivo pilot study. Endoscopy 2003; 35:823–9.

Foutch PG, Zimmerman K. Diverticular bleeding and the pigmented protuberance (sentinel clot): clinical implications, histopathological correlation, and results of endoscopic intervention. Am J Gastroenterol 1996; 91:2589–93.

Janes SE, Meagher A, Frizelle FA. Management of diverticulitis. BMJ 2006; 332:271–5.

Jensen DM, Machicado GA, Jutabha R, Kovacs TO. Urgent colonoscopy for the diagnosis and treatment of severe diverticular hemorrhage. N Engl J Med 2000; 342:78–82.

Khanna A, Ognibene SJ, Koniaris LG. Embolization as first-line therapy for diverticulosis-related massive lower gastrointestinal bleeding: evidence from a meta-analysis. J Gastrointest Surg 2005; 9:343–52.

Petruzziello L, Iacopini F, Bulajic M, Shah S, Costamagna G. Review article: uncomplicated diverticular disease of the colon. Aliment Pharmacol Ther 2006; 23:1379–91.

Salzman H, Lillie D. Diverticular disease: diagnosis and treatment. Am Fam Physician 2005; 72:1229–34.

Simpson PW, Nguyen MH, Lim JK, Soetikno RM. Use of endoclips in the treatment of massive colonic diverticular bleeding. Gastrointest Endosc 2004; 59:433–7.

Stollman N, Raskin JB. Diverticular disease of the colon. Lancet 2004; 363:631–9.

Strate LL, Syngal S. Predictors of utilization of early colonoscopy vs. radiography for severe lower intestinal bleeding. Gastrointest Endosc 2005; 61:46–52.

33 Gastrointestinal Complications of HIV Disease

Afshin Nasoodi, Wallace Dinsmore

Introduction

HIV has been shown to mimic any medical condition and a high index of suspicion should be maintained for its presence. The gastrointestinal tract with, its rich lymphatic tissue plays, a major role in the epidemiology and pathogenesis of HIV infection. Anal acquisition is the primary route of infection in homosexual men and gut-associated lymphoid tissue (GALT) is the suitable medium in the body for virus replication. HIV causes selective depletion of the CD4 population of lymphocytes in GALT and in this way plays a part in the pathogenesis of gastrointestinal opportunistic disorders (OD). The gastrointestinal ODs in acquired immunodeficiency syndrome (AIDS) represent opportunistic infections and neoplastic diseases that could affect the gastrointestinal tract, and include *Candida* esophagitis, cytomegalovirus (CMV) gastrointestinal disease, Herpes simplex virus (HSV) esophagitis, idiopathic esophageal and colonic ulcers, *Mycobacterium avium* complex (MAC), *Cryptosporidium*, *Microsporidium*, Kaposi sarcoma (KS), and non-Hodgkin lymphoma (NHL) [1].

Highly active antiretroviral treatment (HAART) was introduced in 1996. This groundbreaking treatment uses three main groups of drugs: protease inhibitors (PI), a nucleoside reverse transcriptase inhibitor (NRTI) and/or nonnucleoside reverse transcriptase inhibitor drug (NNRTI). Since the introduction of HAART, the prevalence and incidence of most of these ODs have declined. However one must always consider opportunistic disorder in dealing with HIV-positive patients with gastrointestinal problems. Consideration of HAART is part of the management of all gastrointestinal emergencies. The regimens used are constantly changing and up-to-date advice is essential. Patients who are receiving HAART should not have their regimen changed without careful consideration as some drugs, e.g. abacavir, even if stopped for a short time, cannot be restarted. These general points apply to all gastrointestinal emergencies.

If HIV is detected, it is advisable to seek expert opinion regarding the management at the earliest opportunity as this may change investigation and treatment of the condition. Many of the emergencies will be of an infective nature and are again best dealt in joint consultation with specialists. In addition the course of gastrointestinal disease may differ in the presence of HIV.

History and examination

Where there is no history of HIV, patients should be asked about specific risk factors, including homosexual exposure, intravenous drug use and heterosexual exposure in areas of high incidence. It is worth mentioning that a large number of HIV-positive patients will have no risk obvious either to the patient or the clinician. It is essential that HIV testing is discussed with the patient with appropriate counselling before testing. The disclosure of a patient's HIV status requires the consent and participation of the patient. Sometimes it may not be possible to discuss HIV testing with a critically ill patient and HIV testing may be undertaken without consent in some circumstances. This must be in line with General Medical Council Guidelines in UK and advice should be sought. Different advice may apply in other countries.

Gastrointestinal Emergencies, 2nd edition. Edited by Tony Tham, John Collins and Roy Soetikno. © 2009 by Blackwell Publishing, ISBN: 978-1-4051-4634-0.

Table 33.1 Upper gastrointestinal endoscopic findings.

Etiology	Endoscopy
Candida	'Cottage cheese', yellow-white plaques, coating the entire esophagus
CMV	One or more large well-circumscribed ulcers, biopsy from the base
HSV	Diffuse erosive esophagitis or small discrete, superficial volcano ulcers; biopsy from the margins
IEU	One or more well-circumscribed ulcers of variable depth
Leishmania	Variable from normal mucosa to mucosal edema, nodularity, multiple superficial erosions, and ulcers
Syphilis	Diffuse antral erythema and edema, thickened gastric folds, polypoid lesions, and serpiginous ulcerations
Cryptococcus	Multiple well-circumscribed nodules with central erosions or focal areas of gastritis with central erosions
MAC	Diffuse gastropathy with erythematous and nonulcerated lesions resembling angioectasis, mainly in gastric body
Gastric Karposi sarcoma	Multiple raised purple-coloured sessile polyps anywhere in the stomach.
Non-Hodgkin lymphoma	Enlarged gastric folds, the stomach loses its ability to distend (air insufflations), multiple large ulcerated lesions, with a hardened mucosa

CMV cytomegalovirus; HSV Herpes simplex virus; IEU idiopathic esophageal ulcers, MAC *Mycobacterium avium* complex

Concise history-taking of the presenting symptoms is imperative in differentiating between various etiologies as well as the localization of pathologies. For example, severe odynophagia is atypical of *Candida* esophagitis and this condition usually presents with dysphagia.

On physical examination of a patient without known HIV, one should be aware of the occurrence of signs defining AIDS and its treatment; these include wasting of the muscles and lipodystrophy, lymphadenopathy, CMV retinitis in ophthalmoscopy, oral thrush, skin rashes such as Kaposi sarcoma, and anogenital signs of sexually transmitted infections, for example genital warts, herpes, anal fissures, abscesses and fistulas.

Lymphogranuloma venereum should always be considered in the differential diagnosis of genital ulcerations or tender inguinal lymphadenopathy.

Investigations

The diagnosis of AIDS is made on clinical suspicion with laboratory HIV antibody confirmation which may be available in an emergency. Other investigations include blood tests for HIV viral load and CD4 count of lymphocytes. These are predictors of the severity of immunocompromise. Lipid profile, renal and liver function tests to monitor for complications of the HAART, stool cultures and PCR suggested by the history, endoscopy with biopsy (Tables 33.1 and 33.2), histopathologic examinations and contrast as well as cross-sectional imaging may be needed in these patients.

Upper gastrointestinal manifestations of HIV

The most common presentations are dysphagia and retrosternal pain (odynophagia). Other symptoms may include abdominal pain, fever, nausea and vomiting. Less common is the incidence of upper gastrointestinal bleeding with hemetemesis and melena unless in patients with coagulopathy.

Figure 33.1 is an algorithm for the approach to upper gastrointestinal symptoms.

Esophageal disorders

Prior to the use of HAART, esophageal candidosis with or without oral involvement was one of the most common presentations of AIDS. It is still common in patients not yet diagnosed and its presence should alert the physician to the likelihood of immunosuppression or rarely seroconversion. It is important to recognize that the presence of thrush in the oropharynx is not proof that *Candida* causes

Table 33.2 Lower gastrointestinal endoscopic findings.

Etiology	Endoscopy
Common bacterial pathogens (*Salmonella*, *Shigella* and *Campylobacter*)	Erythema, edema, hemorrhagic and ulcerated mucosal lesions which could mimic ulcerative colitis
C. difficile	Erythema, edema and friability of the mucosa covered by yellow-white pseudomembrane
TB	Nodular mucosa with areas of ulceration, mostly localized in proximal colon
MAC	Granular white nodules 2 to 4 mm in diameter with a surrounding rim of erythema, occasionally completely normal
CMV	Colitis without ulcers, ulcers without colitis, normal looking colon, and occasionally a pseudotumor, typically distal colon
HSV	Erythematous areas with small vesicular lesions, small ulcers coalescing to form larger ulcers
Cryptosporidium, *Isospora*	Colonic cryptitis, colitis
E. histolytica	Nonspecific colitis with ulcerations or larger mucosal ulcers associated with yellow-green pseudomembranes
Balantidium	Ulceration with features similar to those of invasive amoebiasis
Histoplasma	Colitis, ulcerations, or most commonly, a mass lesion
Candida albicans	Patchy erythema or discrete ulcers that resemble those caused by CMV
Karposi sarcoma	Violaceous plaque-like macular or nodular lesions, sometimes with central umbilication or ulceration
Lymphoma	Bulky mass lesion, ulcerations, colitis-like picture, and necrotic abscesses

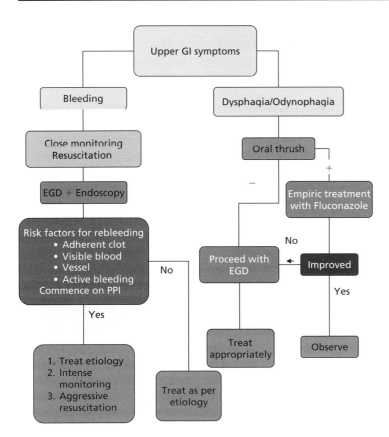

Figure 33.1 Algorithm for the approach to upper gastrointestinal symptoms.

the esophageal symptoms, and oral thrush may be absent in one-third of patients with endoscopy-documented esophagitis. Concurrent esophageal involvement with other pathologies such as CMV or idiopathic esophageal ulcers (IEU) is reported in up to half of the cases [2].

Among the viruses, CMV is the most common cause of esophagitis in patients with AIDS. It more commonly causes ulceration at the lower esophagus, but may also spread to the stomach and duodenum. HSV is the second most common viral cause of esophagitis [1,2]. With HAART a wide range of other less common organisms may cause esophagitis including EBV, human HSV-6, MAC, *Cryptosporidium*, *Aspergillus* and *Leishmania*.

Idiopathic ulcers of the esophagus are also common and frequently associated with aphthous ulcers. They have not been shown to be directly caused by HIV. Drugs used in HAART such as zalcitabine and zidovudine may cause ulceration as well as many other drugs which HIV patients are usually using e.g. NSAIDs [2]. CMV and HSV esophagitis and ideopathic esophageal ulcers occur almost exclusively in severe immunodeficiency with typically CD4 counts of less than 50–100/mm³.

The common conditions of gastroesophageal reflux disease and gastrointestinal disease related to *Helicobacter pylori* are less common in HIV-positive patients and multiple factors including decreased acid production and lack of CD4 lymphocytes have been implicated in such a difference [3].

A normal endoscopy in a patient with normal CD4 should be followed with empiric PPI for non-erosive GERD or a barium swallow to exclude rings or motility disorders.

Finally, it must be remembered that complications such as esophageal strictures are rare in AIDS patients affected by ulcerative esophagitis due to opportunistic infections. However they are amenable to safe dilatation despite the presence of ulceration and multiple biopsies. The appropriate treatment can only be correctly instituted if the right diagnosis through multiple biopsies is made. Attempts at dilatation may prove unsuccessful if ulceration persists [4].

Investigations

Upper gastrointestinal endoscopy with biopsy/culture is the investigation of choice. Different endoscopic features of opportunistic infection (OI) of the upper gastrointestinal tract are presented in Table 33.1. It is important to note that HSV causes shallow ulcers and is located at the edge of the ulcer but CMV is located in the base of the ulcer, where the granulation tissue is present. For those patients with CD4 values above 200/mm³, the indication for endoscopy should be as for other immunocompetent patients. Multiple biopsies of both base and margin of the ulcers, found during an endoscopy, should be taken even if *Candida* is present. *Candida* esophagitis most commonly manifests as multiple plaques or diffuse mucosal irregularity resulting in a 'shaggy' appearance. Herpetic ulceration presents with multiple small ulcerations and both CMV and IEU result in one or multiple well-circumscribed ulcers of variable depth. Fistulas to the mediastinum may result from tuberculosis, MAC or CMV.

Treatment

Oral fluconazole for 10 to 14 days is the usual treatment for *Candida*, starting with a loading dose of 200 mg/d followed by 100 mg/d and may be required intravenously. Sometimes amphotericin B may be required. Low-dose fluconazole or itraconazole may prevent relapse.

In CMV esophagitis, ganciclovir or foscarnet are used for up to 4 weeks and may be needed in combination. Herpes will respond to acyclovir either intravenously or orally.

Different regimens including prednisone 40 mg and thalidomide have been recommended for management of EIU [1].

Gastric diseases

Isolated involvement of the stomach is a less common finding in endoscopic examinations of gastrointestinal tract in HIV-seropositive patients. Individuals with gastric pathologies present with myriad of symptoms including upper abdominal pain, bloating, nausea and vomiting, or upper gastrointestinal bleeding. Gastroscopy with biopsies taken from multiple normal and abnormal sites is the mainstay of diagnosis, as pathologies such as gastric Kaposi sarcoma tend to be submucosal and may be missed in two-third of the cases [5].

The gastrointestinal tract is a common site of involvement with Kaposi sarcoma, and factors such as age, the occurrence of Kaposi sarcoma at or after AIDS onset, the presence of comorbid conditions and immune status as reflected by CD4 count determine its prognosis.

Different organisms have been documented to be involved in OI of the stomach, including *Cryptosporidium*, *Toxoplasma gondii*, *Leishmania*, MAC, *Treponema pallidum* and *Cryptococcus*; however, gastric CMV is the most common infection. Ulcerative and diffuse erosive gastropathies may be complicated by gastrointestinal bleeding whereas the most common presentation of antral and pyloric mucosa is abdominal pain, nausea and vomiting [5].

Radiological tests are mostly in keeping with hypertrophic mucosal folds, nodular filling defects, erosions and ulcers in upper gastrointestinal series and CT studies.

In contrast to HIV-negative patients, chronic active gastritis in HIV patients is usually due to organisms such as CMV and *Cryptosporidium*. However, with more patients on HAART and restored CD4 counts, this trend will change in favor of *H. pylori*.

Finally, extranodal non-Hodgkin lymphoma can be a cause of upper gastrointestinal symptoms in AIDS patients with systemic signs of weight loss and anemia, and may be complicated by massive hematemesis, gastric outlet obstruction and perforation. Gastrointestinal lymphoma and Kaposi sarcoma are common causes of upper gastrointestinal bleeding [5].

Lower gastrointestinal manifestations of HIV

The colon is a common site of gastrointestinal disease in patients with AIDS. Severe diarrhea and weight loss of more than 10% are AIDS-defining conditions. Chronic diarrhea of longer than 1 month, lower gastrointestinal bleeding and abdominal pain are the most common manifestations of HIV/AIDS-related colonic disease.

Chronic diarrhea is considered an independent poor prognostic marker in AIDS patients, who suffer higher morbidity and mortality related to colonic infection. Diarrhea has a huge impact on health care utilization and has been shown to affect the quality of life scores unfavorably in patients with HIV.

Diarrhea is by far the most common reported gastrointestinal symptom in patients with cumulative lifetime incidence of 30–70% in industrialized countries and nearly 100% in developing countries [6].

Toxins play a major role in pathogenicity of diarrhea; therefore agents inhibiting small bowel ion secretion may be effective in decreasing this form of diarrhea. Clinically, diarrhea in patients with AIDS consists of water loss and stools containing little or no bulk.

The isolation of HIV from mucosal cells and expression of p24 antigen have led to the speculation that HIV is responsible for cases of 'pathogen-negative diarrhea', also known as HIV enteropathy. However, minor abnormalities of the villous architecture such as mild villous atrophy or hyperplasia, in the absence of clinical diarrhea are well established in HIV-seropositive persons. Other mechanisms such as bacterial overgrowth, altered and dysfunctional mucosal immune function, increased permeability of the mucosa to foreign antigens and subsequent release of detrimental cytokines and abnormal enteric neural and endocrine function have been implicated in the pathogenicity of this condition [1].

Diarrhea is a well-known side effect of protease inhibitors. The result of studies emphasized that significant diarrhea without obvious pathogen was still present even though more than 75% of patients were on HAART. Other well-known gastrointestinal side effects of protease inhibitors include nausea, vomiting, abdominal pain, anorexia, dyspepsia, and asymptomatic hyperbilirubinemia [6,7].

Generally patients receiving pathogen-specific therapy for HIV-associated diarrhea experience better outcome than patients in whom no pathogen has been identified [7].

Lower gastrointestinal bleeding is uncommon in HIV-infected individuals. It is three times less common than upper gastrointestinal bleeding. The three most common causes of lower gastrointestinal bleeding are CMV colitis, idiopathic colonic ulcers and hemorrhoids. Other causes include lymphoma, colonic Kaposi sarcoma, colonic histoplasmosis and pneumatosis intestinalis.

Diverticulosis, vascular ectasia and colon cancer are relatively uncommon causes of lower gastrointestinal bleeding in patients with AIDS. This difference may well be related to the higher age and different underlying disorders seen in non-HIV-related lower gastrointestinal bleeding [1,8].

The mortality associated with lower gastrointestinal bleeding in HIV/AIDS patients has proven to be above the figures for the general population; however,

Table 33.3 Risk factors for recurrent bleeding.

CMV colitis or lymphoma
Presence of comorbid illness
A hemoglobin level of less than 8 g/dL
A platelet count of less than 100 000/mm^3
The presence of major stigmata of hemorrhage

seropositive individuals carry the same risk of rebleeding, governed by the same risk factors of recurrent bleeding mentioned in Table 33.3 [9,10]. Predictors of mortality are the presence of comorbid illness, recurrent bleeding and surgical interventions.

Abdominal pain is mainly associated with ulcerating colitis, which is commonly caused by CMV, and is accompanied by other signs such as bloody diarrhea and rebound tenderness. The ischemia secondary to arteritis, caused by CMV, may induce abdominal pain via mechanisms such as appendicitis and acalculous cholecystitis as a result of obstruction of bile duct entrance and appendix outlet, respectively.

The diagnosis of perforated CMV ulcers of the colon or CMV-associated appendicitis should be entertained in HIV-positive patients with severe abdominal pain and peritoneal signs, although other pathologies such as Kaposi sarcoma, NHL or adenocarcinoma of the colon may also manifest as colon obstruction or perforation [11].

The other unique cause of abdominal pain in HIV-seropositive patients is AIDS-related sclerosing cholangitis; this complication has been linked to pathogens including *Microsporidium*, CMV and *Cryptosporidium* [12]. The role of sphincterotomy in the management of pain in these patients is unclear.

Investigations

A thorough examination of stool for common enteric pathogens, *C. difficile* toxin and organisms responsible for OI should be carried out. Blood cultures for MAC are warranted, even without clinical indications. Endoscopy plays a crucial part in diagnosis and management of many OI associated with AIDS and panendoscopy with multiple biopsies is considered the gold standard of diagnosis [13]. It also enables the endoscopist to engage in the initial management of bleeding sources through injection of epinephrine with or without electrocoagulation. Due to improvements in laboratory diagnostic tools, availing PCR studies, and enhanced diagnostic

yield associated with trichrome staining of stool specimens in diagnosis of more proximally inhabited organisms such as *Microsporidium*, fewer patients with diarrhea are referred to the endoscopist. The use of aggressive endoscopic workup has been criticized due to the high cost of investigations, the unclear role of many enteric pathogens in causing diarrhea and lack of evidence in favor of improvement in quality of life for patients undergoing such intensive investigations [13].

Figure 33.2 is an algorithm for the approach to lower gastrointestinal symptoms.

However, recent diagnostic and therapeutic developments in the management of opportunistic disorder of the lower gastrointestinal tract and AIDS advocate more extensive investigations. In every case a balanced decision should be made, and risks and benefits of more invasive tests should be weighed up.

The advantage of colonoscopy over flexible sigmoidoscopy lies in its ability to diagnose isolated proximal illness with CMV and has been reported to be as high as 46% in various studies [11.]

Viral, fungal and protozoal infections of the lower gastrointestinal tract

Cytomegalovirus is the most common and the most serious virus affecting the intestine and presents with a spectrum of symptoms including diarrhea with colicky abdominal pain, tenesmus, rebound tenderness, fever, anorexia and weight loss. The endoscopy could be normal in up to 25% of the cases and, with this in mind, biopsies from normal mucosa should be obtained. Colonoscopy is a superior diagnostic test and multiple biopsies are recommended.

Herpes simplex virus is mostly involved in distal colitis or proctitis, where its vesicles may be visible during anal examination, and may be associated with anorectal pain, tenesmus, hematochezia and mild alteration of the bowel habit. Adenovirus is another pathogen with a doubtful role in HIV-induced diarrhea. Its mucosal lesions are limited to the surface and spare the crypt epithelium. CMV is a common coinfection.

Candida albicans has been isolated from colonic ulcers but a causative relation with diarrhea remains to be determined. Intestinal *Histoplasma capsulatum* often occurs secondary to widespread disseminated disease after reactivation of the latent infection.

Microsporidiosis due to *Enterocytozoon bieneusi* and cryptosporidiosis due to *Cryptosporidium parvum* are two

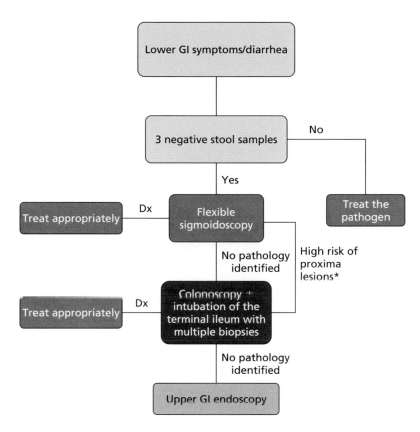

Figure 33.2 Algorithm for the approach to lower gastrointestinal symptoms and diarrhea. *Patient's clinical picture, previous history of opportunistic disorder, state of immunodeficiency, local resources dictates whether to opt for colonoscopy as the first line of investigation in stool-negative patients.

common pathogens with lower gastrointestinal predilection. Affected patients with chronic microsporidiosis and cryptosporidiosis can present with anything from persistent diarrhea, weight loss, abdominal pain and a sclerosing cholangiopathy.

MAC is most commonly encountered in patients with CD4 counts less than $50/mm^3$. It is particular more common in small bowel and its presence should be considered in protracted cases of diarrhea, accompanied with systemic signs of fever, anemia, weight loss and night sweats. *Mycobacterium tuberculosis* can also involve small bowel and the ileocecal region and is included in the differential diagnosis of Crohn's disease.

Penultimately, common enteric pathogens, such as *Salmonella*, *Shigella flexneri*, *Campylobacter jejuni* and *C. difficile* should be considered in immunocompromised patients with whom diarrhea, abdominal cramping and nausea are the common presentations. *Clostridium difficile* can cause a bloody mucoid diarrhea with abdominal pain and fever, with or without history of recent antibiotic treatment.

Finally, the widespread utilization of trimethoprim-sulfamethoxazole for PCP seems to have reduced the incidence of pathogens such as *Salmonella*, *Isospora* and *Cyclosporidium*.

Diagnosis of cryptosporidiosis and microsporidiosis can be made on stool examination. Common enteric pathogens are diagnosed with stool cultures. CMV and HSV infections are diagnosed by immunohistochemical analysis of biopsy specimens obtained during endoscopy, supported by their characteristic intracellular inclusion bodies. Other pathogens are identified by a combination of their endoscopic appearance and biopsy findings with appropriate staining techniques (e.g. Ziehl–Neelson for MAC) [1,11,14].

Treatment

The majority of patients do better on HAART. Pathogen-specific treatments when available should be used to improve the outcome. Treatment of CMV consists of ganciclovir or foscarnet intravenously for at least 3 weeks. Expert advice in complex cases should be sought. Intravenous acyclovir for a week is the best way forward in cases of colonic or anorectal HSV. Infections with *Candida* are usually responsive to oral nystatin but systemic therapy with amphotericin or iatraconazole may be required. Atovaquone and parmomycin have limited efficacy against microsporidiosis and cryptosporidiosis, respectively; however, both pathogens have shown complete and sustained clinical, microbiological and histological response to treatment with HAART. Combined therapy with azithromycin and one other antimycobacterial agent such as rifampin or ethambutol has been recommended by the US Public Health Service Task Force. Appropriate antibacterials should be used for common pathogens and oral metronidazole is the first-line treatment for *C. difficile*. Steroid therapy may aid in the management of bleeding caused by idiopathic colonic ulcers.

Symptomatic treatment with loperamide, opioids and somatostatin analogues are often helpful [1,18].

Miscellaneous gastrointestinal disorders

Anecdotal cases of amyloidosis as a cause of gastrointestinal bleeding, in AIDS patients have been reported. The diagnosis is made by Congo red staining of the rectal or abdominal fat pad biopsy specimens [15]. Acute pancreatitis is an important cause of morbidity and mortality of HIV-infected patients. There is evidence to suggest that the incidence of pancreatitis is increased and this has been associated with factors such as antiretroviral medications, in particular protease inhibitors, other HIV medications (pentamidine), excessive alcohol consumption and opportunistic infections such as CMV, MAC and toxoplasmosis. It is worth mentioning that HIV infection and AIDS per se are not indicative of poor outcome, compared to the non-HIV positive populations [16].

Lactic acidosis secondary to mitochondrial toxicity is a rare yet serious and sometimes fatal complication of the HAART especially NRTIs and can present with malaise, nausea, abdominal discomfort, and sometimes weight loss. Early discontinuation of the treatment should be followed by seeking expert advice on reintroduction of the alternative treatments.

Finally, metabolic abnormalities such as lipodystrophy have been observed to complicate the course of HAART and are also related to mitochondrial toxicity of these drugs [17].

Table 33.4 Causes of increased frequency of opportunistic disorders.

Limited availability of HAART (developing countries)
Low bioavailability of drugs
Undiagnosed, unidentified or late presentations
Drug intolerance or presence of side effects
Poor compliance or complicated treatment regimes
Drug resistance
Incomplete immune restitution and persistent
 immunosuppressant due to dysfunctional CD4 T-cell
 lymphocytes

The impact of HAART on HIV/AIDS management

With the introduction of HAART in HIV, the incidence of OI has reduced and the mortality and progression of HIV-infected patients to overt AIDS decreased. Unfortunately diarrhea (in some studies) appears to have the same frequency (8–10% of patients with CD4 cell count less than 200/mm^3) despite the dramatic drop in the incidence of opportunistic infections in the HAART era [19]. However, a significant difference in the etiologic pattern of diarrhea has been demonstrated and noninfectious causes of diarrhea appear to have risen in incidence.

In summary, advanced diagnostics and improvement in treatment of opportunistic disorder as well as immune modulation with HAART have heralded better outcomes.

Despite reduction in the prevalence of opportunistic disorder of the colon [20], it is important for endoscopists to be familiar with the spectrum of the abnormalities to be able to diagnose and treat them in patients with AIDS. Factors associated with increase in opportunistic disorder despite HAART therapy are presented in Table 33.4.

References

1. Sande MA, Volberding PA. The Medical Management of AIDS, 6th ed. Philidelphia, WB Saunders, 1999; 196–216.

2. Wilcox M. Approach to esophageal disease in AIDS: a primer for the endoscopist. Techniques Gastrointest Endosc 2002; 4:59–65.

3. Chiu H, Ming-Shiang W, Chien-Ching H et al. Low prevalence of *Helicobactor pylori* but high prevalence of cytomegalovirus-associated peptic ulcer disease in AIDS patients: comparative study of symptomatic subjects evaluated by endoscopy and CD4 counts. J Gastroenterol Hepatol 2004; 19:423–8.

4. Wilcox M. Esophageal strictures complicating ulcerative esophagitis in patients with AIDS. Am J Gastroenterol 1999; 94:339–42.

5. Monkemuller KE, Olmos M. Gastric diseases in AIDS. Techniques Gastrointest Endosc 2002; 4:66–9.

6. Call SA, Heudebert G, Saag M, et al. The changing etiology of chronic diarrhea in HIV-infected patients with CD4 counts less than 200 cells/mm^3. Am J Gastroenterol 2000: 95:3142–6.

7. Bini EJ, Cohen J. Impact of protease inhibitors on the outcome of human immunodeficiency virus-infected patients with chronic diarrhea. Am J Gastroenterol 1999; 94:3553–8.

8. Chalasani N, Wilcox CM. Gastrointestinal hemorrage in patients with AIDS. AIDS Patient Care STDs 1999; 13:343–6.

9. Chalasani N, Wilcox CM. Etiology and outcome of lower gastrointestinal bleeding in patients with AIDS. Am J Gastroenterol 1997; 93:175–7.

10. Bini EJ, Weinshel EH and Falkenstein BD. Risk factors for recurrent bleeding and mortality in human immunodeficiency virus-infected patients with acute lower GI hemorrage. Gastrointest Endosc 1999; 49:748–53.

11. Bini EJ, Diehl DL. Colonic disease in patients with AIDS. Techniques Gastrointest Endosc 2002; 4.77–85.

12. Sharpstone D, Gazzard B. Gastrointestinal manifestations of HIV infection. Lancet 1996; 348:379–81.

13. Kearney DJ, Steuerwald M, Koch J et al. A prospective study of endoscopy in HIV-associated diarrhea. Am J Gastroenterol 1999; 94:596–601.

14. Field AS. Light microscope and electron microscope diagnosis of gastrointestinal opportunistic infections in HIV-positive patients. Roy Coll Pathol Australasia 2002; 34:21–34.

15. Chinnakoltla AK, De Luna AM, Thew ST, et al. Syptomatic gastrointestinal amyloidosis in an HIV-infected patient. Am J Gastroenterol 2001; 96:2248–50.

16. Gan I, May G, Raboud J et al. Pancreatitis in HIV infection: predictors of severity. Am J Gastroenterol 1998: 1278–1283.

17. Boyd M, Reiss P. The long-term consequences of antiretroviral therapy: a review. J HIV Ther 2006; 11:26–33.

18. Carr A, Marriott, Field A, Vasak et al. Treatment of HIV-1 associated microsporidiosis and cryptosporidiosis with combination antiretroviral therapy. Lancet 1998; 351:256–9.

19. Monkemuller KE, Lazenby AJ, Lee DH et al. Occurrence of gastrointestinal opportunistic disorders in AIDS despite the use of highly active antiretroviral therapy. Dig Dis Sc 2005; 50:230–4.

20. Monkemuller KE, Call SA, Lazenby AJ et al. Declining prevalence of opportunistic gastrointestinal disease in the era of combination antiretroviral therapy. Am J Gastroenterol 2000; 95:457–61.

Index

Index

Index

Index